T0317609

Identifying Perinatal Depression and Anxiety

Identifying Perinatal Depression and Anxiety

Evidence-Based Practice in Screening, Psychosocial Assessment, and Management

Edited by

Jeannette Milgrom and Alan W. Gemmill

WILEY Blackwell

This edition first published 2015
© 2015 John Wiley & Sons, Ltd.

Registered Office
John Wiley & Sons, Ltd., The Atrium, Southern Gate, Chichester, West Sussex, PO19 8SQ, UK

Editorial Offices
350 Main Street, Malden, MA 02148-5020, USA
9600 Garsington Road, Oxford, OX4 2DQ, UK
The Atrium, Southern Gate, Chichester, West Sussex, PO19 8SQ, UK

For details of our global editorial offices, for customer services, and for information about how
to apply for permission to reuse the copyright material in this book please see our website at
www.wiley.com/wiley-blackwell.

Library of Congress Cataloging-in-Publication Data

Identifying perinatal depression and anxiety : evidence-based practice in screening, psychosocial assessment and
management / edited by Jeannette Milgrom, Alan W. Gemmill.
    p. ; cm.
  Includes bibliographical references and index.
  ISBN 978-1-118-50965-4 (hb) – ISBN 978-1-118-50969-2 (pb)
I. Milgrom, Jeannette, editor.   II. Gemmill, Alan, editor.
[DNLM: 1. Depression, Postpartum–diagnosis.   2. Anxiety Disorders–diagnosis.
3. Anxiety Disorders–psychology.   4. Depression, Postpartum–psychology.   5. Evidence-Based
Medicine–methods.   6. Internationality. WQ 500]
  RC537
  616.85′27–dc23
                                   2014048416

A catalogue record for this book is available from the British Library.

Cover image: Cracked White Marble © LordRunar / iStockphoto; Vector silhouette of family
© majivecka / iStockphoto

Set in 10/12pt MinionPro by SPi Global, Pondicherry, India

1   2015

Contents

About the Editors   vii
About the Contributors   viii
Foreword   xvi

Introduction: Current Issues in Identifying Perinatal Depression: An Overview   1
Jeannette Milgrom and Alan W. Gemmill

1 Is Population-Based Identification of Perinatal Depression
   and Anxiety Desirable?: A Public Health Perspective on the Perinatal
   Depression Care Continuum   11
   Norma I. Gavin, Samantha Meltzer-Brody, Vivette Glover,
   and Bradley N. Gaynes

2 When Screening Is Policy, How Do We Make It Work?   32
   Barbara P. Yawn, Elizabeth M. LaRusso, Susan L. Bertram,
   and William V. Bobo

3 Acceptability, Attitudes, and Overcoming Stigma   51
   Anne Buist, Heather O'Mahen, and Rosanna Rooney

4 How to Use the EPDS and Maximize Its Usefulness in the Consultation
   Process: A Clinician's Guide   63
   Carol Henshaw and Jennifer Ericksen

5 Screening Tools and Methods of Identifying Perinatal Depression   76
   Rachel Mann and Jonathan Evans

6 Identifying Perinatal Anxiety   93
   Susan Ayers, Rose Coates, and Stephen Matthey

7 Diagnostic Assessment of Depression, Anxiety, and Related Disorders   108
   Arianna Di Florio, John Seeley, and Ian Jones

8 Psychosocial Assessment and Integrated Perinatal Care   121
   Marie-Paule Austin, Jane Fisher, and Nicole Reilly

9   Postnatal Depression, Mother–Infant Interactions, and Child Development:
    Prospects for Screening and Treatment   139
    Lynne Murray, Pasco Fearon, and Peter Cooper

10 Fathers' Perinatal Mental Health   165
    Richard Fletcher, Craig F. Garfield, and Stephen Matthey

11 Evidence-Based Treatments and Pathways to Care   177
    Michael W. O'Hara, Cindy-Lee Dennis, Jennifer E. McCabe,
    and Megan Galbally

12 International Approaches to Perinatal Mental Health Screening
    as a Public Health Priority   193
    Katherine L. Wisner, Marie-Paule Austin, Angela Bowen, Roch Cantwell,
    and Nine M.-C. Glangeaud-Freudenthal

13 Training Health-Care Professionals for the Assessment and Management
    of Perinatal Depression and Anxiety   210
    C. Jane Morrell, Jan Cubison, Tom Ricketts, Anne Sved Williams,
    and Pauline Hall

14 An Overview of Health Economic Aspects of Perinatal Depression   228
    Stavros Petrou, C. Jane Morrell, and Martin Knapp

15 The Future of Perinatal Depression Identification: Can Information
    and Communication Technology Optimize Effectiveness?   240
    Tara Donker, Pim Cuijpers, David Stanley, and Brian Danaher

16 Conclusion: Perinatal Depression: Looking Back, Moving Forward   256
    Alan W. Gemmill, Jeannette Milgrom, and Nicole Highet

Index   266

About the Editors

Alan W. Gemmill is Senior Research Fellow at the Parent-Infant Research Institute in Melbourne, Australia. He has worked in perinatal mental health research for 14 years and has a special interest in clinical research studies and preventive intervention programs for maternal mental health difficulties. He has had a lead role in several randomized treatment trials for perinatal depression and has published widely on such topics as the neurodevelopmental benefits of early stress reduction for premature infants, the prevention of perinatal mood disorders and parenting difficulty, the major risk factors for perinatal depression and anxiety, and the predictive value of screening instruments for perinatal mood disorders.

Jeannette Milgrom is Professor of Psychology in the Melbourne School of Psychological Sciences at the University of Melbourne, Director of Clinical and Health Psychology at Austin Health, and Founder and Director of the Parent-Infant Research Institute, Australia. She is internationally recognized for her work with mothers and babies and is currently President of the Marcé Society for Perinatal Mental Health. She is the author of six books, and over 116 scientific articles and chapters. Her research and clinical practice focuses on high-risk infants and early intervention, ante- and postnatal depression, neurodevelopment of premature infants, and screening and developing psychological treatments. Her books on treating and preventing postnatal depression have been translated into Italian and French. She has had a major role with beyondblue and the National Perinatal Depression Initiative since 2001.

About the Contributors

Marie-Paule Austin is the chair of Perinatal and Women's Mental Health at the University of New South Wales; director at St John of God Health Care Mother–Baby Unit; and psychiatrist at the Royal Hospital for Women, Sydney. Professor Austin has long been at the forefront of research into models of universal psychosocial assessment in the perinatal period, and both her clinical and population-based researches have been instrumental in shaping the development of policy and practice in perinatal mental health across Australia.

Susan Ayers is a professor in the Centre for Maternal and Child Health Research at City University London and visiting professor at the University of Sussex, United Kingdom. Susan's research focuses on women's psychological well-being and mental health during pregnancy and after birth. Susan is an author of *Psychology for Medicine* (2011) and editor of the Cambridge *Handbook of Psychology, Health and Medicine*, 2nd Ed. (2007). She was awarded the Annual Lecturer Prize by the Society for Reproductive and Infant Psychology in 2012.

Susan L. Bertram, BSN RN MSN, is trained as a psychiatric clinical nurse specialist. She has worked as a lead study coordinator for the past 20 years with Dr. Barbara Yawn in the Olmsted Medical Center, Department of Research. She served as the lead coordinator and project manager for the recently completed TRIPPD 5-year trial assessing the outcomes of implementing postnatal depression screening, diagnosis, and management in family medicine offices.

William V. Bobo, MD MPH, is a psychiatrist and researcher, associate professor of psychiatry at the Mayo Medical School, and medical director of the Mayo Clinic Mood Program. His research is focused on the effectiveness, safety, and clinical use of treatments for severe mood disorders. Dr. Bobo has special interest in the perinatal management of these disorders and use of psychotropic medications during pregnancy.

Angela Bowen, RN, PhD, is an associate professor in the College of Nursing and the Department of Psychiatry at the University of Saskatchewan. Recent research includes a longitudinal study and epidemiological study of antenatal depression in progress, evaluation of maternal mental health programs, and policy development. She is the lead of the

Maternal Mental Health Strategy group, which developed and is implementing policy recommendations to address antenatal and postpartum depression (PPD) in Saskatchewan, Canada.

Anne Buist, MBBS, MMed, MD, FRANZCP, is the professor/director of Women's Mental Health at the University of Melbourne and Austin Health and has clinical and research experience in perinatal mental illness, its association with childhood abuse, and long-term outcomes. She led the beyondblue Postnatal Depression Program that resulted in screening implementation throughout Australia.

Rose Coates is a doctoral researcher in the School of Psychology, University of Sussex, United Kingdom. Her research is on optimal ways of conceptualizing and screening for postnatal psychological distress such as anxiety, depression, and posttraumatic stress following birth. She has published on anxiety measurement, symptoms of perinatal distress, and intervention.

Roch Cantwell is a consultant perinatal psychiatrist with Greater Glasgow and Clyde Health Board, United Kingdom, and honorary senior clinical lecturer at Glasgow University. He is past chair of the RCPsych Perinatal Section and lead psychiatric assessor for the UK Confidential Enquiries into Maternal Deaths. He chaired the SIGN Perinatal Mood Disorders Guideline Development Group and was joint author of the RCOG Good Practice Guideline on Mental Health Issues in Pregnancy.

Peter Cooper is a research professor in psychopathology at the University of Reading and codirector, with Lynne Murray, of the Winnicott Research Unit. He is also professor extraordinaire at Stellenbosch University in South Africa. He has conducted epidemiological, experimental, longitudinal, and intervention research in a range of areas, including eating disorders, depression, and child anxiety. His current work, in collaboration with Lynne Murray, principally concerns the development and evaluation of early interventions to improve child outcomes in the developing world. He is the editor of the Constable & Robinson *Overcoming* series of self-help books for psychological disorders.

Jan Cubison is a clinical service manager, Sheffield Perinatal Mental Health Service. Jan provided the introductory day health visitor training for the PoNDER trial. Research outputs include screening for postnatal depression in primary care, in *Screening for Perinatal Depression* (eds C. Henshaw and S. Elliott, 2005), and *Thoughts of infanticide* (Marcé International Conference, September 2006). Expert advisory work includes independent inquiry on Daksha Emson (2003); NICE Guidelines, *Pregnancy and complex social factors* (2010); *Service user experience in adult mental health* (2011); and NHS England, Clinical Reference Group for specialized perinatal mental health services (current).

Dr. Pim Cuijpers is a professor of clinical psychology at the VU University Amsterdam (the Netherlands) and head of the Department of Clinical Psychology. Since 2009, he has published more than 475 papers, chapters, reports, and professional publications, including more than 300 papers in peer-reviewed international scientific journals.

Dr. Brian Danaher is a senior research scientist at Oregon Research Institute (Eugene, OR, United States). Recent grant-funded research projects and publications have focused on development and evaluation of technology-delivered behavioral interventions (including use of web and mobile phone methods) for treatment of tobacco and postnatal depression.

Cindy-Lee Dennis is a professor of nursing and psychiatry at the University of Toronto and a senior scientist at Women's College Research Institute. She simultaneously holds the Canada Research Chair in Perinatal Community Health and the Shirley Brown Chair in Women's Mental Health Research. She has published widely in the area of perinatal depression and has completed five Cochrane systematic reviews. Her research focuses on evaluating telephone-based interventions for the prevention and treatment of PPD.

Arianna Di Florio is a clinical research fellow at the Department of Psychological Medicine and Clinical Neurosciences at Cardiff University (United Kingdom). After obtaining her undergraduate qualification in medicine at the University of Padua (Italy), she specialized in psychiatry. She completed her PhD at Cardiff University with a thesis on bipolar disorder in pregnancy and postpartum. She has recently been awarded a Marie Curie International Outgoing Fellowship to visit the Center for Women's Mood Disorders at the University of North Carolina at Chapel Hill (United States), where she will develop predictive models for postnatal depression and psychosis.

Dr. Tara Donker is a research fellow at the Black Dog Institute, University of New South Wales, Australia. Her research areas include online screening, early intervention, and prevention of depression, anxiety, and suicide, with a special interest in e-mental health.

Jennifer Ericksen is a clinical psychologist and manager of Perinatal Mental Health Services and Training, Parent–Infant Research Institute, Austin Health. The institute is a large treatment center for perinatal depression and anxiety specializing in developing and evaluating clinical interventions. She also provides professional development sessions to maternal and child health nurses, psychologists, general practitioners and midwives. She has contributed to many intervention programs and academic publications.

Jonathan Evans is a senior lecturer, University of Bristol, Bristol, UK, and honorary consultant psychiatrist. His research has focused on parental depression and consequences for offspring particularly using data from the Avon Longitudinal Study of Parents and Children. He has a particular interest in identifying and treating depression during pregnancy and has conducted one of the few randomized trials for antenatal depression.

Pasco Fearon is a professor of developmental psychopathology at University College London (UCL) and joint director of UCL's doctoral training program in clinical psychology. He is a developmental and clinical psychologist, and his research focuses on the role of relationships in early child development. His work integrates social and biological perspectives, particularly the role of parenting and attachment on the one hand and genetics and physiology on the other.

Jane Fisher is a professor of women's health and the director of the Jean Hailes Research Unit in the School of Public Health and Preventive Medicine at Monash University. She is an academic clinical and health psychologist with long-standing interests in public health perspectives on the links between women's reproductive health and mental health including during pregnancy, birth, and the postpartum period. She has been consultant clinical psychologist to Masada Private Hospital Mother–Baby Unit since 1996.

Richard Fletcher, PhD, is a senior lecturer in the Family Action Centre, Faculty of Health, the University of Newcastle, NSW, and convenor of the Australian Fatherhood Research Network. He is currently researching the effects of paternal play on children's self-regulation and video-feedback processes for addressing father–infant and father–child attachment and identifying practice and policy components to reduce paternal perinatal depression. His book *The Dad Factor* has been translated into Spanish, Korean, German, and Chinese.

Megan Galbally is a consultant psychiatrist and head of unit, Perinatal Mental Health, at Mercy Hospital for Women and a clinical associate professor in the Department of Obstetrics and Gynaecology, University of Melbourne. Dr Galbally's research focus is on the effects of exposure to maternal mental illness and pharmacological treatments in pregnancy on pregnancy, neonatal, and child developmental outcomes.

Craig F. Garfield, MD, MAPP, is an associate professor at the Northwestern University Feinberg School of Medicine in the Departments of Pediatrics and Medical Social Sciences. His research focuses on the role families play in optimizing and promoting the well-being of children, with current research projects examining the role of fathers in health care, using technology to support families with children, and the effect of workplace policies on family well-being.

Norma I. Gavin, PhD, is a senior research economist in RTI International's Division of Health Services and Social Policy Research. Dr. Gavin has more than 30 years of experience in policy analysis and health services research. Her research has focused on the access to and quality of health care for vulnerable populations, particularly low-income pregnant women and children, and includes a widely cited systematic evidence review of the prevalence and incidence of perinatal depression.

Bradley N. Gaynes, MD, MPH, is a professor of psychiatry at the University of North Carolina and the associate chair of Research Training and Education. Dr. Gaynes works at the crossroads between clinical trials research and mental health services research, focusing his clinical and research efforts on mental health–primary care integration and health-care delivery in real-world nonpsychiatric settings. His primary research interests involve assessing and managing depressive illness in primary care settings, HIV settings, and obstetrical/gynecological settings.

Nine M.-C. Glangeaud-Freudenthal, PhD, is a senior researcher in the field of perinatal mental health and is working in an epidemiological research unit on perinatal health and women's and children's health. She is a Marcé Society past president and a founder of the Francophone group of this society. She has published papers on PPD and postpartum blues and on the analysis of a 10-year database on mother–baby inpatient units in France, Belgium, and Luxembourg. Nine Glangeaud-Freudenthal wishes to thank and acknowledge Bénédicte Coulm, Christine Rainelli, Michel Dugnat, and Anne Laure Sutter-Dallay for useful discussions and input to the section of Chapter 10 dealing with best-practice guidelines in France.

Vivette Glover, MA, PhD, DSc, is a professor of perinatal psychobiology, Imperial College London. In recent years, Dr. Glover has applied her expertise in biological psychiatry to the problems of mothers and babies. Projects include studies showing maternal prenatal stress increases the probability for a range of adverse neurodevelopmental outcomes for the child. Her group is also studying the underlying biological mechanisms. She has published over 400 papers and been awarded the Marcé Society Medal.

Dr. Pauline Hall is a training coordinator and clinician at the National Perinatal Depression Initiative in South Australia. Research interests include ego-dystonic intrusive thoughts after childbirth and implementation of universal perinatal screening for depression. Publications relevant to this book include Hall, P.L. (2012) (*Current considerations of the effects of untreated maternal perinatal depression and the National Perinatal Depression Initiative. Journal of Developmental Origins of Health and Disease* 3, 293–295) and Hall, P.L. (2013) (*Normalisation of negative thoughts after childbirth. Interaction* 31, 9–12).

Carol Henshaw is a consultant in perinatal mental health at Liverpool Women's Hospital, honorary senior lecturer at the University of Liverpool, and honorary visiting fellow at Staffordshire University, United Kingdom. Her research has focused on the long-term follow-up of postpartum blues and depression and systematic reviews. She has edited, written, and contributed to books on screening for perinatal depression, the Edinburgh Postnatal Depression Scale, and perinatal psychiatry.

Nicole Highet is the Founder and Executive Director of COPE: Centre of Perinatal Excellence, Australia. Nicole has played a significant role in perinatal mental health reform, providing national leadership and advocacy for the establishment and implementation of Australia's $85M National Perinatal Depression Initiative (NPDI). Nicole has also co-chaired the development of Australia's first Clinical Practice Guidelines and has had oversight of national and local campaigns and approaches to mental health promotion and stigma reduction.

Ian Jones is a professor of psychiatry and director of the National Centre for Mental Health (www.NCMH.info) at Cardiff University, Wales. He is the director of the Bipolar Education Programme Cymru which was named Innovation in Medicine Team of the Year at the British Medical Journal Awards 2014. His research involves clinical and molecular genetic studies of bipolar disorder and postpartum psychosis. He has authored or coauthored over 200 publications and book chapters in the fields of mood disorder genetics and perinatal psychiatry. He has been awarded the Marcé Medal for his research on postpartum psychosis and was named Academic Psychiatrist of the Year at the RCPsych Awards 2013.

Martin Knapp is an academic researcher working in the areas of health and social care policy and practice. He is now based full time at the London School of Economics and Political Science (LSE), United Kingdom, after also working for more than 20 years as professor of health economics at King's College London. At LSE, he has been professor of social policy and director of the Personal Social Services Research Unit since 1996. He has also been codirector of LSE Health and Social Care since this overarching center was set up in 2000. Since 2009, he has been director of the School for Social Care Research, funded by the National Institute for Health Research in England. Martin's research in recent years has mainly been in the areas of mental health, dementia, autism, and long-term care. Most of this work has had a particular focus on economic issues. He has authored or edited

16 books, more than 450 papers in peer-reviewed journals, and many book chapters and reports. His work has fed through to have an impact on policy and practice discussions in the mental health and long-term care areas, both in the United Kingdom and elsewhere.

Elizabeth M. LaRusso, MD, is a perinatal and reproductive psychiatrist at Allina Health and Children's Hospitals and Clinics of Minnesota. Her clinical work is focused on women with psychiatric issues during the perinatal period and her publications focus on perinatal mood disorders. She is also the director of the Mother–Baby Mental Health Program at Allina Health and Children's Hospitals and Clinics of Minnesota.

Rachel Mann, research fellow, University of York, York, UK, has a background in nursing and completed her PhD in health sciences at the University of York on the validity and acceptability of case-finding questions to identify perinatal depression. She has worked on two mental health projects including an HTA-funded review of screening for postnatal depression in primary care. Prior to joining the University of York, she was a visiting scholar at the global headquarters of Merck & Co., Inc., United States.

Stephen Matthey is a senior clinical psychologist and researcher in the Department of Health in NSW, Australia. He is also an adjunct associate professor in the School of Psychology, University of Sydney, Australia (but note: I'm English!). He has published around 100 papers in peer-reviewed journals on a range of topics, including child and adult treatment, educational psychology, cross-cultural psychology, perinatal mental health, psychological assessment, questionnaire development, statistics, brain injury, fathers, parenting programs, and the evaluation of clinical services. He loves playing football, riding his motorbike, learning Italian, and playing the violin.

Jennifer E. McCabe is a graduate student at the University of Iowa. She is a doctoral candidate in the clinical psychology program under the advisement of Dr. Michael O'Hara. Her research broadly pertains to the effects of maternal mental health on mother–child interactions and child development. She has a particular interest in maternal "distress tolerance" and its impact on the developing mother–child relationship.

Samantha Meltzer-Brody, MD, MPH, is an associate professor and director of the Perinatal Psychiatry Program of the UNC Center for Women's Mood Disorders. Her research is focused on pathophysiological and genetic models of PPD and lactation failure, and she has established an international PPD genetics consortium examining the biomarker signature of PPD. Dr. Meltzer-Brody maintains an active clinical practice in perinatal psychiatry and has published numerous manuscripts on women's reproductive mood disorders.

Dr. C. Jane Morrell is associate professor in health research, University of Nottingham, United Kingdom. She was principal investigator in randomized controlled trials and economic evaluations examining the cost-effectiveness of postnatal social support and examining the cost-effectiveness of training health visitors in the prevention and management of postnatal depression (the PoNDER trial). Jane is chief investigator for the National Institute for Health Research, Health Technology Assessment 11/95/03, "Evidence synthesis, meta-analysis and decision analytic modelling following a systematic review of quantitative and qualitative studies evaluating the effectiveness, cost-effectiveness, safety and acceptability of interventions to prevent postnatal depression."

Lynne Murray is research professor in developmental psychopathology at the University of Reading and codirector, with Peter Cooper, of the Winnicott Research Unit. She is also professor extraordinaire at Stellenbosch University in South Africa. Her work principally concerns the development of children growing up in the context of adversity: this includes children of post-natally depressed, and anxious, mothers, children of parents facing extreme socioeconomic adversity, and children with congenital difficulties such as difficult temperament and cleft lip. Her research with these populations has included longitudinal prospective studies, experimental investigations, and treatment trials. She is coeditor, with Peter Cooper, of *Postpartum Depression and Child Development* (1997) and the author of *The Social Baby* (2000) and *The Psychology of Babies: How Relationships Support Development from Birth to Two* (2014).

Michael W. O'Hara is a professor of psychology at the University of Iowa. He has published extensively in the area of perinatal depression for over 30 years. His principal interests are in interventions for perinatal depression, particularly in the use of interpersonal psychotherapy. He recently coedited an issue of *Best Practice & Research Clinical Obstetrics & Gynaecology* entitled "Perinatal mental health: Guidance for the obstetrician-gynaecologist."

Heather O'Mahen, PhD, is a senior lecturer/assistant professor in clinical psychology in the Mood Disorders Centre at the University of Exeter, United Kingdom. Dr. O'Mahen conducts research on identifying and modifying factors to increase access to psychological treatments for perinatal mental illness. She has specific interests in using technology to augment delivery of perinatal treatments. She has recently published several clinical trials investigating treatments for perinatal depression, including an online behavioral activation treatment for postnatal depression.

Stavros Petrou is a professor of health economics within Warwick Medical School, University of Warwick, United Kingdom. He leads a research group conducting high-quality economic evaluations and research alongside large phase III clinical trials and within health technology appraisal reviews. In recent years, he has pursued a methodological and applied research agenda largely focused on economic aspects of perinatal and pediatric health care. Prior to his appointment by the University of Warwick in 2010, Stavros was employed for 13 years as a health economist by the University of Oxford. During that period, he held an MRC Senior Non-Clinical Research Fellowship and conducted several research projects on economic aspects of perinatal depression. He remains a research associate at the Nuffield Department of Population Health, University of Oxford.

Nicole Reilly is a senior research associate at the Perinatal and Women's Mental Health Unit, St John of God Health Care, and lecturer (conjoint) at the University of New South Wales. She has worked in the field of perinatal mental health for 10 years and has a particular interest in the role of policy initiatives in improving outcomes for women and families and in the use of population-based data to examine these issues.

Dr. Tom Ricketts is a nurse consultant in psychotherapy within the NHS in England. He has extensive experience in delivering cognitive behavioral psychotherapies and the training and supervision of others delivering those therapies. Tom designed and evaluated the health visitor training in the PoNDER trial. His research interests include psychological therapies for longer-term depression, the effectiveness of routine NHS psychotherapies, and the impact of training and clinical supervision on outcomes. He is an honorary research fellow within the University of Sheffield School of Health and Related Research.

Dr. Rosanna Rooney is the director of clinical psychology at Curtin University and codirector of Aussie Optimism funded by the Mental Health Commission (Western Australia). She specializes in depression and cross-cultural mental health and, along with her colleagues, has held over three million dollars worth of grants in the areas of postnatal depression across cultures and preventing and reducing anxiety and depression in children. She has been instrumental in writing guidelines for reducing the stigma of mental illness in communities with culturally and linguistically diverse (CALD) backgrounds.

Dr. John Seeley is a senior research scientist at the Oregon Research Institute (ORI) with a special interest in mood and disruptive behavior disorders, behavioral health intervention, research design and program evaluation, and health-related technology. He has over 25 years of experience conducting epidemiologic and intervention research on depressive disorders and as the lead methodologist on many large efficacy and effectiveness trials. His current emphasis is on general methodological issues in research involving web-based behavioral interventions, as well as evaluations of programs that target specific issues such as depression, parenting, physical activity, grief, and tobacco cessation.

David Stanley is the founding director of Convenience Advertising, an international public health agency that over the past twenty-nine years has developed the field of narrowcasting. In the past thirteen years, through preventionXpress, David has focused on the development of preventative health screening using digital and touch screen technology and working in collaboration with health professionals and researchers.

Dr. Anne Sved Williams is a director, Perinatal and Infant Mental Health Services, Women's and Children's Health Network, South Australia, and clinical senior lecturer, University of Adelaide. Anne's work in psychiatry has included the development and delivery of teaching packages in perinatal and infant mental health in many parts of Australia. Publications include coediting *Infants of Parents with Mental Illness: Developmental, Clinical, Cultural and Personal Perspectives* (2008). Current research focuses on borderline personality disorder in perinatal populations.

Katherine L. Wisner, MD, MS, is the Norman and Helen Asher professor of psychiatry and behavioral sciences and obstetrics and gynecology and director of the Asher Center for the Study and Treatment of Depressive Disorders at the Northwestern University Feinberg School of Medicine. She is internationally recognized as an expert in mood disorders across childbearing. She has published a screening study of 10,000 women with follow-up home visits and assessment across the first postpartum year.

Barbara P. Yawn, MD, MSc, is a family physician researcher, director of research at the Olmsted Medical Center, and adjunct professor in the Department of Family and Community Health at the University of Minnesota. She focuses her work on areas of screening, screening outcomes, and implementation research. She has worked on issues in the perinatal period for more than 20 years and recently completed a 5-year clinical trial of postnatal depression screening and management in primary care. Dr. Yawn has served as a member of the US Preventive Services Task Force and five National Institutes of Health guideline panels, published over 300 papers in peer-reviewed journals, edited three books, and authored numerous book chapters.

Foreword

To screen or not to screen, that is the question! This timely book provides the reader with a scholarly examination of how to answer this important public health question—and above all how to implement the answer. Of course, as the contributors have made plain, the answer will vary across the world according to the resources available and the relative prominence of scientific and folk beliefs about explanatory models of perinatal mental health.

I recently concluded a plenary lecture at the Health Visitor's Institute in London by saying, "Of course you should screen for perinatal mental disorder—you are skilled health professionals." There should, I believe, be no debate about whether, even in the fast-paced, underresourced milieu of a community health service, we should devise ways of identifying those mothers with severe perinatal mental disorders. The EPDS was first developed because it was self-evident in Scotland that women with moderate or severe depression were being missed by primary care services and that screening tools were therefore necessary to reduce the chances of a calamitous outcome for the whole family.

The reader must, however, decide whether *universal* screening for perinatal mental disorder, or even nationally implemented targeted screening that can be sustained over time, is desirable, ethical, and practical. The authoritative contributors do not beat about the bush in this regard—nor have the editors avoided consideration of the need for the specific diagnostic and management skills of psychiatrists and other professionals or the need for a cogent differential diagnosis as a component of any screening pathway.

The decision to implement screening may in part depend on whether a national committee or ministry of health regards screening for mental disorder as having parity of importance with screening for diabetes, bowel cancer, or hypertension. I believe it should—and the scientific scrutiny of the evidence should be no *less, and no more*, than that applied to screening for prostate or breast cancer, for example. Applying rigorously the UK's National Screening Committees criteria for targeted screening program (e.g., sensitivity of the test, nature of the disorder, availability of cost effective treatments, and risk of harm) would have halted many of the screening programs for these conditions currently being implemented in the United Kingdom. The use of screening tools such as the EPDS or the PHQ and the interpretation of their scores require the participation of a trained health worker in the same way as the prostate-specific antigen test, fecal occult blood, and a random blood pressure check.

Paradoxically, this fully referenced book highlights the continued limitations of DSM-5, which has failed to categorize adequately the puerperal psychoses and the perinatal nonpsychotic mood disorders; the disorders that are the target of the screening programs discussed by the contributors of this volume. Let us hope that ICD-11 may yet fulfill more satisfactorily this crucial public health task.

This is a landmark book that should be read around the world. The scholarly editors of this volume have shown that multidisciplinary approaches to perinatal mental health are essential and that the Marcé Society (which cradled the EPDS) will therefore continue to motivate researchers and clinicians and inspire the burgeoning advocacy groups which are demanding improved services for childbearing mothers and their families.

John Cox
Professor Emeritus, Keele University, Staffordshire, UK

Introduction

Current Issues in Identifying Perinatal Depression
An Overview

Jeannette Milgrom and Alan W. Gemmill

The idea behind this new book on the identification and management of perinatal depression is to provide researchers and practitioners with an up-to-the-minute reference text on how and whether to undertake active identification in the context of the latest research and expert opinion. We believe that the value in such a publication lies in allowing a regrouping and updating of various disparate sources of guidance and information on perinatal depression identification.

As editors, we asked contributors to consider what would be needed for screening programs to achieve clinical efficacy, to reflect upon what aspects of the field require specific future work, and to speculate on future developments and applications.

To our delight and surprise, this relatively simple idea immediately took on a life of its own. The project was clearly timely and with the input of many, its structure took shape. As editors, we quickly realized that one of the great strengths of the book would be the number of distinguished clinicians/researchers involved as authors and the insights they would bring on what the field needs in order to advance. The editorial process was deliberately iterative to give us the opportunity to engage in productive discussions with contributors about the most relevant topics and emphases for each chapter. While we endeavored to edit a coherent book with some consistent messages, we tried also to encourage in-depth coverage of some complex issues and some that are likely to remain contentious for some time.

What has emerged is more than a collection of up-to-date information on identification of perinatal depression and offers a fuller and (we think) deeper treatment of many issues, some of which have not previously been expounded fully in the literature. As such, the contributions to this book offer original and high-quality insight on areas of both consensus and controversy.

Identifying Perinatal Depression and Anxiety: Evidence-Based Practice in Screening, Psychosocial Assessment, and Management, First Edition. Edited by Jeannette Milgrom and Alan W. Gemmill.
© 2015 John Wiley & Sons, Ltd. Published 2015 by John Wiley & Sons, Ltd.

The Screening Conundrum

Definitions

This book, entitled *Identifying Perinatal Depression and Anxiety*, considers the current knowledge and issues regarding evidence-based screening, assessment, and management. Interestingly, given that a major focus of the book is evidence-based practice in screening for perinatal depression, few authors sought to define the term "screening." While various definitions exist, the UK National Screening Committee (NSC) provides a comprehensive and useful framework for understanding issues around screening in general (NSC website: http://www.screening.nhs.uk/screening). The NSC defines a screening *test* as "*A test or inquiry used on people who do not have or have not recognised the signs or symptoms of the condition being tested for. It divides people into low and higher risk groups.*" This is consistent with the global description of "screening for depression" by Thombs and colleagues (2012). However, the NSC definition also emphasizes that screening *tests* are only one necessary aspect of screening *programs* which take place in a specific *context*: namely, the allocation of resources to apply a screening test in a population of apparently healthy individuals who have not been previously identified with the target condition. This is carried out with a view to appropriately further assessing and managing those individuals (while taking into account other existing conditions). Furthermore, screening *programs* are designed for a specific *purpose* which is usually to reduce risk/improve outcome through early identification and management/treatment inside the program. Occasionally, however, screening serves a worthwhile purpose purely by providing information, as in the case of prenatal screening for some (nontreatable) genetic abnormalities. In the mental health area, this potentially could be helpful, for instance, by raising awareness among women with mild symptoms.

Importantly, in order to be effective, a screening *program* needs to be a *process* that, on balance, is doing more good than harm given the properties of the particular test and the context and purpose of the screening program. Potential harms attached to perinatal mental health screening that are often cited include distress resulting from being asked about one's emotional state, stigma arising from a positive screen, diversion of resources from other mental health services, and the possibility that screening tests may be misused as diagnostic tools resulting in unnecessary or inappropriate treatment. Crucial to achieving a balance is demonstrating benefits that outweigh resource implications. Such a process can only be expected to work if the process represents a "coordinated quality assured system of care" which has resource implications.

In editing this book, we have tried to adopt a terminology that is consistent with the NSC framework, by identifying a minimum set of sequential elements in a perinatal depression *screening program*: (i) a screening **test**, (ii) information about test results plus a **diagnostic procedure** following all positive test results, (iii) **management** options for diagnosed cases based on the screening test and consideration of the woman's context (broader psychosocial assessment defined here to include past and present mental health history, other mental health conditions especially anxiety, risk factors such as abuse or interpersonal violence, and social factors including impact on the infant and partner), and (iv) **sufficient treatment resources** for all diagnosed individuals wanting treatment (which requires sufficient training of health professionals). Points (iii) and (iv) are necessary for any increase in identified cases achieved by points (i) and (ii) to translate into better outcomes for those screened.

The various chapters provide food for thought on how to minimize potential harms and improve outcomes and benefits.

Enduring controversies

An enduring area of controversy in perinatal mental health is whether there is currently sufficient evidence to recommend (either universal or targeted) depression screening programs. For sure, we have screening *tests* that are capable of dividing people *"into low- and higher-risk groups"*. For example, a positive score on the Edinburgh Postnatal Depression Scale (EPDS) defines a subgroup with a prevalence of depression between 5 and 17 times higher than in the unscreened population (Milgrom, Mendelsohn, & Gemmill, 2011). But the questions remain: does this initial numerical advantage offered by depression screening feed through to increased treatment and a corresponding increase in remission and recovery? If so, how many individuals would need to be screened in order that one extra case of depression be treated successfully? What would the cumulative steps needed to achieve that result add up to in terms of costs? Are there ethical implications about basing such decisions on cost?

Certainly, perinatal depression meets most of the central prerequisites for considering the implementation of a screening program (the condition is serious, prevalent, and treatable, most cases go undetected in current best-practice care, and an acceptable screening test of known accuracy is available: Hill, 2010; Milgrom & Gemmill, 2014). It therefore seems all the more remarkable that the most important prerequisite remains frustratingly difficult to evaluate—we still lack sufficient good-quality evidence with which to weigh the potential benefits of perinatal depression screening against the potential costs and harms. The main stumbling block remains the rarity of suitably designed effectiveness trials (Thombs et al., 2014). While the conclusions of recent reviews acknowledge the slowly emerging body of evidence supporting the benefits of screening (judged low-to-moderate strength in the latest Comparative Effectiveness Review by the AHRQ: Myers et al., 2013), none have found sufficient grounds to recommend systematic screening at this time. This is not to say that screening has been established as ineffective, overcostly, or harmful, only that close scrutiny of the available facts has revealed a gaping absence of evidence on both costs and benefits. There are only five published studies which, taken together, may provide low-to-moderate strength of evidence in favor of the clinical efficacy of screening programs in reducing depression morbidity among postpartum women (Myers et al., 2013). While on this basis it is difficult for policy makers to make recommendations with any confidence that scarce health system resources be allocated to perinatal depression screening programs, international guidelines developed largely by academics and clinicians have taken various positions regarding the application of current knowledge (reviewed in this book). The justified skepticism regarding the state of the evidence base coexists in uneasy tension with a general consensus that timely identification and treatment of perinatal mental disorders is and should be a desirable aim. Good-quality perinatal health care perinatal health care needs to address the fact that depression in particular is highly prevalent, serious in its impact, and, although treatable, help-seeking is poor).

What to do now?

In practice, resources into current practice processes that lead incidentally to identification (including investment in education aimed at increased clinician awareness of mental health) to (iii) opting to deploy screening tests universally since, at least, they ask standardized questions and their properties and limitations are well circumscribed and hoping that their mandatory application may help to ensure that, at an absolute minimum, every woman's mental health is at least considered by her perinatal health-care providers (Chaudron & Wisner, 2014; Gemmill, 2014; Thombs & Stewart, 2014). Currently, none of these alternatives, including the continuance of current standard practices, can be rigorously supported by evidence-based arguments—together, they represent the diversity of expert opinion informed by both clinical experience and research.

In seeking a possible interim resolution to this impasse, it is worth noting that (i) these alternatives are not entirely mutually exclusive, (ii) there is scope for harm through nonidentification, (iii) the clinical guidelines in one jurisdiction can differ from those in other jurisdictions and may officially mandate for or against the use of screening tests, and (iv) the strongest evidence for the benefits of perinatal depression screening comes mainly from three cluster trials of *combined identification and treatment*, which demonstrated improvement in maternal mental health in well-integrated screening and management programs supported by specific health professional training. Indeed, it would be surprising if there was *any* evidence that merely deploying a screening test in isolation from a well-integrated program had any positive impact. A "good" screening program would support the chain of necessary steps outlined earlier (diagnosis, treatment) for an integrated system of care, also reducing the scope for harm through misdiagnosis. In brief, when considering deploying a perinatal depression screening *test*, the *context* of screening must be able support a *process* of "coordinated quality assured care" (which includes resources for further assessment and treatment as well as training) in order to achieve the *purpose* of improving outcomes at a tolerable cost (including the balancing of resource implications and potential discomforts to the patient).

In most health-care systems, clinical considerations may be overshadowed by the lack of availability of information on cost-effectiveness. The robustness and structure of such analyses also have some ethical implications in the perinatal context. For example, is it acceptable to make such judgments based solely around the outcomes for "patients" (depressed mothers) when we know that perinatal depression and anxiety also have big impacts on the future health and development of infants? Questions such as these arise from the content presented in this book.

The Contributed Chapters

In this book, we challenged authors to consider what would be needed to make screening a viable approach in order to improve the identification of not only perinatally depressed women but their infants and partners.

The first two chapters tackle the question of whether systematic, population-level screening for perinatal depression and anxiety is desirable and the conditions are required for maximizing its impact in improving outcomes. Chapter 1 introduces the clinical presentations and adverse consequences of not only perinatal depression but also anxiety, particularly the negative impact during pregnancy on the developing fetus. The chapter introduces the enduring controversy that recurs throughout the book: the need for better-quality research evidence on how screening programs affect the outcomes of those women screened.

Nevertheless, an innovative model assesses the extent to which a strategy of increased initial identification can lead to improvement in women's final outcomes. This leads to a confronting analysis of the ultimate effectiveness of current care processes—few depressed women are treated at all, even fewer are treated adequately, and ultimately, only a fraction of cases receive treatment that leads to remission. The conclusion is that the lamentably low rate of *initial identification* represents the weakest link in the perinatal "care continuum" so that concentrating on this critical step may have the biggest impact on outcomes.

The screening program

In Chapter 2, clear principles are derived for the construction and operation of a successful perinatal depression screening program with recommendations of who should implement screening, with what tools (tests), where, when, and the steps that should follow a screening test (including the importance of how to ensure effective management of suicidal ideation). It is concluded that among perinatal mental disorders, it is only for depression that we have sufficient evidence to begin formulating screening and management programs. Screening tests and processes for perinatal anxiety require further investigation prior to recommendations for widespread use. This leaves us with a dilemma of how to best identify anxious women within a depression screening program, an issue expanded in detail in Chapter 6. The answer may lie in a recurring theme of this book—that screening and management programs are most successful when the screening, diagnostic, assessment, management, and treatment components are provided in an integrated system of care (resources therefore become a rate-limiting step).

Chapters 3, 4, and 5 provide a detailed resource for practitioners regarding practical issues of implementation. Chapter 4 is conceived as a guide to delivering the most common screening tool, the EPDS (Cox, Holden, & Sagovsky, 1987), in practice from the point of view of clinicians in the field. The interpretation and sensitive feeding back of test results are clearly articulated with reference to particular configurations of scores on individual items, such as those indicating anxiety and thoughts of self-harm. Throughout, the contributors take great care to caution against the various possible inappropriate applications of the test and against simplistic interpretations of results. A helpful demonstration of a screening program and process is detailed and how potential misuses of the test, such as inaccurate feedback to women, or treatment commencement based only on a positive screening score can be minimized in practice. Central to this is maintaining a woman-centered focus that remains sensitive to the woman's personal situation as well as her social and cultural context.

A range of potential hindrances to each stage of identification, referral, and treatment are tackled in Chapter 3. The contributors aim to provide a review that can inform strategies aimed at overcoming these barriers to better outcomes for depressed women. The evidence surrounding many practical, cultural, and attitudinal barriers is carefully covered. An important conclusion is that the interaction of patient and provider attitudes is critical at all stages of the identification and management continuum. For example, the authors stress the importance of both patient and clinician recognizing that depression is a stigmatized condition in many societies and cultures. Provision of culturally sensitive, nonjudgmental information, advice, and support can engender more confident, informed and empowered help-seeking choices by women.

In Chapter 5, the contributors provide an impressive and exhaustive review of the purposes, technical properties, and comparative utilities of available screening instruments for depression in the perinatal period. Two broad classes exist: generic depression instruments and those designed for use in the perinatal context. The potential benefits of using ultra-brief case-finding tests as a triage approach within clinical settings are also explored.

Available instruments are compared in terms of their false-positive and false-negative rates, their content validity for perinatal women, and the length of time required for administration. The conclusion reached is that generic instruments have been insufficiently evaluated in the perinatal context and that testing in antenatal populations is a particularly underresearched area. In agreement with previous reviews of the area, the EPDS is again identified as the perinatal-specific instrument that has been most widely validated and whose properties are best understood.

Chapter 6 reviews the difficulties in initial identification of anxiety. Though little information on the clinical effectiveness of perinatal anxiety screening is available, the prevalence, comorbidity with depression, and potential impact on the health of women and their infants lend urgency to research into reliable identification during pregnancy and in the postnatal period. The message of the chapter concerns the importance of being clear about what we are screening for when considering the use of a screening test—focusing our attention on the possible importance of both subsyndromal levels of anxiety and more generalized experiences of emotional "distress." A range of diagnosable anxiety disorders are discussed, and the question is posed whether fulfillment of diagnostic criteria is the most relevant route to supporting women with regard to perinatal anxiety. The authors outline the different generic and pregnancy-specific anxiety instruments and again conclude that screening for anxiety is an underdeveloped area encompassing a diverse array of symptoms, presentations, and classifications. Much future research is required to develop and validate appropriate tools in this area.

Given the importance of following a screening test with further assessment to determine whether an individual is clinically depressed and in need of treatment, Chapter 7 addresses formal diagnostic identification of perinatal mood disorders. The value of a structured approach to diagnosis is discussed along with current challenges in this area in respect of perinatal populations. Importantly, the range of potential disorders occurring in the post-partum, which require appropriate identification, is highlighted. Conditions such as bipolar disorders, while not highly prevalent, necessitate immediate management.

A strong argument is mounted in Chapter 8 supporting the idea that psychosocial assessment holds intrinsic value in starting a conversation about wider issues impacting on families and in raising awareness. The usefulness of a broad focus of inquiry, at the same time as using a screening test for depression and anxiety, is highlighted. The use of struc-tured questionnaires on past and current risk to provide a standardized starting point for integrated psychosocial assessment and intervention programs is described. Establishing such programs in primary care settings requires collaborative, multidisciplinary involve-ment, supported by suitable training and a set of decision-making rules to aid clinicians.

Complex issues around psychosocial assessment in resource-constrained settings emerge in this chapter. While the prevalence of perinatal mental disorders may be considerably higher in low-income countries, their recognition is generally very low. Further, the experi-ence of responding to a screening test can be alien in many cultures, the disclosure of neg-ative emotional states may be socially unacceptable, and/or there may be little or no health system infrastructure to support women identified. The authors poignantly add: "*There are risks that using psychopathological labels to describe the social suffering that is associated with poverty and gender-based violence increases the risk of marginalization and discrimination.*" However, the authors argue that opting to do nothing about perinatal assessment of psychosocial issues in such settings is not an acceptable response. Their conclusions point optimistically to the emerging results of community-based approaches to perinatal mental health in resource-constrained settings. They urge capacity-building partnerships drawing support by nonspecialist health workers and the development of perinatal mental health-care models built on the basis of local culture and evidence about prevalence, assessment, and identification methods.

Chapters 9 and 10 expand the concept of a wider inquiry and turn to the questions of whether screening and assessment for perinatal mental health can be usefully extended to parent–infant relationships and to fathers. Chapter 9 represents the only real existing synthesis of the relevant literature with a view to informing screening and treatment to ameliorate impact on infants. Importantly, the negative impact of postnatal depression on the infant's development is examined in terms of the possible mechanisms and opportunities to intervene early. Treating maternal depression alone is not necessarily associated with improvements in child outcome, and both interventions targeting difficulties in parenting and the development of reliable measures to identify problems are discussed. Similarly, in Chapter 10, the lack of existing tools to identify difficulties experienced by fathers is covered in the context of the need for more research and targeting a broader range of emotional difficulties and presentations.

The final step in a successful perinatal depression screening program is the provision of effective management and treatment options for the women identified as requiring help. In Chapter 11, the contributors give an up-to-date account of psychological, pharmacological, and complementary approaches for depression and anxiety. The evidence base particularly for psychological approaches confirms that where resources are sufficient, identified women can be offered effective treatments.

Existing guidelines and the need for training

Taking together the information regarding the need for screening, evidence about screening tools for depression and anxiety, and consideration of further assessment and available treatments, several countries have now developed extensive guidelines on management of perinatal mental health. These include positions on the use of screening tests. In Chapter 12, a systematic comparison of the approach in six different countries is provided, with the fascinating conclusion that the same evidence base has been interpreted in various ways regarding its implications for good practice. Leading academics and clinicians on the "front line" from Australia, the United Kingdom, Scotland, France, Canada, and the United States provide a synthesis regarding the development and implementation of national guidelines. The authors stress that differences in guidelines no doubt reflect varying practices in assessment and treatment and intercountry differences in societal values (and views of motherhood), attitudes, as well as resource availability. There is, however, a clear international consensus that identifying perinatal women who are depressed or have other psychiatric or psychosocial issues is important. Nevertheless, recommendations are mixed and not always evidence based.

Australian guidelines recommend universal screening, including using the EPDS, accompanied by a broader psychosocial assessment, although the latter is not supported by an extensive evidence base. UK guidelines have a clear focus on the service organization and do not endorse what they define as "screening"—past history and early identification, particularly of severe postpartum illness, are the preferred language. Paradoxically, it is recommended that *all* women be asked the two standardized "Whooley questions" (Whooley, Avins, & Miranda, 1997) that inquire about symptoms of depressed mood despite little evidence validating this instrument in perinatal populations.

Scottish guidelines also focus on early intervention and risk reduction but do not recommend use of a universal "screening" test for postnatal depression due to insufficient evidence. The picture in Canada's provinces is varied. No existing national guidelines have been formulated, and there are no national recommendations concerning use of screening test, of case-finding questions, or of psychosocial assessment. Nonetheless, some health-care services deploy screening tests, and some provinces have developed guidelines. In France, we see a leading focus on the importance of early mother–infant attachment and training professionals in perinatal mental health disorders. At the same time, implementation appears fragmented. Similarly, while we see no unifying US national guidelines, there are a number of developments at the state and national levels. Most notably, the Mother's Act requires health insurance coverage for depression screening and the introduction of mandatory perinatal depression screening in New Jersey. The most recent report from the United States (Myers et al., 2013) recommends that deploying screening tests can be useful in well-resourced health service settings in the context of integrated care.

A diverse range of health-care professionals may be involved in the identification and management of perinatal depression and anxiety, such as midwives, health visitors (HVs), child and family health nurses, clinical psychologists, psychiatrists, community mental health nurses, mental health social workers, counselors, general practitioners, and nurse practitioners.

Chapter 13 describes the principles of training health-care professionals and gives as examples the UK PoNDER trial (Morrell et al., 2011) which showed benefits in terms of cost-effectiveness and improvement in outcomes for women in the clusters whose HV had been trained (as well as a universal preventive effect). The Australian National Perinatal Depression Initiative (NPDI) also has developed training for screening which is "well embedded" into routine practice. While there is widespread access to training, particularly at the level of "basic knowledge," there are still areas where training has not been comprehensive, and there are remaining implementation challenges including time pressures in busy nursing centers.

Interestingly, educational interventions do not necessarily result in the necessary changes to attitudes, skills, and behavior needed to improve care. These are more likely to occur when teaching is integrated as part of an organizational intervention using a range of strategies, including collaborative care, particularly when offered in conjunction with the trainers.

Concluding Issues

Chapter 14 turns to the important issue of the economic consequences of screening for perinatal depression with a focus on the postnatal period as there are no studies during pregnancy and the intrapartum period. Existing studies during the postnatal period tend to be limited in perspective and timescale. For example, in some studies aiming to evaluate economic benefits, screening was accompanied by additional enhancements to health care, and consequently, it was not possible to estimate the cost-effectiveness of the screening component per se (e.g., Morrell et al., 2011; Petrou, Cooper, Murray, & Davidson, 2006). Another approach has been to develop decision-analytic models investigating the EPDS as a strategy for identifying women with postnatal depression; relaxing some of the base assumptions in sensitivity analyses, there is a suggestion screening may approach cost-effectiveness under some circumstances. The chapter highlights the need to obtain new estimates of health utilities directly from depressed perinatal women, extend the time horizons of economic evaluations, and find ways to include infant outcomes in modeling.

Finally, Chapter 15 addresses innovative methods now available through information technology that may have the potential "*to further optimize effectiveness of both identification and treatment of perinatal depression and can facilitate the dissemination of therapies among the public.*" These programs offer a source for population-based approaches to reducing perinatal depression in the community. This may lead to earlier detection, increased awareness, and recognition of symptoms although interpretation should be cautious, given the limitations of online screening without professional input. Online screening shares potential harms from "traditional" routine screening for depression including, among others, the labeling of depression in patients who are incorrectly identified as having the disorder. The usefulness of computer-based depression screening may well be enhanced by combining computer-based screening with decision support systems and use of online diagnostic instruments.

This chapter also describes online interventions for perinatal depression and concludes with recommendations for further research.

Final Comments

The contributors to the book have certainly not minimized the scale of the challenges involved in successfully increasing early identification and treatment rates for perinatal depression and anxiety. At the same time, the enormous body of work reviewed and synthesized here demonstrates some tremendous advances and an ongoing upsurge of interest in the field. Enjoy the book.

References

Chaudron, L.H. & Wisner, K. (2014) Perinatal depression screening: Let's not throw the baby out with the bathwater!. *Journal of Psychosomatic Research, 76*, 489–491.

Cox, J., Holden, J. & Sagovsky, R. (1987) Detection of postnatal depression: Development of a 10 item postnatal depression scale. *The British Journal of Psychiatry: The Journal of Mental Science, 150*, 782–786.

Gemmill, A. W. (2014). The long gestation of screening programmes for perinatal depressive disorders. *Journal of Psychosomatic Research, 77*, 242–243. doi:http://dx.doi.org/10.1016/j.jpsychores.2014.06.017.

Hill, C. (2010). *An Evaluation of Screening for Postnatal Depression Against NSC Criteria*. London, UK: UK National Screening Committee. Retrieved from http://www.screening.nhs.uk/postnataldepression

Milgrom, J. & Gemmill, A.W. (2014) Screening for perinatal depression. *Best Practice & Research. Clinical Obstetrics & Gynaecology, 28* (1), 13–23. doi: 10.1016/j.bpobgyn.2013.08.014.

Milgrom, J., Mendelsohn, J. & Gemmill, A.W. (2011) Does postnatal depression screening work? Throwing out the bathwater, keeping the baby. *Journal of Affective Disorders, 132* (3), 301–310.

Morrell, C.J., Ricketts, T., Tudor, K., Williams, C., Curran, J. & Barkham, M. (2011) Training health visitors in cognitive behavioural and person-centred approaches for depression in postnatal women as part of a cluster randomised trial and economic evaluation in primary care: The

PoNDER trial. *Primary Health Care Research & Development, 12* (1), 11–20. doi: 10.1017/s1463423610000344.

Myers, E., Aubuchon-Endsley N, Bastian LA, Gierisch JM, Kemper AR, Swamy GK,...Sanders GD. (2013). *Efficacy and Safety of Screening for Postpartum Depression. Comparative Effectiveness Review 106.* Rockville, MD: Agency for Healthcare Research and Quality.

Petrou, S., Cooper, P., Murray, L. & Davidson, L.L. (2006) Cost-effectiveness of a preventive counseling and support package for postnatal depression. *International Journal of Technology Assessment in Health Care, 22* (4), 443–453.

Thombs, B.D., Arthurs, E., Coronado-Montoya, S., Roseman, M., Delisle, V.C. & Leavens, A. (2014) Depression screening and patient outcomes in pregnancy or postpartum: A systematic review. *Journal of Psychosomatic Research, 76,* 433–446.

Thombs, B. D., Coyne, J. C., Cuijpers, P., de Jonge, P., Gilbody, S., Ionnidis, J. P. A.,...Ziegelstein, R. C. (2012). Rethinking recommendations for screening for depression in primary care. *CMAJ: Canadian Medical Association Journal, 184,* 413–418.

Thombs, B.D. & Stewart, D.E. (2014) Depression screening in pregnancy and postpartum: Who needs evidence? *Journal of Psychosomatic Research, 76,* 492–493.

Whooley, M., Avins, A. & Miranda, J. (1997) Case-finding instruments for depression: Two questions are as good as many. *Journal of General Internal Medicine, 12,* 439–445.

1

Is Population-Based Identification of Perinatal Depression and Anxiety Desirable?

A Public Health Perspective on the Perinatal Depression Care Continuum

Norma I. Gavin, Samantha Meltzer-Brody, Vivette Glover, and Bradley N. Gaynes

Introduction

The perinatal period is a profound time of transition for women and their families; a myriad of determinants—including social, psychological, behavioral, environmental, and biological forces—shape pregnancy and the postpartum course (Misra, Guyer, & Allston, 2003). Due to the complexity of this vulnerable time, psychiatric complications such as maternal depression and anxiety are common during the perinatal period (Wisner et al., 2013). The longitudinal course of depressive and anxiety disorders that manifest during pregnancy and the postpartum period and the management of the disorders are active areas of investigation. In particular, the study of whether systematic, population-level screening and case identification of perinatal depression and anxiety are desirable is an important area of controversy.

Although screening for current disorders has been widely promoted based on the serious adverse consequences of untreated maternal depression and anxiety, population-based screening has significant resource implications (Austin, Middleton, Reilly, & Highet, 2013; Henshaw & Elliott, 2005; National Institute for Health and Clinical Excellence [NICE], 2007; Shakespeare, 2005). In many settings, the successful implementation and maintenance of a population-based screening program would require additional provider training, increased provider workloads, and improved patient access to

Identifying Perinatal Depression and Anxiety: Evidence-Based Practice in Screening, Psychosocial Assessment, and Management, First Edition. Edited by Jeannette Milgrom and Alan W. Gemmill.
© 2015 John Wiley & Sons, Ltd. Published 2015 by John Wiley & Sons, Ltd.

health services. Barriers to screening for existing disorders and the evidence base are covered in following chapters.

In this chapter, we investigate the case for population-based screening of perinatal depression and anxiety using a public health-care continuum model that takes the reader through the sequential steps from the identification and management of perinatal depression and anxiety to successful health outcomes. The conditions required for successful population-based screening are presented, and the current evidence in Western industrialized countries on each of these conditions is summarized.

Although we discuss both perinatal depression and anxiety, the literature on perinatal depression, and postnatal depression in particular, is more comprehensive and well developed than the literature on perinatal anxiety disorders. As a result, our discussion in this chapter, which primarily addresses perinatal depression but refers to perinatal anxiety where possible, reflects the current state of the literature. Moreover, because anxiety is often a common clinical symptom in women with perinatal mood disorders, it can be difficult to tease apart the difference between perinatal depression with anxious features and a completely separate perinatal anxiety disorder.

The chapter begins with a description of the clinical presentation of perinatal depression and anxiety followed by a description of the care continuum model and current evidence supporting each of the model's components. We conclude with implications for policy and future research.

Clinical Presentation of Perinatal Depression and Anxiety

Perinatal depression and anxiety are clinical syndromes commonly described as the onset of a major depressive episode (MDE) or significant anxiety symptoms occurring during pregnancy and/or in the postpartum period (Gavin et al., 2005; O'Hara & Swain, 1996; Wisner et al., 2013). Symptom onset during pregnancy is often referred to as antenatal or prenatal depression or anxiety. Onset of symptoms in the postpartum period is usually described as postpartum/postnatal depression (PND) or postnatal anxiety.

PND has been the most widely studied perinatal psychiatric illness, although controversy exists regarding how best to define the onset of symptoms in the postpartum period (Elliott, 2000; Wisner, Moses-Kolko, & Sit, 2010). For example, the DSM-IV postpartum specifier strictly defined an MDE with onset of symptoms within 4 weeks after delivery (DSM-IV, 1994). DSM-5 instead provides a "peripartum" specifier expanded to include onset of symptoms during pregnancy (American Psychiatric Association, 2013). In ICD-10, postpartum onset is considered to be within 6 weeks after childbirth (Cox, 2004). A common broader definition of the term "perinatal depression" includes onset of mood and anxiety symptoms that occur during pregnancy and through one year postpartum (Gavin et al., 2005; Gaynes et al., 2005a). Subthreshold depressive symptoms are often considered important by clinicians and researchers. However, because more information is available on MDEs, our focus in this chapter is on major depression.

In addition to PND, the development of a new-onset anxiety disorder in the postpartum period or exacerbation of an existing anxiety disorder have been documented in the literature including, but not limited to, generalized anxiety disorder (GAD) (Prenoveau et al., 2013) and postpartum obsessive–compulsive disorder (PP-OCD) (Abramowitz et al., 2010; Fairbrother & Abramowitz, 2007; Prenoveau et al., 2013). GAD is characterized by excessive worry that interferes in multiple domains of the person's life. Because symptoms must be present for 6 months before a diagnosis can be made, criteria for new-onset GAD are unlikely to be met during the 9 months of pregnancy or the early postpartum period (Ross & McLean, 2006). In contrast to ruminating symptoms, PP-OCD is characterized by persistent, and unwanted, obsessional thoughts and the implementation of compulsive rituals and behaviors aimed at neutralizing or managing the intrusive thoughts (Abramowitz et al., 2010; DSM-IV, 1994). The literature documents an increased incidence of both obsessive–compulsive symptoms and a clinical diagnosis of OCD in postpartum women, although controversy exists in the field regarding whether PP-OCD is a distinct clinical entity (Abramowitz et al., 2010; Altemus et al., 2012; McGuinness, Blissett, & Jones, 2011; Uguz, Akman, Kaya, & Cilli, 2007). Postpartum posttraumatic stress disorder (PP-PTSD) also occurs (Cohen, Ansara, Schei, Stuckless, & Stewart, 2004; Olde, van der Hart, Kleber, & van Son, 2006: but note that PTSD is no longer listed as an anxiety disorder in DSM-5).The primary trigger for the development of PP-PTSD is the women's subjective experience of a negative or traumatic birth (Garthus-Niegel, von Soest, Vollrath, & Eberhard-Gran, 2013). A history of sexual trauma and a preexisting anxiety sensitivity have also been associated as risk factors for developing PTSD after childbirth (Verreault et al., 2012).

Depressive symptoms occur on a continuum of severity, and not all women will meet diagnostic categories. The clinical presentation of perinatal depression is often characterized by mood symptoms that cause significant distress to the perinatal woman (Bernstein et al., 2008; Cooper & Murray, 1997). Sadness, weepiness, low mood, irritability, impaired concentration, and feeling overwhelmed are commonly reported symptoms (Hendrick, Altshuler, Strouse, & Grosser, 2000). Moreover, anxiety or agitation is often a distinguishing feature of perinatal depression and can take the form of ruminating and obsessional thoughts, often about the pregnancy or the infant (Abramowitz et al., 2010; Bernstein et al., 2008). In the postpartum period, women with PND can demonstrate severe hypervigilance about the baby and will be unable to sleep at night, even when the baby is sleeping, due to concerns about the infant's well-being (Leckman et al., 1999; Wisner, Peindl, Gigliotti, & Hanusa, 1999). Alternatively, some women will report feeling detached from the infant and/or will exhibit a lack of interest in holding, interacting, or caring for their baby. Importantly, most women with perinatal mood symptoms report feelings of guilt that they are not able to enjoy the baby (Beck, 1996b; Yonkers, Vigod, & Ross, 2011). Diagnostic criteria for MDEs and other specified depressive disorders are covered in Chapter 7.

Care Continuum

Strategies for screening and case identification (including standardized perinatal depression screens) have been promoted but remain controversial (Austin et al., 2013; Henshaw & Elliott, 2005; National Institute for Health and Clinical Excellence [NICE], 2007; Shakespeare, 2005), with arguments against screening including that the potential additional costs of managing women falsely identified as depressed or anxious are not cost-effective (Paulden, Palmer, Hewitt, & Gilbody, 2009).

To determine whether population-based identification of perinatal depression and anxiety is desirable, we consider a model that assesses whether a strategy of screening ultimately leads to improved outcome. In the model, the identification and management of perinatal depression follow along a "treatment cascade" or "care continuum," which involves multiple sequential steps that can lead to a successful outcome (Figure 1.1) (Gardner, McLees, Steiner, Del Rio, & Burman, 2011; Pence, O'Donnell, & Gaynes, 2012). The model posits that to

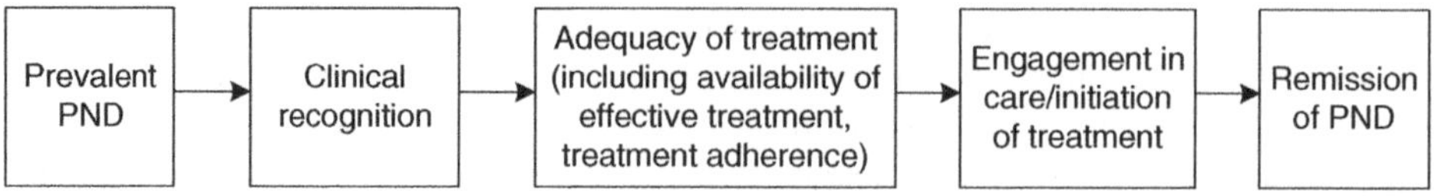

Figure 1.1   Care continuum for perinatal depression and anxiety.

achieve successful treatment, both patient and her clinician must be aware of the diagnosis; effective care must be available and accessible; and the patient must be engaged in care, remain in care, and adhere to treatment (Mugavero, Norton, & Saag, 2011). This model requires active participation by both the patient and the provider. Attrition of the population at any of these steps may worsen health outcomes for both the patient and the child.

At any point along the care continuum, strategies can be developed and applied to strengthen the likelihood of remission. For example, clinical recognition can be increased with population-based screening and both clinical and patient education efforts, and the likelihood that providers adhere to treatment guidelines and patients comply with treatment recommendations can be increased through education and various patient support systems.

Within this framework, a number of conditions are necessary to make population-based identification desirable:

1   *The condition must be common.* Enough women must suffer from perinatal depression or anxiety that general screening among a population of pregnant and postpartum women would yield enough cases to make screening worthwhile.

2   *The condition must have bad consequences.* The harmful effects on the woman and her child of unrecognized and untreated perinatal depression and anxiety must be significant enough to outweigh the costs of screening and treatment.

3   *Screening must identify a significant number of otherwise unrecognized cases.* The screening instrument and procedures must be sensitive enough to correctly identify most of the women suffering from perinatal depression or anxiety and specific enough to identify only a few false positives.

4   *An effective treatment must exist.* Management, whether pharmacologic or psychotherapeutic, has to be able to reduce or eliminate the poor outcomes of the depressive or anxious episode and minimize adverse effects of treatment in a cost-effective manner.

5   *Effective treatment must be available to the affected population.* The population targeted for screening must have access to the treatment.

6   *Effective treatment must be followed.* Treatment guidelines must be easily followed by most providers, and women must seek and follow up recommended treatment.

Evidence on whether each of these conditions is met for perinatal depression and anxiety in Western industrialized countries is summarized in what follows.

Prevalence and Incidence

Depression is a common complication of pregnancy and the postpartum period. As many as 20% of women in industrialized countries meet the criteria for a diagnosis of major or minor depression sometime during pregnancy, with a similar or higher percentage meeting these criteria sometime during the first year postpartum (Gavin et al., 2005). Major depression accounts for 20–50% of diagnosed depression during the perinatal period (Dietz et al., 2007; Reck et al., 2008). Furthermore, one-third or more of perinatal women with depression have been found to have a concurrent diagnosis of anxiety (Austin et al., 2010; Miller, Pallant, & Negri, 2006; Reck et al., 2008; Wisner et al., 2013), and another 9–10% of postpartum women have been found to have anxiety alone (Miller et al., 2006; Reck et al., 2008). Estimates vary depending on the definition of anxiety used, the population studied, and the time period at which the diagnosis is assessed.

Most definitions of anxiety in the research literature include some combination of GAD, panic disorder, social phobia, specific phobias, and generalized panic disorder. Studies in Western industrialized countries have found 8.5% of pregnant women in their third trimester (Sutter-Dallay, Giaconne-Marcesche, Glatigny-Dallay, & Verdoux, 2004) and 4.4–8.2% of postpartum women (Wenzel, Haugen, Jackson, & Brendle, 2005; Wenzel, Haugen, Jackson, & Robinson, 2003) to have GAD, 1.3–5.6% of postpartum women to have PTSD (Olde et al., 2006; Soderquist, Wijma, Thorbert, & Wijma, 2009; Verreault et al., 2012), and 1.2–1.6% of pregnant women (Andersson et al., 2003; Borri et al., 2008; Grigoriadis et al., 2011; Sutter-Dallay et al., 2004) and 2.7–3.9% of postpartum women (Grigoriadis et al., 2011; Wenzel, Gorman, O'Hara, & Stuart, 2001; Wenzel et al., 2005) to have OCD.

Although recent studies have discredited the notion that depression is more prevalent among women of childbearing age during pregnancy compared to other times (Dietz et al., 2007; Ko, Farr, Dietz, & Robbins, 2012; Loxton & Lucke, 2009; Najman, Andersen, Bor, O'Callaghan, & Williams, 2000; Schmied et al., 2013), the prevalence of depression, GAD, and OCD during the postpartum period is consistently estimated to be higher than at other times of a woman's life (Dave, Petersen, Sherr, & Nazareth, 2010; Gavin et al., 2005; Ross & McLean, 2006; Vesga-Lopez et al., 2008; Wisner et al., 2013).

Certain subgroups of women are at higher risk of perinatal depression and anxiety. A prior episode of depression is consistently the strongest predictor of depression during pregnancy and the postpartum period (Dennis, Heaman, & Vigod, 2012; Flynn, Davis, Marcus, Cunningham, & Blow, 2004; Leigh & Milgrom, 2008; Meltzer-Brody et al., 2013; Milgrom et al., 2008; Rich-Edwards et al., 2006; Schmied et al., 2013). Recent research by Di Florio et al. reported that more than 70% of parous women with a history of a mood disorder will experience at least one perinatal mood episode in relation to pregnancy and childbirth (Di Florio et al., 2013). Other significant risk factors for perinatal depression include antenatal anxiety (Leigh & Milgrom, 2008), poor partner relationship (Milgrom et al., 2008; Schmied et al., 2013), low social support (Dennis et al., 2012; Leigh & Milgrom, 2008; Schmied et al., 2013), stressful life events (Dennis et al., 2012; Schmied et al., 2013), low socioeconomic status (Dennis et al., 2012; Rich-Edwards et al., 2006; Schmied et al., 2013), and unwanted pregnancy (Rich-Edwards et al., 2006; Schmied et al., 2013). Studies have found similar risk factors for anxiety disorders. In addition, complications in pregnancy and delivery were found to increase the incidence of both PP-PTSD and PP-OCD (Verreault et al., 2012; Zambaldi et al., 2009).

Adverse Health Effects

Untreated perinatal depression and anxiety are associated with serious short- and long-term, adverse consequences for the mother, her baby and the family (Flynn et al., 2004; Marcus et al., 2011; O'Hara & Swain, 1996; Stowe, Hostetter, & Newport, 2005; Wisner, Parry, & Piontek, 2002).

During pregnancy, women with antenatal depression and anxiety have an amplification of reported physical symptoms including complaints of gastrointestinal distress, headaches, dizziness, shortness of breath, and cardiac symptoms (Kelly, Russo, & Katon, 2001). More importantly, antenatal depression increases the risk of poor obstetrical outcomes, such as preterm birth and low birth weight (Diego et al., 2004, 2009; Fransson, Ortenstrand, & Hjelmstedt, 2011; Grote et al., 2010; Halbreich, 2005; Ibanez et al., 2012). Evidence has shown that this is partly due to decreased prenatal care, decreased practice of recommended health behaviors during pregnancy, and increased risk of smoking and substance use in the perinatal period (Flynn et al., 2004). Antenatal anxiety symptoms (with or without mood symptoms) have also been associated with increased risk of preterm birth and low birth weight (Halbreich, 2005; Martini, Knappe, Beesdo-Baum, Lieb, & Wittchen, 2010).

During the perinatal period, women with depression are at increased risk of maternal suicide. In the postnatal period, there is increased risk of infanticide, and decreased maternal sensitivity and attachment with the infant (Campbell et al., 2004; Lindahl, Pearson, & Colpe, 2005; McLearn, Minkovitz, Strobino, Marks, & Hou, 2006; Paulson, Dauber, & Leiferman, 2006). Maternal depression has also been associated with the decreased practice of recommended parenting behaviors such as engaging in enriching interactions with the child (e.g., reading or singing) (Network NECCR, 1999). In addition, postpartum anxiety has been associated with increased maternal health-care utilization and reduced duration of breastfeeding (Paul, Downs, Schaefer, Beiler, & Weisman, 2013; Stuebe, Grewen, & Meltzer-Brody, 2013).

The mechanisms through which maternal depression and anxiety affect the fetus are likely to be biological in pregnancy, whereas postnatally, the mechanisms are more likely psychological. Considerable evidence shows that if the mother is anxious, depressed, or stressed during pregnancy, her child is more likely to experience neurodevelopmental and other problems (Talge et al., 2007). Fetal exposure to suicide attempts during pregnancy has been associated with mental retardation and congenital abnormalities (Gentile, 2011; Gidai, Acs, Banhidy, & Czeizel, 2010; Petik, Czeizel, Banhidy, & Czeizel, 2011).

Infants and toddlers born to anxious/depressed mothers have more difficult temperament and sleep problems. Older children have more emotional difficulties, symptoms of ADHD, and conduct disorder, as well as lower cognitive function. Debate continues as to the extent that this association is causal. However, studies that have taken into account a wide range of potential confounders, including paternal mood and maternal postnatal mood and parenting, still find a substantial prenatal component. Children of mothers in the top 15% for anxiety or depression in a general population in the United Kingdom had double the risk of a probable mental disorder at age 13 (O'Donnell, Glover, Barker, & O'Connor, in press). Prenatal depression and anxiety may contribute 10–15% of the attributable load to behavioral outcome (Talge et al., 2007). The literature provides little consistency as to the most sensitive time in gestation for these altered outcomes. However, several studies have found effects in later gestation (Glover, 2014), so interventions at any stage of pregnancy are likely to be beneficial.

Considerable evidence also shows that PND is associated with different types of difficulty in parenting, particularly the early mother–infant interaction that are, in turn, associated with different problems among children (Milgrom, Westley, & Gemmill, 2004). These overlapping difficulties can be characterized in three groups (Murray et al., 2010): withdrawn interactions, hostile and intrusive interactions, and general sadness and insensitivity. These in turn are associated with an increased risk of worse child emotional, behavioral, and cognitive outcomes. For example, where a depressed mother's vocal interactions signal sadness and she appears insensitive to the baby's attachment needs, there is a more than fourfold increase in the risk of the child developing emotional problems in adolescence (Murray et al., 2011).

The relation between maternal depression and paternal mood symptoms is also important and has critical implications for family health and functioning (Goodman, 2004; Paulson & Bazemore, 2010; Paulson et al., 2006). Maternal perinatal depression has been identified as one of the strongest predictors of paternal depression with estimates that 24–50% of men whose partners are depressed also meet the criteria for minor or major depression (Areias, Kumar, Barros, & Figueiredo, 1996; Goodman, 2004). Perinatal depression in either the mother or father can negatively impact the couple's relationship, leading to increased marital discord and a decrease in marital satisfaction (Beck, 1996a).

Clinical Recognition

Clinical recognition of perinatal depression and anxiety can occur in family practice or general medical settings (Buist et al., 2005; Hickie et al., 2001), obstetrical settings (Austin et al., 2013; Miller et al., 2012), pediatric settings (Earls & Committee on Psychosocial Aspects of Child and Family Health American Academy of Pediatrics, 2010) and at contacts with maternal and child health nurses. Recognition of perinatal depression and anxiety is often poor. Although clinicians are generally supportive of screening for perinatal depression (Dietrich et al., 2003; LaRocco-Cockburn, Melville, Bell, & Katon, 2003), these attitudes do not consistently translate into practice. In the United States, less than half of women are formally screened for perinatal depression (Seehusen, Baldwin, Runkle, & Clark, 2005), even in settings with active perinatal depression screening programs (Kim et al., 2009). Consistent with such efforts, less than 50% of PND cases are detected in routine clinical practice, with prenatal recognition rates reported at 41% (Goodman & Tyer-Viola, 2010) and postnatal rates ranging from 29% (Fairbrother & Abramowitz, 2007) to 43% (Hearn et al., 1998). Chapter 12 describes the variation in screening policies and practices internationally.

A number of effective, easy-to-administer screening tools, including the Edinburgh Postnatal Depression Scale (EPDS: Cox, Holden, & Sagovsky, 1987) and more generic tools such as the Beck Depression Inventory, are available to screen for perinatal depression (Austin et al., 2013; Gaynes et al., 2005a; Paulden et al., 2009). Chapters 5 and 6 describe depression screening tools and anxiety identification, respectively. Population-based perinatal depression screening with such tools can improve health outcomes when the infrastructure to monitor and respond to at-risk patients is available (Gordon, Cardone, Kim, Gordon, & Silver, 2006). A recent systematic evidence review found that across a variety of low-intensity interventions, screening was associated with modest improvements in depression (Myers et al., 2013). These tools can identify perinatal depression, most accurately major depression; their accuracy appears similar to what is found with depression screeners in primary care settings (Gaynes et al., 2005b). These tools can reduce the number of cases of missed perinatal depression (Paulden et al., 2009).

Commonly used and validated screening instruments for anxiety have also been used in the perinatal period. The Generalized Anxiety Disorder Scale (GAD-7) is a brief, seven-item screening tool to assess the presence of GAD validated in primary care populations (Spitzer, Kroenke, Williams, & Lowe, 2006; Swinson, 2006). The Spielberger State-Trait

Anxiety Inventory has been validated for use in perinatal populations (Meades & Ayers, 2011). The trait inventory provides a stable measure of anxiety, whereas the state inventory captures perceived stress "right now" (Spielberger, 1983). In addition, the new Tilburg Pregnancy Distress Scale was developed to assess pregnancy distress and also includes an important subscale measuring perceived partner involvement (Pop et al., 2011). Furthermore, the anxiety subscale of the EPDS has emerging evidence showing its reliability and validity as an anxiety screen (Swalm, Brooks, Doherty, Nathan, & Jacques, 2010). Further details on screening tools are found in Chapters 5 and 6.

Effective Treatment

For pregnant and postpartum women with mild to moderate depressive illness or anxiety, psychological or behavioral treatments without medication therapy are recommended as a first-line treatment option (Yonkers et al., 2009, 2011). Solid evidence exists on the efficacy of a wide range of psychological interventions including, but not limited to, interpersonal psychotherapy (Brandon et al., 2012; Grote et al., 2009; Stuart & O'Hara, 1995; Zlotnick, Miller, Pearlstein, Howard, & Sweeney, 2006), cognitive behavioral therapy (Chabrol et al., 2002; Cooper, Murray, Wilson, & Romaniuk, 2003), and group psychoeducation (Honey, Bennett, & Morgan, 2002; Morgan, Matthey, Barnett, & Richardson, 1997). Importantly, the type of therapeutic modality must be tailored to the primary presenting symptoms of the patient and is the reason why a broad psychosocial assessment is recommended (as detailed later in the book). For example, women who report a negative or traumatic birth experience as a trigger for onset of symptoms may be best served by participating in psychotherapy that integrates trauma recovery work.

For more severe depressive and anxiety symptoms, pharmacotherapy is considered an appropriate and efficacious treatment option (Einarson, 2010; Yonkers et al., 2009). A recent large systematic review and meta-analysis found the absolute risks associated with antidepressant exposure during pregnancy to be small (Einarson, Choi, Einarson, & Koren, 2009; Ross et al., 2013). Evidence also exists for the efficacy of both newer antidepressants (selective serotonin reuptake inhibitors—SSRIs) and older tricyclic antidepressants in the treatment of perinatal depression and anxiety (Newport, Hostetter, Arnold, & Stowe, 2002; Wisner et al., 2006). The benzodiazepines may also used for treatment of anxiety during pregnancy and lactation and are generally considered safe in the perinatal period after careful weighing of the potential risks and benefits (Buist, Norman, & Dennerstein, 1990; Burt et al., 2001; Kelly, Poon, Madadi, & Koren, 2012; see Chapter 11 for a fuller discussion).

Other evidence-based treatment modalities for perinatal depression and anxiety (though the evidence for some is limited) include hormonal therapy (Moses-Kolko, Berga, Kalro, Sit, & Wisner, 2009), such as the use of the estrogen patch in the prevention and treatment of PND and bright light therapy in antenatal depression (Epperson et al., 2004; Oren et al., 2002; Wirz-Justice et al., 2011) and the administration of repetitive transcranial magnetic stimulation (rTMS) during pregnancy (Kim et al., 2011; Zhang, Liu, Sun, & Zheng, 2010) and the postpartum period (Garcia, Flynn, Pierce, & Caudle, 2010; Myczkowski et al., 2012).

Overall, treatment for perinatal depression and anxiety is associated with some improvement in maternal functioning and improved maternal interaction with her baby, partner, and overall family health (Miller, Shade, & Vasireddy, 2009; Yonkers et al., 2011).

Availability of and Barriers to Access of Treatment

Despite the existence of sensitive screening instruments, effective treatment, and frequent interactions with the health-care system during pregnancy and the first year postpartum, many pregnant women and new mothers with depression or anxiety remain undiagnosed and untreated (Vesga-Lopez et al., 2008). Women's help-seeking behaviors, their lack of financial resources, and the lack of available services all contribute to this treatment gap.

At 9 months postpartum, one-third of the 1385 Australian women participating in the Maternal Health Study who were experiencing depressive symptoms and more than one-half of those who were experiencing anxiety had not spoken to a health professional about their symptoms (Woolhouse, Brown, Krastev, Perlen, & Gunn, 2009). Reasons included a belief that they could handle their condition on their own, that their feelings were normal or not a medical issue, or that health professionals could not help them. The women also noted that they were too busy or too embarrassed to seek care (e.g., social stigma). Women experiencing anxiety symptoms, either with or without depression, were more likely to say that they felt too embarrassed to seek help (Woolhouse et al., 2009).

Other studies have found that even when health-care professionals detect perinatal anxiety or depression, many women do not receive treatment (typically less than 50%: Dennis & Chung-Lee, 2006; Farr, Dietz, Williams, Gibbs, & Tregear, 2011; Patel & Wisner, 2011). Treatment rates for clinics serving less well-resourced populations are likely lower than in well-educated, high socioeconomic status settings (Goodman & Tyer-Viola, 2010); Kohn, Saxena, Levav, & Saraceno, 2004; Pence et al., 2012; Saxena, Thornicroft, Knapp, & Whiteford, 2007).

Barriers to care described in the literature include both maternal and professional and health system factors and are explored in detail in Chapter 3. Maternal factors include structural barriers, such as an inability to pay and lack of transportation or child care, lack of motivation and social stigma, and fear of adverse reproductive outcomes or of losing custody of their child or children (Bonari et al., 2005; Dennis & Chung-Lee, 2006; Goodman, 2009). At the same time, many health-care providers, including obstetricians and pediatricians, do not see the diagnosis and treatment of maternal depression or anxiety as their responsibility and frequently lack the training and time required (Olson, Dietrich, Prazar, & Hurley, 2006; National Institute for Health Care Management [NIHCM], 2010).

Moreover, mental health resources are often scarce and/or inequitably distributed between communities, countries, and regions. Populations with high rates of socioeconomic deprivation may have the highest need for mental health care but the lowest access to it (Saxena et al., 2007). Depressed women continuously enrolled in a large health plan in the United States had high rates of treatment (93.4%), suggesting a willingness of perinatal women to accept treatment when it is available (Dietz et al., 2007).

Adherence to Best Practices

Once treatment is sought, providers must adhere to treatment guidelines and best practices when prescribing care, and patients must comply with treatment recommended by their providers. For example, abrupt discontinuation of medication treatment during pregnancy has been associated with both a significant risk of relapse of major depression and significant economic costs (Cohen et al., 2006; O'Brien, Laporte, & Koren, 2009).

Compliance among pregnant and postpartum women is often complicated by women's preferences and by social stigma. Pregnant and postpartum women suffering from depression or anxiety may experience significant stigma associated with having a mental illness during what is commonly viewed as a "happy time of life." The stigma of mental illness causes unique difficulties for women with depression who must weigh the pros and cons of treatment options during pregnancy and/or lactation. However, because effective and safe treatments for both mother and baby are available, overcoming stigma is critically important and should always include a careful discussion of risks and benefits of treatment options with the patient, family, and health-care providers.

Little is known about the proportion of perinatally depressed or anxious patients who receive adequate treatment. For perinatal depression, adequate treatment is defined as "receiving at least eight psychotherapy visits or at least four medication monitoring visits in the prior year" (Kessler et al., 2003) and consists of moderately dosed treatment for at least 6–8 weeks (Gaynes et al., 2009). This regimen allows for many breakdowns in compliance. For depression care in nonspecialty mental health settings, the likelihood of adequate treatment is approximately 40% for the general population (Pence et al., 2012).

Finally, even when receiving adequate treatment, rates of remission (i.e., full recovery from the depression, which is the goal of depression treatment) remain low. In real-world primary care settings, the likelihood of remission following aggressive treatment is approximately 30% (Trivedi et al., 2006), and, for example, only about two-thirds of individuals in trials of cognitive behavioral therapy are no longer diagnosed with depressive disorders at follow-up (Gloaguen, Cottraux, Cucherat, & Blackburn, 1998).

Discussion

In most areas, conditions necessary for successful adoption of population-based screening for perinatal depression and anxiety are met in Western industrialized countries. Perinatal depression and anxiety are common and have serious adverse consequences for the patient and her child and family. Clinical recognition is poor, and accurate screening tools are available that can assist in identification of unrecognized cases. Effective treatments, both pharmacologic and psychotherapeutic, exist and can be followed and, for the most part, are accessible by the affected population.

Summary estimates of the evidence on each major step in the perinatal depression and anxiety care continuum can be graphed to help clarify where gaps exist and to underscore the role of screening (see Figure 1.2). Based on the literature review provided previously and assuming a best-case scenario among prevalent perinatal depression cases, approximately 40% are recognized clinically, and of those recognized, approximately 60% receive treatment (or 24% of the overall cases). Of those treated, 40% will be adequately treated, and of those adequately treated, 30–66% may sufficiently recover to have measureable impact on health outcomes. Accordingly, approximately 3–6% of prevalent perinatal depression cases will be treated and achieve remission. (How many cases would achieve remission without treatment is unknown; however, the clinical trial literature cited previously suggests that lack of treatment would likely lead to longer and more severe episodes.) The largest drop-off in the perinatal depression care continuum is between prevalent cases and clinical recognition, a step that population-based screening can address.

The evidence base for the effectiveness of population-based screening to improve identification of depressive or anxiety disorders and to subsequently improve health outcomes is

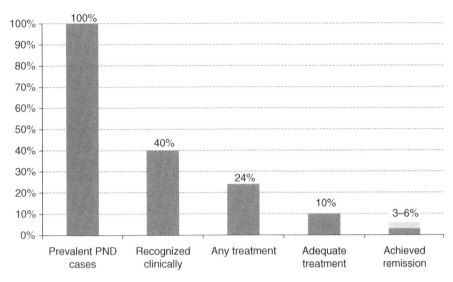

Figure 1.2 Perinatal depression care continuum. Recognized clinically: prenatal, 41% (Goodman & Tyer-Viola, 2010); postpartum, 29% (Heneghan, Silver, Bauman, & Stein, 2000) to 43% (Hearn et al., 1998). Best-case scenario, 40%. Any treatment: prenatal, 58% of those identified received treatment in clinic or accepted referral to mental health in well-educated, high SES setting (27/46); postpartum, 82% (9/11) in well-educated, high SES setting. In general, in primary care nonpsychiatric settings (high and low SES), 50% (Pence et al., 2012). Average, 60%. Adequate treatment, 40% (likely best-case scenario) for depression care in a nonspecialty mental health setting (Pence et al., 2012). Achieved remission, 30% (in real-world primary care setting following aggressive treatment) (Trivedi et al., 2006) to 66% (in clinical trials) (Gloaguen et al., 1998).

growing (Myers et al., 2013). However, the cost of such a strategy remains a concern. Little work has been done in this area. One study found the costs of universal screening with the EPDS at cut points of 12–16 to be £40,000 and £60,000 per quality-adjusted life year (QALY), which does not meet the NICE threshold of £20,000–30,000 per QALY (Paulden et al., 2009). Most of the excess cost was driven by the costs of treating false-positive patients. The authors had assumed that these women would receive supportive care of four 45 minute visits from a health visitor and one 1 hour home visit from a community psychiatric nurse. In sensitivity analyses, they found that if these costs were replaced by the cost of a single visit with a general practitioner, who would then immediately make the correct diagnosis, that universal screening with an EPDS cut point of 10 was borderline cost-effective, with an incremental cost-effectiveness ratio of £29,186 per QALY. They also considered the scenario of the home visitor taking 30 minutes to administer a structured clinical interview for DSM-IV axis I disorders (SCID) to confirm the diagnosis among women with a positive screen and found an incremental cost-effectiveness ratio of £33,776 per QALY compared with routine care at an EPDS cut point of 13. However, the authors did not consider the possibility of medication treatment in place of psychological therapy nor did they consider costs beyond the first year postpartum or the potentially very important impact that successful identification and subsequent management might have had on the infant or other family members. Further, the authors did not consider that false positives might instead indicate women who had anxiety disorders (Austin, 2004) or low-intensity, low-cost treatment options such as group treatment or Internet treatment with telephone support, which could change the cost-effectiveness ratios. Consideration of how best to weigh the potential costs and benefits of screening paradigms remains a critical consideration in decisions to adopt population-based perinatal depression and anxiety screening.

Further, the case for population-based screening must be assessed at a country, region, or community level. Important factors to consider include whether adequate resources are available for diagnosis and treatment and whether women have the means to access care and are willing to accept care. Medical institutions and governments may need to first engage in mental health-care capacity building and public awareness campaigns aimed at reducing the stigma of depression and anxiety during pregnancy and early motherhood.

Additional research is needed to confirm the link between screening for perinatal depression and anxiety and improved health outcomes. As a field, perinatal psychiatry is attempting to disentangle the biological, genetic, and psychological contributions that determine prognosis and long-term outcomes, including (i) identification of women at risk, (ii) how best to screen, (iii) symptom severity threshold that leads to intervention (i.e., DSM-based diagnoses vs. subsyndromal disorders), (iv) longitudinal course of illness, (v) risk of recurrence in subsequent pregnancies, (vi) differentiation of subtype of perinatal psychiatric illness, (vii) the interrelationship between anxiety and depressive disorders, (viii) the effects on the fetus and the child, and (ix) partner support. As our understanding of the pathophysiology of perinatal mood and anxiety disorders grows, our ability to provide evidence-based diagnostic and treatment recommendations will also improve. Improved knowledge on these dimensions will help weigh the case for population-based screening.

In sum, the evidence (though much is limited to high-income countries) suggests that population-based screening can be an important first step toward identifying those women suffering from perinatal mood and anxiety disorders who would otherwise remain undiagnosed and untreated. The care continuum model presented in this chapter discusses the conditions that are needed to make population-based screening programs successful. Examples of successful programs exist that can serve as models for widespread dissemination and will help address the vital mental health needs of mothers and their children (Buist et al., 2007; Earls & Committee on Psychosocial Aspects of Child and Family Health American Academy of Pediatrics, 2010; Leung et al., 2011; Segre, O'Hara, Brock, & Taylor, 2012; Yawn et al., 2012). Of note is a clinical trial of health visitor training in psychologically informed approaches for depression identification, prevention, and management of postnatal women that was found to be both effective and cost-effective among patients of general practices in Trent, England (Morrell et al., 2009). The remainder of the book addresses key issues that will aid in the decision-making process.

References

Abzramowitz, J. S., Meltzer-Brody, S., Leserman, J., Killenberg, S., Rinaldi, K., Mahaffey, B. L., & Pedersen, C. (2010). Obsessional thoughts and compulsive behaviors in a sample of women with postpartum mood symptoms. *Archives of Women's Mental Health, 13*(6), 523–530.

Altemus, M., Neeb, C. C., Davis, A., Occhiogrosso, M., Nguyen, T., & Bleiberg, K. L. (2012). Phenotypic differences between pregnancy-onset and postpartum-onset major depressive disorder. *Journal of Clinical Psychiatry, 73*(12), e1485–e1491. doi:10.4088/JCP.12m07693.

American Psychiatric Association. (2013). *Diagnostic and statistical manual of mental disorders* (5th ed.). Arlington, VA: Author.

Andersson, L., Sundstrom-Poromaa, I., Bixo, M., Wulff, M., Bondestam, K., & åStrom, M. (2003). Point prevalence of psychiatric disorders during the second trimester of pregnancy: A population-based study. *American Journal of Obstetrics and Gynecology, 189*(1), 148–154.

Areias, M. E., Kumar, R., Barros, H., & Figueiredo, E. (1996). Correlates of postnatal depression in mothers and fathers. *British Journal of Psychiatry, 169*(1), 36–41.

Austin, M. P. (2004). Antenatal screening and early intervention for "perinatal" distress, depression and anxiety: Where to from here? *Archives of Women's Mental Health, 7*(1), 1–6. doi:10.1007/s00737-003-0034-4.

Austin, M. P., Hadzi-Pavlovic, D., Priest, S. R., Reilly, N., Wilhelm, K., Saint, K., & Parker, G. (2010). Depressive and anxiety disorders in the postpartum period: How prevalent are they and can we improve their detection? *Archives of Women's Mental Health, 13*(5), 395–401. doi:10.1007/s00737-010-0153-7.

Austin, M. P., Middleton, P., Reilly, N. M., & Highet, N. J. (2013). Detection and management of mood disorders in the maternity setting: The Australian Clinical Practice Guidelines. *Women Birth, 26*(1), 2–9. doi:10.1016/j.wombi.2011.12.001.

Beck, C. T. (1996a). A meta-analysis of predictors of postpartum depression. *Nursing Research, 45*(5), 297–303.

Beck, C. T. (1996b). Postpartum depressed mothers' experiences interacting with their children. *Nursing Research, 45*(2), 98–104.

Bernstein, I. H., Rush, A. J., Yonkers, K., Carmody, T. J., Woo, A., McConnell, K., & Trivedi, M. H. (2008). Symptom features of postpartum depression: Are they distinct? *Depression and Anxiety, 25*(1), 20–26.

Bonari, L., Koren, G., Einarson, T. R., Jasper, J. D., Taddio, A., & Einarson, A. (2005). Use of antidepressants by pregnant women: Evaluation of perception of risk, efficacy of evidence based counseling and determinants of decision making. *Archives of Women's Mental Health, 8*(4), 214–220. doi:10.1007/s00737-005-0094-8.

Borri, C., Mauri, M., Oppo, A., Banti, S., Rambelli, C. , Ramacciotti, D., … Cassano, G. B. (2008). Axis I psychopathology and functional impairment at the third month of pregnancy: Results from the Perinatal Depression-Research and Screening Unit (PND-ReScU) study. *Journal of Clinical Psychiatry, 69*(10), 1617–1624.

Brandon, A. R., Ceccotti, N., Hynan, L. S., Shivakumar, G., Johnson, N., & Jarrett, R. B. (2012). Proof of concept: Partner-Assisted Interpersonal Psychotherapy for perinatal depression. *Archives of Women's Mental Health, 15*(6), 469–480. doi:10.1007/s00737-012-0311-1.

Buist, A., Bilszta, J., Barnett, B., Milgrom, J., Ericksen, J., Condon, J., … Brooks, J. (2005). Recognition and management of perinatal depression in general practice—a survey of GPs and postnatal women. *Australian Family Physician, 34*(9), 787–790.

Buist, A., Ellwood, D., Brooks, J., Milgrom, J., Hayes, B. A., Sved-Williams, A., … Bilszta, J. (2007). National program for depression associated with childbirth: The Australian experience. *Best Practice & Research in Clinical Obstetrics & Gynaecology, 21*(2), 193–206. doi:10.1016/j.bpobgyn.2006.11.003.

Buist, A., Norman, T. R., & Dennerstein, L. (1990). Breastfeeding and the use of psychotropic medication: A review. *Journal of Affective Disorders, 19*(3), 197–206.

Burt, V. K., Suri, R., Altshuler, L., Stowe, Z., Hendrick, V. C., & Muntean, E. (2001). The use of psychotropic medications during breast-feeding. *American Journal of Psychiatry, 158*(7), 1001–1009.

Campbell, S. B., Brownell, C. A., Hungerford, A., Spieker, S. I., Mohan, R., & Blessing, J. S. (2004). The course of maternal depressive symptoms and maternal sensitivity as predictors of attachment security at 36 months. *Development and Psychopathology, 16*(2), 231–252.

Chabrol, H., Teissedre, F., Saint-Jean, M., Teisseyre, N., Roge, B., & Mullet, E. (2002). Prevention and treatment of post-partum depression: A controlled randomized study on women at risk. *Psychological Medicine, 32*(6), 1039–1047.

Cohen, L. S., Altshuler, L. L., Harlow, B. L., Nonacs, R., Newport, D. J., Viguera, A. C., … Stowe, Z. N. (2006). Relapse of major depression during pregnancy in women who maintain or discontinue antidepressant treatment. *Journal of the American Medical Association, 295*(5), 499–507. doi:10.1001/jama.295.5.499.

Cohen, M. M., Ansara, D., Schei, B., Stuckless, N., & Stewart, D. E. (2004). Posttraumatic stress disorder after pregnancy, labor, and delivery. *Journal of Women's Health, 13*(3), 315–324. doi:10.1089/154099904323016473.

Cooper, P., & Murray, L. (1997). Prediction, detection, and treatment of postnatal depression. *Archives of Disease in Childhood, 77*(2), 97–99.

Cooper, P. J., Murray, L., Wilson, A., & Romaniuk, H. (2003). Controlled trial of the short- and long-term effect of psychological treatment of post-partum depression. I. Impact on maternal mood. *British Journal of Psychiatry. 182*:412–419.

Cox, J. (2004). Postnatal mental disorder: Towards ICD-11. *World Psychiatry, 3*(2), 96–97.

Cox, J., Holden, J., & Sagovsky, R. Detection of postnatal depression: Development of a 10 item postnatal depression scale. *British Journal of Psychiatry 150*(1987), 782–786.

Dave, S., Petersen, I., Sherr, L., & Nazareth, I. (2010). Incidence of maternal and paternal depression in primary care: A cohort study using a primary care database. *Archives of Pediatrics and Adolescent Medicine, 164*(11), 1038–1044. doi:10.1001/archpediatrics.2010.184.

Dennis, C. L., & Chung-Lee, L. (2006). Postpartum depression help-seeking barriers and maternal treatment preferences: A qualitative systematic review. *Birth, 33*(4), 323–331. doi:10.1111/j.1523-536X.2006.00130.x.

Dennis, C. L., Heaman, M., & Vigod, S. (2012). Epidemiology of postpartum depressive symptoms among Canadian women: Regional and national results from a cross-sectional survey. *Canadian Journal of Psychiatry, 57*(9), 537–546.

Di Florio, A., Forty, L., Gordon-Smith, K., Heron, J., Jones, L., N. Craddock, & Jones, I. (2013). Perinatal episodes across the mood disorder spectrum. *Journal of the American Medical Association Psychiatry, 70*(2), 168–175. doi:10.1001/jamapsychiatry.2013.279.

Diego, M. A., Field, T., Hernandez-Reif, M., Cullen, C., Schanberg, S., & Kuhn, C. (2004). Prepartum, postpartum, and chronic depression effects on newborns. *Psychiatry, 67*(1), 63–80.

Diego, M. A., Field, T., Hernandez-Reif, M., Schanberg, S., Kuhn, C., & Gonzalez-Quintero, V. H. (2009). Prenatal depression restricts fetal growth. *Early Human Development, 85*(1), 65–70. doi:10.1016/j.earlhumdev.2008.07.002.

Dietrich, A. J., Williams, J. W., Jr., Ciotti, M. C., Schulkin, J., Stotland, N., Rost, K., … Cornell, J. (2003). Depression care attitudes and practices of newer obstetrician-gynecologists: A national survey. *American Journal of Obstetrics and Gynecology, 189*(1), 267–273.

Dietz, P. M., Williams, S. B., Callaghan, W. M., Bachman, D. J., Whitlock, E. P., & Hornbrook, M. C. (2007). Clinically identified maternal depression before, during, and after pregnancies ending in live births. *American Journal of Psychiatry, 164*(10), 1515–1520. doi:10.1176/appi.ajp.2007.06111893.

DSM-IV (Ed.). (1994). *Diagnostic and statistical manual of mental disorders (DSM-IV)* (4th ed.) Washington, DC: American Psychiatric Association.

Earls, M. F., & Committee on Psychosocial Aspects of Child and Family Health American Academy of Pediatrics. (2010). Incorporating recognition and management of perinatal and post-partum depression into pediatric practice. *Pediatrics, 126*(5), 1032–1039. doi:10.1542/peds.2010-2348.

Einarson, A. (2010). Antidepressants and pregnancy: Complexities of producing evidence-based information. *Canadian Medical Association Journal, 182*(10), 1017–1018. doi:10.1503/cmaj.100507.

Einarson, A., Choi, J., Einarson, T. R., & Koren, G. (2009). Incidence of major malformations in infants following antidepressant exposure in pregnancy: Results of a large prospective cohort study. *Canadian Journal of Psychiatry, 54*(4), 242–246.

Elliott, S. (2000). Report on the satra bruk workshop on classification of postnatal mental disorders on November 7-10, 1999. Convened by Birgitta Wickberg, Philip Hwang and John Cox. *Archives of Women's Mental Health, 3*:27–33.

Epperson, C. N., Terman, M., Terman, J. S., Hanusa, B. H., Oren, D. A., Peindl, K. S., & Wisner, K. L. (2004). Randomized clinical trial of bright light therapy for antepartum depression: Preliminary findings. *Journal of Clinical Psychiatry, 65*(3), 421–425.

Fairbrother, N., & Abramowitz, J. S. (2007). New parenthood as a risk factor for the development of obsessional problems. *Behaviour Research and Therapy, 45*(9), 2155–2163. doi:10.1016/j.brat.2006.09.019.

Farr, S. L., Dietz, P. M., Williams, J. R., Gibbs, F. A., & Tregear, S. (2011). Depression screening and treatment among nonpregnant women of reproductive age in the United States, 1990–2010. *Preventing Chronic Disease, 8*(6), A122.

Flynn, H. A., Davis, M., Marcus, S. M., Cunningham, R., & Blow, F. C. (2004). Rates of maternal depression in pediatric emergency department and relationship to child service utilization. *General Hospital Psychiatry, 26*(4), 316–322. doi:10.1016/j.genhosppsych.2004.03.009.

Fransson, E., Ortenstrand, A., & Hjelmstedt, A. (2011). Antenatal depressive symptoms and preterm birth: A prospective study of a Swedish national sample. *Birth, 38*(1), 10–16. doi:10.1111/j.1523-536X.2010.00441.x.

Garcia, K. S., Flynn, P., Pierce, K. J., & Caudle, M. (2010). Repetitive transcranial magnetic stimulation treats postpartum depression. *Brain Stimulation, 3*(1), 36–41. doi:10.1016/j.brs.2009.06.001.

Gardner, E. M., McLees, M. P., Steiner, J. F., Del Rio, C., & Burman, W. J. (2011). The spectrum of engagement in HIV care and its relevance to test-and-treat strategies for prevention of HIV infection. *Clinical Infectious Diseases, 52*(6), 793–800. doi:10.1093/cid/ciq243.

Garthus-Niegel, S., von Soest, T., Vollrath, M. E., & Eberhard-Gran, M. (2013). The impact of subjective birth experiences on post-traumatic stress symptoms: A longitudinal study. *Archives of Women's Mental Health, 16*(1), 1–10. doi:10.1007/s00737-012-0301-3.

Gavin, N. I., Gaynes, B. N., Lohr, K. N., Meltzer-Brody, S., Gartlehner, G., & Swinson, T. (2005). Perinatal depression: A systematic review of prevalence and incidence. *Obstetrics and Gynecology, 106*(5 Pt 1), 1071–1083. doi:10.1097/01.AOG.0000183597.31630.db.

Gaynes, B. N., Gavin, N., Meltzer-Brody, S., Lohr, K. N., Swinson, T., Gartlehner, G., … Miller, W. C. (2005a). Perinatal depression: Prevalence, screening accuracy, and screening outcomes. *Evidence Report Technology Assessment (Summary), 119*(119), 1–8.

Gaynes, B. N., Gavin, N., Meltzer-Brody, S., Lohr, K. N., Swinson, T., Gartlehner, G., … Miller, W. C. (2005b). Perinatal depression: Prevalence, screening accuracy, and screening outcomes. Rockville, MD: Evidence Report/Technology Assessment No. 119. (Prepared by the RTI-University of North Carolina Evidence-based Practice Center, under Contract No. 290-02-0016.)

Gaynes, B. N., Warden, D., Trivedi, M. H., Wisniewski, S. R., Fava, M., & A. J. Rush. 2009. What did STAR*D teach us? Results from a large-scale, practical, clinical trial for patients with depression. *Psychiatric Services, 60*(11), 1439–1445. doi:10.1176/appi.ps.60.11.1439.

Gentile, S. (2011). Suicidal mothers. *Journal of Injury and Violence Research, 3*(2), 90–97. doi:10.5249/jivr.v3i2.98.

Gidai, J., Acs, N., Banhidy, F., & Czeizel, A. E. (2010). Congenital abnormalities in children of 43 pregnant women who attempted suicide with large doses of nitrazepam. *Pharmacoepidemiology and Drug Safety, 19*(2), 175–182. doi:10.1002/pds.1885.

Gloaguen, V., Cottraux, J., Cucherat, M., & Blackburn, I. M. (1998). A meta-analysis of the effects of cognitive therapy in depressed patients. *Journal of Affective Disorders, 49*(1), 59–72.

Glover, V. (2014). Maternal depression, anxiety and stress during pregnancy and child outcome; what needs to be done. *Best Practice & Research Clinical Obstetrics & Gynaecology, 28*(1), 25–35.

Goodman, J. H. (2004). Paternal postpartum depression, its relationship to maternal postpartum depression, and implications for family health. *Journal of Advanced Nursing, 45*(1), 26–35.

Goodman, J. H. (2009). Women's attitudes, preferences, and perceived barriers to treatment for perinatal depression. *Birth, 36*(1), 60–69. doi:10.1111/j.1523-536X.2008.00296.x.

Goodman, J. H., & Tyer-Viola, L. (2010). Detection, treatment, and referral of perinatal depression and anxiety by obstetrical providers. *Journal of Women's Health, 19*(3), 477–490. doi:10.1089/jwh.2008.1352.

Gordon, T. E., Cardone, I. A., Kim, J. J., Gordon, S. M., & Silver, R. K. (2006). Universal perinatal depression screening in an Academic Medical Center. *Obstetrics and Gynecology, 107*(2 Pt 1), 342–347. doi:10.1097/01.AOG.0000194080.18261.92.

Grigoriadis, S., de Camps Meschino, D., Barrons, E., Bradley, L., Eady, A., Fishell, A., … Ross, L. E. (2011). Mood and anxiety disorders in a sample of Canadian perinatal women referred for psychiatric care. *Archives of Women's Mental Health, 14*(4), 325–333. doi:10.1007/s00737-011-0223-5.

Grote, N. K., Bridge, J. A., Gavin, A. R., Melville, J. L., Iyengar, S., & Katon, W. J. (2010). A meta-analysis of depression during pregnancy and the risk of preterm birth, low birth weight, and intrauterine growth restriction. *Archives of General Psychiatry, 67*(10), 1012–1024. doi:10.1001/archgenpsychiatry.2010.111.

Grote, N. K., Swartz, H. A., Geibel, S. L., Zuckoff, A., Houck, P. R., & Frank, E. (2009). A randomized controlled trial of culturally relevant, brief interpersonal psychotherapy for perinatal depression. *Psychiatric Services, 60*(3), 313–321. doi:10.1176/appi.ps.60.3.313.

Halbreich, U. (2005). The association between pregnancy processes, preterm delivery, low birth weight, and postpartum depressions—the need for interdisciplinary integration. *American Journal of Obstetrics and Gynecology, 193*(4), 1312–1322. doi:10.1016/j.ajog.2005.02.103.

Hearn, G., Iliff, A., Jones, I., Kirby, A., Ormiston, P., Parr, P., … Wardman, L. (1998). Postnatal depression in the community. *British Journal of General Practice, 48*(428), 1064–1066.

Hendrick, V., Altshuler, L., Strouse, T., & Grosser, S. (2000). Postpartum and nonpostpartum depression: Differences in presentation and response to pharmacologic treatment. *Depression and Anxiety, 11*(2), 66–72.

Heneghan, A. M., Silver, E. J., Bauman, L. J., & Stein, R. E. (2000). Do pediatricians recognize mothers with depressive symptoms? *Pediatrics, 106*(6), 1367–1373.

Henshaw, C., & Elliott, S. (Eds.). (2005). *Screening for perinatal depression*. London, UK: Jessica Kingsley Publishers.

Hickie, I. B., Davenport, T. A., Scott, E. M., Hadzi-Pavlovic, D. , Naismith, S. L., & Koschera, A. (2001). Unmet need for recognition of common mental disorders in Australian general practice. *The Medical Journal of Australia, 175* Suppl:S18–S24.

Honey, K. L., Bennett, P., & Morgan, M. (2002). A brief psycho-educational group intervention for postnatal depression. *British Journal of Clinical Psychology, 41*(Pt 4), 405–409.

Ibanez, G., Charles, M. A., Forhan, A., Magnin, G., Thiebaugeorges, O., Kaminski, M., & Saurel-Cubizolles, M. J. (2012). Depression and anxiety in women during pregnancy and neonatal outcome: Data from the EDEN mother-child cohort. *Early Human Development, 88*(8), 643–649. doi:10.1016/j.earlhumdev.2012.01.014.

Kelly, L. E., Poon, S., Madadi, P., & Koren, G. (2012). Neonatal benzodiazepines exposure during breastfeeding. *Journal of Pediatrics, 161*(3), 448–451. doi:10.1016/j.jpeds.2012.03.003.

Kelly, R. H., Russo, J., & Katon, W. (2001). Somatic complaints among pregnant women cared for in obstetrics: Normal pregnancy or depressive and anxiety symptom amplification revisited? *General Hospital Psychiatry, 23*(3), 107–113.

Kessler, R. C., Berglund, P., Demler, O., Jin, R., Koretz, D., Merikangas, K. R., … Replication National Comorbidity Survey. (2003). The epidemiology of major depressive disorder: Results from the National Comorbidity Survey Replication (NCS-R). *Journal of the American Medical Association, 289*(23), 3095–3105. doi:10.1001/jama.289.23.3095.

Kim, J. J., La Porte, L. M., Adams, M. G., Gordon, T. E., Kuendig, J. M., & Silver, R. K. 2009. Obstetric care provider engagement in a perinatal depression screening program. *Archives of Women's Mental Health, 12*(3), 167–172. doi:10.1007/s00737-009-0057-6.

Kim, D. R., Sockol, L., Barber, J. P., Moseley, M., Lamprou, L., Rickels, K., … & Epperson, C. N. (2011). A survey of patient acceptability of repetitive transcranial magnetic stimulation (TMS) during pregnancy. *Journal of Affective Disorders, 129*(1–3), 385–390. doi:10.1016/j.jad.2010.08.027.

Ko, J. Y., Farr, S. L., Dietz, P. M., & Robbins, C. L. (2012). Depression and treatment among U.S. pregnant and nonpregnant women of reproductive age, 2005–2009. *Journal of Women's Health, 21*(8), 830–836. doi:10.1089/jwh.2011.3466.

Kohn, R., Saxena, S., Levav, I., & Saraceno, B. (2004). The treatment gap in mental health care. *Bulletin of the World Health Organization, 82*(11), 858–866. doi:10.1590/s0042-96862004001100011.

LaRocco-Cockburn, A., Melville, J., Bell, M., & Katon, W. (2003). Depression screening attitudes and practices among obstetrician-gynecologists. *Obstetrics and Gynecology, 101*(5 Pt 1), 892–898.

Leckman, J. F., Mayes, L. C., Feldman, R., Evans, D. W., King, R. A., & Cohen, D. J. (1999). Early parental preoccupations and behaviors and their possible relationship to the symptoms of obsessive-compulsive disorder. *Acta Psychiatrica Scandinavica. Supplementum, 396*:1–26.

Leigh, B., & Milgrom, J. (2008). Risk factors for antenatal depression, postnatal depression and parenting stress. *BMC Psychiatry, 8*:24. doi:10.1186/1471-244X-8-24.

Leung, S. S., Leung, C., Lam, T. H., Hung, S. F., Chan, R., Yeung, T., ... Lee, D. T. (2011). Outcome of a postnatal depression screening programme using the Edinburgh Postnatal Depression Scale: A randomized controlled trial. *Journal of Public Health, 33*(2), 292–301. doi:10.1093/pubmed/fdq075.

Lindahl, V., Pearson, J. L., & Colpe, L. (2005). Prevalence of suicidality during pregnancy and the postpartum. *Archives of Women's Mental Health, 8*(2), 77–87. doi:10.1007/s00737-005-0080-1.

Loxton, D., & Lucke, J. (2009). *Reproductive health: findings from the Australian longitudinal study of Women's Health*. University of Queensland & University of Newcastle. Retrieved from http://www.alswh.org.au/Reports/OtherReportsPDF/MajorReportD2010.pdf. Accessed November 22, 2014.

Marcus, S., Lopez, J. F., McDonough, S., Mackenzie, M. J., Flynn, H., Neal, C. R., ... Vazquez, D. M. (2011). Depressive symptoms during pregnancy: Impact on neuroendocrine and neonatal outcomes. *Infant Behavior and Development, 34*(1), 26–34. doi:10.1016/j.infbeh.2010.07.002.

Martini, J., Knappe, S., Beesdo-Baum, K., Lieb, R., & Wittchen, H. U. (2010). Anxiety disorders before birth and self-perceived distress during pregnancy: Associations with maternal depression and obstetric, neonatal and early childhood outcomes. *Early Human Development, 86*(5), 305–310. doi:10.1016/j.earlhumdev.2010.04.004.

McGuinness, M., Blissett, J., & Jones, C. (2011). OCD in the perinatal period: Is postpartum OCD (ppOCD) a distinct subtype? A review of the literature. *Behavioural and Cognitive Psychotherapy, 39*(3), 285–310. doi:10.1017/S1352465810000718.

McLearn, K. T., Minkovitz, C. S., Strobino, D. M., Marks, E., & Hou, W. (2006). The timing of maternal depressive symptoms and mothers' parenting practices with young children: Implications for pediatric practice. *Pediatrics, 118*(1), e174–e182.

Meades, R., & Ayers, S. (2011). Anxiety measures validated in perinatal populations: A systematic review. *Journal of Affective Disorders, 133*(1–2), 1–15. doi:10.1016/j.jad.2010.10.009.

Meltzer-Brody, S., Bledsoe-Mansori, S. E., Johnson, N., Killian, C., Hamer, R. M., Jackson, C., ... Thorp, J. (2013). A prospective study of perinatal depression and trauma history in pregnant minority adolescents. *American Journal of Obstetrics and Gynecology, 208*(3), 211e1–211e7. doi:10.1016/j.ajog.2012.12.020.

Milgrom, J., Gemmill, A. W., Bilszta, J. L., Hayes, B., Barnett, B., Brooks, J., ... Buist, A. (2008). Antenatal risk factors for postnatal depression: A large prospective study. *Journal of Affective Disorders, 108*(1–2), 147–157. doi:10.1016/j.jad.2007.10.014.

Milgrom, J., Westley, D. T., & Gemmill, A. W. (2004). The mediating role of maternal responsiveness in some longer term effects of postnatal depression on infant development. *Infant Behavior and Development, 27*(4), 443–454. doi:10.1016/j.infbeh.2004.03.003.

Miller, L. J., McGlynn, A., Suberlak, K., Rubin, L. H., Miller, M., & Pirec, V. (2012). Now what? Effects of on-site assessment on treatment entry after perinatal depression screening. *Journal of Women's Health, 21*(10), 1046–1052. doi:10.1089/jwh.2012.3641.

Miller, R. L., Pallant, J. F., & Negri, L. M. (2006). Anxiety and stress in the postpartum: Is there more to postnatal distress than depression? *BMC Psychiatry, 6*:12. doi:10.1186/1471-244X-6-12.

Miller, L., Shade, M., & Vasireddy, V. (2009). Beyond screening: Assessment of perinatal depression in a perinatal care setting. *Archives of Women's Mental Health, 12*(5), 329–334. doi:10.1007/s00737-009-0082-5.

Misra, D. P., Guyer, B., & Allston, A. (2003). Integrated perinatal health framework. A multiple determinants model with a life span approach. *American Journal of Preventive Medicine, 25*(1), 65–75.

Morgan, M., Matthey, S., Barnett, B., & Richardson, C. (1997). A group programme for postnatally distressed women and their partners. *Journal of Advanced Nursing, 26*(5), 913–920.

Morrell, C. J., Warner, R., Slade, P., Dixon, S., Walters, S., Paley, G., & Brugha, T. (2009). Psychological interventions for postnatal depression: Cluster randomised trial and economic evaluation. The PoNDER trial. *Health Technology Assessment, 3*(30), iii–iv, xi–xiii, 1–153. doi:10.3310/hta13300.

Moses-Kolko, E. L., Berga, S. L., Kalro, B., Sit, D. K., & Wisner, K. L. (2009). Transdermal estradiol for postpartum depression: A promising treatment option. *Clinical Obstetrics and Gynecology, 52*(3), 516–529. doi:10.1097/GRF.0b013e3181b5a395.

Mugavero, M. J., Norton, W. E., & Saag, M. S. (2011). Health care system and policy factors influencing engagement in HIV medical care: Piecing together the fragments of a fractured health care delivery system. *Clinical Infectious Diseases, 52* Suppl 2:S238–S246. doi:10.1093/cid/ciq048.

Murray, L., Arteche, A., Fearon, P., Halligan, S., Croudace, T., & Cooper, P. (2010). The effects of maternal postnatal depression and child sex on academic performance at age 16 years: A developmental approach. *Journal of Child Psychology and Psychiatry, 51*(10), 1150–1159. doi:10.1111/j.1469-7610.2010.02259.x.

Murray, L., Arteche, A., Fearon, P., Halligan, S., Goodyer, I., & Cooper, P. (2011). Maternal postnatal depression and the development of depression in offspring up to 16 years of age. *Journal of the American Academy of Child and Adolescent Psychiatry, 50*(5), 460–470. doi:10.1016/j.jaac.2011.02.001.

Myczkowski, M. L., Dias, A. M., Luvisotto, T., Arnaut, D., Bellini, B. B., Mansur, C. G., … Marcolin, M. A. (2012). Effects of repetitive transcranial magnetic stimulation on clinical, social, and cognitive performance in postpartum depression. *Neuropsychiatric Disease and Treatment, 8*:491–500. doi:10.2147/NDT.S33851.

Myers, E. R., Aubuchon-Endsley, N., Bastian, L. A., Gierisch, J. M., Kemper, A. R., Swamy, G. K., … Sanders, G. D. (2013). *Efficacy and safety of screening for postpartum depression. comparative effectiveness review 106.* Rockville, MD: Agency for Healthcare Research and Quality.

Najman, J. M., Andersen, M. J., Bor, W., O'Callaghan, M. J., & Williams, G. M. (2000). Postnatal depression-myth and reality: Maternal depression before and after the birth of a child. *Social Psychiatry and Psychiatric Epidemiology, 35*(1), 19–27.

National Institute for Health and Clinical Excellence [NICE]. (2007). *Antenatal and postnatal mental health: The NICE guideline on clinical management and service guidance.* Leicester, UK: British Psychological Society.

National Institute for Health Care Management [NIHCM]. (2010). Identifying and treating maternal depression: Strategies and considerations for health plans (NIHCM Foundation Issue Brief). Washington, DC: National Institute for Health Care Management. Retrieved from www.nihcm.org/pdf/FINAL_MaternalDepression6-7.pdf. Accessed December 15, 2014.

Network NECCR. (1999). Chronicity of maternal depressive symptoms, maternal sensitivity, and child functioning at 36 months. NICHD Early Child Care Research Network. *Developmental Psychology, 35*(5), 1297–1310.

Newport, D. J., Hostetter, A., Arnold, A., & Stowe, Z. N. (2002). The treatment of postpartum depression: Minimizing infant exposures. *Journal of Clinical Psychiatry, 63*(Suppl 7), 31–44.

O'Brien, L., Laporte, A., & Koren, G. (2009). Estimating the economic costs of antidepressant discontinuation during pregnancy. *Canadian Journal of Psychiatry, 54*(6), 399–408.

O'Donnell, K. J., Glover, V., Barker, E. D, & O'Connor, T. G. (in press). The persisting effect of maternal mood in pregnancy on childhood psychopathology. *Development and Psychopathology, 26*(2), 393–403.

O'Hara, M. W., & Swain, A. M. (1996). Rates and risk of postpartum depression—A meta-analysis. *International Review of Psychiatry, 8*(1), 37–54.

Olde, E., van der Hart, O., Kleber, R., & van Son, M. (2006). Posttraumatic stress following childbirth: A review. *Clinical Psychology Review, 26*(1), 1–16. doi:10.1016/j.cpr.2005.07.002.

Olson, A. L., Dietrich, A. J., Prazar, G., & Hurley, J. (2006). Brief maternal depression screening at well-child visits. *Pediatrics, 118*(1), 207–216. doi:10.1542/peds.2005-2346.

Oren, D. A., Wisner, K. L., Spinelli, M., Epperson, C. N., Peindl, K. S., Terman, J. S., & Terman, M. (2002). An open trial of morning light therapy for treatment of antepartum depression. *The American Journal of Psychiatry, 159*(4), 666–669.

Patel, S. R., & Wisner, K. L. (2011). Decision making for depression treatment during pregnancy and the postpartum period. *Depression and Anxiety, 28*(7), 589–595. doi:10.1002/da.20844.

Paul, I. M., Downs, D. S., Schaefer, E. W., Beiler, J. S., & Weisman, C. S. (2013). Postpartum anxiety and maternal-infant health outcomes. *Pediatrics, 131*(4), e1218–e1224. doi:10.1542/peds.2012-2147.

Paulden, M., Palmer, S., Hewitt, C., & Gilbody, S. (2009). Screening for postnatal depression in primary care: Cost effectiveness analysis. *British Medical Journal, 339*(dec22 1), b5203. doi:10.1136/bmj.b5203.

Paulson, J. F., & Bazemore, S. D. (2010). Prenatal and postpartum depression in fathers and its association with maternal depression: A meta-analysis. *Journal of the American Medical Association, 303*(19), 1961–1969. doi:10.1001/jama.2010.605.

Paulson, J. F., Dauber, S., & Leiferman, J. A. (2006). Individual and combined effects of postpartum depression in mothers and fathers on parenting behavior. *Pediatrics, 118*(2), 659–668.

Pence, B. W., O'Donnell, J. K., & Gaynes, B. N. (2012). The depression treatment cascade in primary care: A public health perspective. *Current Psychiatry Report, 14*(4), 328–335. doi:10.1007/s11920-012-0274-y.

Petik, D., Czeizel, B., Banhidy, F., & Czeizel, A. E. (2011). A study of the risk of mental retardation among children of pregnant women who have attempted suicide by means of a drug overdose. *Journal of Injury and Violence Research, 4*, 10–19. doi:10.5249/jivr.v4i1.85.

Pop, V. J., Pommer, A. M., Pop-Purceleanu, M., Wijnen, H. A., Bergink, V., & Pouwer, F. (2011). Development of the Tilburg Pregnancy Distress Scale: The TPDS. *BMC Pregnancy Childbirth, 11*, 80. doi:10.1186/1471-2393-11-80.

Prenoveau, J., Craske, M., Counsell, N., West, V., Davies, B., Cooper, P., … Stein, A. (2013). Postpartum gad is a risk factor for postpartum mdd: The course and longitudinal relationships of postpartum GAD and MDD. *Depression and Anxiety, 30*(6), 506–514. doi:10.1002/da.22040.

Reck, C., Struben, K., Backenstrass, M., Stefenelli, U., Reinig, K., Fuchs, T., … Mundt, C. (2008). Prevalence, onset and comorbidity of postpartum anxiety and depressive disorders. *Acta Psychiatrica Scandinavica, 118*(6), 459–468. doi:10.1111/j.1600-0447.2008.01264.x.

Rich-Edwards, J. W., Kleinman, K., Abrams, A., Harlow, B. L., McLaughlin, T. J., Joffe, H., & Gillman, M. W. (2006). Sociodemographic predictors of antenatal and postpartum depressive symptoms among women in a medical group practice. *Journal of Epidemiology and Community Health, 60*(3), 221–227. doi:10.1136/jech.2005.039370.

Ross, L. E., Grigoriadis, Mamisashvili, L., Vonderporten, E. H., Roerecke, M., Rehm, J., … Cheung, A. (2013). Selected pregnancy and delivery outcomes after exposure to antidepressant medication: A systematic review and meta-analysis. *Journal of the American Medical Association Psychiatry, 70*(4), 436–443. doi:10.1001/jamapsychiatry.2013.684.

Ross, L. E., & McLean, L. M. (2006). Anxiety disorders during pregnancy and the postpartum period: A systematic review. *Journal of Clinical Psychiatry, 67*(8), 1285–1298.

Saxena, S., Thornicroft, G., Knapp, M., & Whiteford, H. (2007). Resources for mental health: Scarcity, inequity, and inefficiency. *The Lancet, 370*(9590), 878–889. doi:10.1016/s0140-6736(07)61239-2.

Schmied, V., Johnson, M., Naidoo, N., Austin, M. P., Matthey, S., Kemp, L., … Yeo, A. (2013). Maternal mental health in Australia and New Zealand: A review of longitudinal studies. *Women Birth*. doi:10.1016/j.wombi.2013.02.006.

Seehusen, D. A., Baldwin, L. M., Runkle, G. P., & Clark, G. (2005). Are family physicians appropriately screening for postpartum depression? *Journal of the American Board of Family Practice, 18*(2), 104–112.

Segre, L. S., O'Hara, M. W., Brock, R. L., & Taylor, D. (2012). Depression screening of perinatal women by the Des Moines Healthy Start Project: Program description and evaluation. *Psychiatric Services, 63*(3), 250–255. doi:10.1176/appi.ps.201100247.

Shakespeare, J. (2005). Screening: The role and recommendations of the UK National Screening Committee. In C. Henshaw & S. Elliott (Eds.), *Screening for perinatal depression* (pp. 21–33). London, UK: Jessica Kingsley Publishers.

Soderquist, J., Wijma, B., Thorbert, G., & Wijma, K. (2009). Risk factors in pregnancy for post-traumatic stress and depression after childbirth. *British Journal of Obstetrics and Gynaecology, 116*(5), 672–680. doi:10.1111/j.1471-0528.2008.02083.x.

Spielberger, C. (1983). *Manual for the state-trait anxiety inventory.* Palo Alto, CA: Consulting Psychologists Press.

Spitzer, R. L., Kroenke, K., Williams, J. B., & Lowe, B. (2006). A brief measure for assessing generalized anxiety disorder: The GAD-7. *Archives of Internal Medicine, 166*(10), 1092–1097. doi:10.1001/archinte.166.10.1092.

Stowe, Z. N., Hostetter, A. L., & Newport, D. J. (2005). The onset of postpartum depression: Implications for clinical screening in obstetrical and primary care. *American Journal of Obstetrics and Gynecology, 192*(2), 522–526.

Stuart, S., & O'Hara, M. W. (1995). Treatment of postpartum depression with interpersonal psycho-therapy. *Archives of General Psychiatry, 52*(1), 75–76.

Stuebe, A. M., Grewen, K., & Meltzer-Brody, S. (2013). Association between maternal mood and oxytocin response to breastfeeding. *Journal of Women's Health, 22*(4), 352–361. doi:10.1089/jwh.2012.3768.

Sutter-Dallay, A. L., Giaconne-Marcesche, V., Glatigny-Dallay, E., & Verdoux, H. (2004). Women with anxiety disorders during pregnancy are at increased risk of intense postnatal depressive symp-toms: A prospective survey of the MATQUID cohort. *European Psychiatry, 19*(8), 459–463. doi:10.1016/j.eurpsy.2004.09.025.

Swalm, D., Brooks, J., Doherty, D., Nathan, E., & Jacques, A. (2010). Using the Edinburgh postnatal depression scale to screen for perinatal anxiety. *Archives of Women's Mental Health, 13*(6), 515–522.

Swinson, R. P. (2006). The GAD-7 scale was accurate for diagnosing generalised anxiety disorder. *Evidence-Based Medicine, 11*(6), 184. doi:10.1136/ebm.11.6.184.

Talge, N. M., Neal, C., Glover, V., & Translational Research Early Stress, Fetal Prevention Science Network, Child Neonatal Experience on, and Health Adolescent Mental. (2007). Antenatal maternal stress and long-term effects on child neurodevelopment: How and why? *Journal of Child Psychology and Psychiatry and Allied Disciplines, 48*(3–4), 245–261. doi:10.1111/j.1469-7610.2006.01714.x.

Trivedi, M. H., Rush, A. J., Wisniewski, S. R., Nierenberg, A. A., Warden, D., Ritz, L., … Star D. Study Team. (2006). Evaluation of outcomes with citalopram for depression using measurement-based care in STAR*D: Implications for clinical practice. *American Journal of Psychiatry, 163*(1), 28–40. doi:10.1176/appi.ajp.163.1.28.

Uguz, F., Akman, C., Kaya, N., & Cilli, A. S. (2007). Postpartum-onset obsessive-compulsive disorder: Incidence, clinical features, and related factors. *Journal of Clinical Psychiatry, 68*(1), 132–138.

Verreault, N., Da Costa, D., Marchand, A., Ireland, K., Banack, H., Dritsa, M., & Khalife, S. (2012). PTSD following childbirth: A prospective study of incidence and risk factors in Canadian women. *Journal of Psychosomatic Research, 73*(4), 257–263. doi:10.1016/j.jpsychores.2012.07.010.

Vesga-Lopez, O., Blanco, C., Keyes, K., Olfson, M., Grant, B. F., & Hasin, D. S. (2008). Psychiatric dis-orders in pregnant and postpartum women in the United States. *Archives of General Psychiatry, 65*(7), 805–815. doi:10.1001/archpsyc.65.7.805.

Wenzel, A., Gorman, L. L., O'Hara, M. W., & Stuart, S. (2001). The occurrence of panic and obsessive compulsive symptoms in women with postpartum dysphoria: A prospective study. *Archives of Women's Mental Health, 4*:5–12.

Wenzel, A., Haugen, E. N., Jackson, L. C., & Brendle, J. R. (2005). Anxiety symptoms and disorders at eight weeks postpartum. *Journal of Anxiety Disorders, 19*(3), 295–311. doi:10.1016/j.janxdis.2004.04.001.

Wenzel, A., Haugen, E. N., Jackson, L. C., & Robinson, K. (2003). Prevalence of generalized anxiety at eight weeks postpartum. *Archives of Women's Mental Health, 6*(1), 43–49. doi:10.1007/s00737-002-0154-2.

Wirz-Justice, A., Bader, A., Frisch, U., Stieglitz, R. D., Alder, J., Bitzer, J., … Riecher-Rossler, A. (2011). A randomized, double-blind, placebo-controlled study of light therapy for antepartum depression. *Journal of Clinical Psychiatry, 72*(7), 986–993. doi:10.4088/JCP.10m06188blu.

Wisner, K. L., Hanusa, B. H., Perel, J. M., Peindl, K. S., Piontek, C. M., Sit, D. K., … Moses-Kolko, E. L. (2006). Postpartum depression: A randomized trial of sertraline versus nortriptyline. *Journal of Clinical Psychopharmacology, 26*(4), 353–360. doi:10.1097/01.jcp.0000227706.56870.dd.

Wisner, K. L., Moses-Kolko, E. L., & Sit, D. K. (2010). Postpartum depression: A disorder in search of a definition. *Archives of Women's Mental Health, 13*(1), 37–40.

Wisner, K. L., Parry, B. L., & Piontek, C. M. (2002). Clinical practice. Postpartum depression. *New England Journal of Medicine, 347*(3), 194–199. doi:10.1056/NEJMcp011542.

Wisner, K. L., Peindl, K. S., Gigliotti, T., & Hanusa, B. H. (1999). Obsessions and compulsions in women with postpartum depression. *Journal of Clinical Psychiatry, 60*(3), 176–180.

Wisner, K. L., Sit, D. K., McShea, M. C., Rizzo, D. M., Zoretich, R. A., Hughes, C. L., … Hanusa, B. H. (2013). Onset timing, thoughts of self-harm, and diagnoses in postpartum women with screen-positive depression findings. *Journal of the American Medical Association Psychiatry, 70*(5), 490–498. doi:10.1001/jamapsychiatry.2013.87.

Woolhouse, H., Brown, S., Krastev, A., Perlen, S., & Gunn, J. (2009). Seeking help for anxiety and depression after childbirth: Results of the Maternal Health Study. *Archives of Women's Mental Health, 12*(2), 75–83. doi:10.1007/s00737-009-0049-6.

Yawn, B. P., Dietrich, A. J., Wollan, P., Bertram, S., Graham, D., Huff, J., … Trippd Practices. (2012). TRIPPD: A practice-based network effectiveness study of postpartum depression screening and management. *Annals of Family Medicine, 10*(4), 320–329. doi:10.1370/afm.1418.

Yonkers, K. A., Vigod, S., & Ross, L. E. (2011). Diagnosis, pathophysiology, and management of mood disorders in pregnant and postpartum women. *Obstetrics and Gynecology, 117*(4), 961–977. doi:10.1097/AOG.0b013e31821187a7.

Yonkers, K. A., Wisner, K. L., Stewart, D. E., Oberlander, T. F., Dell, D. L., Stotland, N., … Lockwood, C. (2009). The management of depression during pregnancy: A report from the American Psychiatric Association and the American College of Obstetricians and Gynecologists. *Obstetrics and Gynecology, 114*(3), 703–713.

Zambaldi, C. F., Cantilino, A., Montenegro, A. C., Paes, J. A., de Albuquerque, T. L., & Sougey, E. B. (2009). Postpartum obsessive-compulsive disorder: Prevalence and clinical characteristics. *Comprehensive Psychiatry, 50*(6), 503–509. doi:10.1016/j.comppsych.2008.11.014.

Zhang, X., Liu, K., Sun, J., & Zheng, Z. (2010). Safety and feasibility of repetitive transcranial magnetic stimulation (rTMS) as a treatment for major depression during pregnancy. *Archives of women's mental health, 13*(4), 369–370. doi:10.1007/s00737-010-0163-5.

Zlotnick, C., Miller, I. W., Pearlstein, T., Howard, M., & Sweeney, P. (2006). A preventive intervention for pregnant women on public assistance at risk for postpartum depression. *American Journal of Psychiatry, 163*(8), 1443–1445. doi:10.1176/appi.ajp.163.8.1443.

2

When Screening Is Policy, How Do We Make It Work?

Barbara P. Yawn, Elizabeth M. LaRusso,
Susan L. Bertram, and William V. Bobo

Introduction

Routine or universal screening for postnatal depression (PND) has become a policy in US states such as Illinois (Illinois Chapter, American Academy of Pediatrics, 2008) and New Jersey (University of Minnesota, 2012) and in Australia (Austin, Middleton, Reilly, & Highet, 2013; Hough, 2013; Rhodes & Segre, 2013). In the United Kingdom, the recommendations are less clear. In 2011, the National Health Services UK National Screening Committee reaffirmed its initial recommendation against systematic screening for PND (UK National Screening Committee, 2011) but refers to the National Institute for Health and Clinical Excellence (NICE) practice guidelines that recommend "case finding" by questioning all postnatal women about feelings of being down or depressed and having little interest or pleasure in doing things (National Collaborating Center for Mental Health (UK), 2007). The American Academy of Pediatrics (AAP; Hagan, Shaw, & Duncan, 2008) and the Australian Midwifery Association recommend routine PND screening (Price, Corder-Mabe, & Austin, 2012), while the American College of Obstetrics and Gynecologists (ACOG, 2012; Yonkers et al., 2009b), the US Agency for Healthcare Research and Quality (AHRQ, 2012), and the US Preventive Services Task Force (USPSTF) (2009) state that evidence remains insufficient to recommend universal PND screening (see Chapter 12 for further coverage of international approaches to screening).

Evidence that routine PND screening improves rates of diagnosis and that appropriate treatment can improve depression outcomes does not mean that screening alone improves outcomes. There must be a chain of evidence beginning with screening, going through the subsequent steps (evaluation, diagnosis, therapy initiation, follow-up, and monitoring), and resulting in improvement in maternal depressive symptoms or amelioration of the negative outcomes for infants (Apter-Levy, Feldman, Vakart, Ebstein, & Feldman, 2013; O'Higgins, Rober, Glover, & Taylor, 2013; Quevedo et al., 2012) and families (Letourneau et al., 2012)

Identifying Perinatal Depression and Anxiety: Evidence-Based Practice in Screening, Psychosocial Assessment, and Management, First Edition. Edited by Jeannette Milgrom and Alan W. Gemmill.
© 2015 John Wiley & Sons, Ltd. Published 2015 by John Wiley & Sons, Ltd.

related to maternal PND (ACOG, 2012; Rosenfield, 2007; USPSTF, 2009; Yawn et al., 2012a, 2012b). The chain of evidence required and the existing evidence for improving outcomes in PND are outlined in Chapter 1 and are further elaborated here.

Despite limited evidence, several groups have published "best practices" for PND screening (Horowitz, Murphy, Gregory, & Wojcik, 2009; Liberto, 2012; Peindl, Wisner, & Hanusa, 2004; Sit et al., 2009). In general, these "best practices" are limited to screening methods to identify women at high risk of PND, with referral to mental health professionals for further evaluation of elevated screening scores. Yet, multiple studies have shown that referral is an ineffective manner of providing care for women who screen positive for PND (Kozhimannil, Adams, Soumerai, Busch, & Huskamp, 2011; Rollans, Schmied, Kemp, & Meade, 2013; Yawn et al., 2012b; Yonkers et al., 2009a). This chapter will address the steps of implementation in the context of screening programs that have provided evidence of improved depression outcomes at 6–18 months postpartum (Leung et al., 2011; Morrell et al., 2011; Yawn et al., 2012a) and highlight the need to develop policies based on evidence rather than clinical lore or dogma.

The chapter is presented in sections dealing with each of the steps that should be considered when implementing perinatal mood disorder screening and management programs. Most of the material deals with PND since that is the condition that has been most widely studied and reported upon.

The Basic Questions to Address When Implementing Perinatal Mood Screening Policies

Addressing the common steps of how, who, when, where, what, and why can facilitate program development among groups struggling to implement perinatal depression and anxiety screening policies (Table 2.1).

Table 2.1   Questions to answer before implementing perinatal depression screening

Basic question	Simplistic answer	Answer presented in context of program to improve outcomes
Why should screening be done?	To increase identification	To improve outcomes. Screening and identification are not ends in and of themselves
Who should implement screening?	Any group with access to women	Groups who have the ability to provide adequate on-site services for most women
What screening tools should be used?	Short and simple tools	Tools with high sensitivity and follow-up with tools with high specificity
Where should screening take place?	Any setting where women are available	Settings that are acceptable to women and have facilities that can deal with mental health emergencies (e.g., suicidal ideation) and have the infrastructure and tools for follow-up services
When should screening occur?	Any time prenatally or postpartum	Prenatally—timing still unclear. Postpartum, 4–12 weeks postpartum
What needs to be available if screening is implemented?	Care for depression	A plan and resources for diagnosis, management, and follow-up that does not rely primarily on referral to off-site services

Why implement universal screening versus targeted screening?

Many risk factors have been identified for PND (Georgiopoulos, Bryan, Wollan, & Yawn, 2001; Janssen, Heaman, Urquila, O'Campo, & Thiessen, 2012; Mercier, Garrett, Thorp, & Siega-Riz, 2013; Shapiro, Fraser, & Seguin, 2012; Wu, Chen, & Xu, 2012). However, even when combined, these risk factors predict only about 50–60% of cases of PND (Sword, Clark, Hegadoren, Brooks, & Kingston, 2012). Identification based on clinical judgment has likewise been shown to miss many cases (Georgiopoulos et al., 2001). Routine or universal PND screening can circumvent some of these problems and has been shown to increase rates of diagnosis and therapy initiation (Gjerdingen, McGovern, & Center, 2011; Yawn et al., 2012b). Women report high satisfaction with questions from health professionals about their postpartum mood (Buist, 2006; Smith et al., 2009), and routine PND screening, when offered, is refused by few women (Yawn et al., 2012a).

Summary recommendation: Targeted screening has been demonstrated to miss many women with depression. Screening programs should include routine, universal screening.

Who should screen and where?

Many individuals provide support, care, or services to women in the perinatal period, and in principle, any of them could initiate screening (Austin, Reilly, Milgrom, & Barnett, 2010; Dietrich et al., 2003b, Dietrich, Oxman, & Williams, 2003a; Jones, Creedy, & Gamble, 2013; Leung et al., 2011; Morrell et al., 2011; Olson, Dietrich, Prazar, & Hurley, 2006). Yet without additional training some health professionals may be uncomfortable asking women about depression and may worry that some women will even react negatively (Bertram et al., 2013). This concern should not be taken lightly. In Australia, universal screening has been recommended for over 13 years, yet only 68% of midwives report ever screening for PND (Jones et al., 2013). Therefore, the decision of who should screen for PND requires consideration of willingness and comfort on the part of the proposed screener as well as the setting in which the screening will occur.

Screening needs to occur at a site that explains and offers follow-up services (Castle, Schweitzer, & Tiller, 2009; Dietrich et al., 2004; Katon et al., 2010; Yawn et al., 2012b). Studies consistently report that screening and then referring high-risk women for further evaluation result in many unevaluated and untreated women. Anywhere from 17.6% to 47% of women referred for further evaluation or treatment for high screening scores actually complete that referral (Goodman & Tyer-Viola, 2010; Kelly, Zatzik, & Anders, 2001; Nelson, Freeman, Johnson, McIntire, & Levano, 2013; Rowan, Greisinger, Brehm, Smith, & McReynolds, 2012; Segre, O'Hara, Brock, & Taylor, 2012). Screening sites that are unable to offer on-site follow-up services for diagnosis or treatment are likely to have less ability to improve outcomes (Gjerdingen, Katon, & Rich, 2008; Hagan et al., 2008; Kozhimannil et al., 2011; Yawn et al., 2012a, 2012b; Yonkers et al., 2009a). Collaborative care which includes adult care clinicians within the same clinic may be an alternative approach for pediatricians or other care centers that provide limited types of services to postnatal women such as the US Women, Infant, and Children (WIC) program that provides food vouchers, basic parenting education, and infant assessments (Dietrich et al., 2003a; O'Hara & McCabe, 2013; Truitt, Pina, Person-Rennell, & Angstman, 2013). However, studies of collaborative care for PND are rare.

Even for sites that have the required screening, diagnostic, treatment, and follow-up services available, barriers to full implementation still exist including lack of time, inadequate funding, absence of referral resources for complex cases, and lack of training (Dietrich et al., 2003a; Miller et al., 2012). To provide financial incentives, the state of Illinois offers $4 for PND screening, a potentially appropriate public health strategy (Illinois Chapter, American Academy of Pediatrics, 2008; Kozhimannil et al., 2011). However, this also incentivizes nonclinical sites to provide screening without any direct access to clinical care. Women with elevated screening scores are referred to the woman's primary care site that does not receive the additional funding for the screening but must deal with the results by appropriately assessing, diagnosing, and managing patients. The pragmatic and ethical considerations of paying sites that are unable to intervene beyond administering the screening assessment need to be discussed openly and with a careful assessment of benefits and risk of harms.

For 3–15% of women in industrialized countries (higher rates in developing countries) who do not attend postpartum visits (Georgiopoulos et al., 2001), PND screening in sites outside of health-care facilities, perhaps even self-screening, may be necessary.

Summary recommendation: Screening should be conducted by health professionals that are comfortable with screening and can complete the screening at a site that women are likely to attend such as scheduled antenatal, postnatal, or home visits. Screening completed at a site that requires referral, especially off-site referral after initial screening and scoring of the screening tool, has not been shown to lead to improved patient outcomes.

What tool or tools should be used for screening?

As described in detail in chapter 5, there are multiple depression screening tools available for use. An important consideration is the time required for completion of the screening tools which ranges from less than 1 min to as high as 20 min (Table 2.2). Sensitivities of PND screening tools are highly relevant as these should be very high in order to maximize identification of possible cases. Sensitivities of individual depression screening instruments

Table 2.2 Comparison of characteristics of PND screening tools

Screening tool	Number of items	Time to complete (min)	Sensitivity/ specificity (%)	Self- administered	Other language
Edinburgh Postnatal Depression Scale (EPDS)	10	<5	Sensitivity: 59–100 Specificity: 49–100	Yes	Yes
Postpartum Depression Screening Scale (PDSS)	35	10–20	Sensitivity: 91–94 Specificity: 72–98	No	Yes
Patient Health Questionnaire-9 (PHQ-9)	9	<5	Sensitivity: 75 Specificity: 90	Yes	Yes
Patient Health Questionnaire-2 (PHQ-2)	2	<1	Sensitivity: 85 Specificity: 49	Yes	Yes
Beck Depression Inventory II (BDI-II)	21	5–10	Sensitivity: 56–57 Specificity: 97–100	Yes	Yes
Zung Self-Rating Depression Scale (Zung SDS)	20	5–10	Sensitivity: 45–89 Specificity: 77–88	Yes	No
NICE case-finding questions	3	<2	Sensitivity: 78 Specificity: 58	Yes	No

range widely and are highly dependent on the cutoff values used to define an "elevated" or "positive" score (Davis, Pearlstein, Stuart, O'Hara, & Zlotnick, 2013). The Edinburgh Postnatal Depression Scale (EPDS; Cox, Chapman, Murray, & Jones, 1996) with a cutoff value of >12 yields sensitivities of ~60%, while lower cutoffs recommended for population screening have sensitivities close to 100% (Boyd, Le, & Somberg, 2005; Gaynes et al., 2005; Sharp & Lipsky, 2002; Yawn et al., 2009a). Specificities of the various PND screening tools range from 77% to 100%, with lower cutoff scores having lower specificities. Tools such as the EPDS (described more fully in chapter 5, as the most widely researched tool), the Patient Health Questionnaire-9 (PHQ-9; Spitzer, Kroenke, & Williams, 1999), and the Beck Depression Inventory II (BDI-II; Beck, 2002) have been validated across several ethnic populations. Most of the tools are available in non-English translations (Augusto, Kumar, Calheiros, Matos, & Figueiredo, 1996; Jadresic, Araya, & Jara, 1995; Nhiwatiwa, Patel, & Acuda, 1998; O'Hara et al., 2012; Wickberg & Hwang, 1996).

The PHQ-9 has been used as both a primary screening tool and as a confirmatory test in women with elevated EPDS scores (≥10) to help confirm elevated risk and severity of depression. The PHQ-9 has also been used to monitor response to therapy through comparison of baseline and follow-up scores (Johanson, Chapman, Murray, Johnson, & Cox, 2000; McGill, Burrows, Holland, Langer, & Sweet, 1995; Yawn et al., 2012a). The sensitivity of the PHQ-9 to changes in depression severity (including PND severity) during treatment increases its potential value. Providing a baseline assessment of severity of depression can also guide treatment selection (Lowe, Kroenke, Herzog, & Grafe, 2004) and facilitate follow-up management, especially in the primary care setting (Yawn et al., 2012a). In addition, the PHQ-9 has been used by many US primary care practices to meet the USPSTF recommendation for routine screening of all adults for depression (USPSTF, 2009). This recommendation has increased the comfort and familiarity of US primary care practices with the use and interpretation of the PHQ-9, which may be an important consideration when determining which PND screening tool to use. The shortened two-question form of the PHQ-9, called the PHQ-2, may also be considered as a first step in screening, but elevated scores should always be followed by administration of the full PHQ-9 (Chae, Chae, Tyndall, Ramirez, & Winter, 2012; Kroenke, Spitzer & Williams, 2001; Gjerdingen et al., 2011).

Recently, subscales of the Pregnancy Report and Monitoring Survey (PRAMS) have been shown to identify women at high risk of clinically significant depression and possibly anxiety (Davis et al., 2013; O'Hara et al., 2012). They are currently used for depression and anxiety disorder surveillance during pregnancy. As currently used, these tools have no value for PND or postnatal anxiety screening since they are not scored immediately and therefore cannot be used to initiate action for clinical care (Liu & Tronick, 2013).

Investigators in the United Kingdom have developed a two-item tool based on the PHQ-2 but with a time frame of 4 rather than 2 weeks and scored only as yes/no responses (Mann, Adamson, & Gilbody, 2012; Whooley, Avins, Browner, & Miranda, 1997). The tool adds a third question asking women if they desire help for their symptoms. This question was reported to have a sensitivity of 60% or less and a specificity of about 90% for PND which must be appended to the values for the two-question screener, making it less sensitive and less specific than most other tools. How the third question impacts outcomes has not been studied.

Tools to assess perinatal anxiety have had less evaluation in the perinatal period. The Generalized Anxiety Disorder-7 (GAD-7) screening tool is reported to be acceptable for use during and after pregnancy (O'Hara et al., 2012). A subset of the EPDS, specifically questions 4 and 5, has also been reported to be useful for anxiety screening (Petrozzi & Gagliardi, 2013). In addition, McDonald and colleagues (2012) report they have successfully used a combination of psychosocial factors to predict anxiety at 16 weeks postpartum. Due to lack of evidence of impact of screening, no anxiety screening is recommended currently except in the context of well-designed clinical studies (see also chapter 6).

Maternal suicide and infanticide are two of the most severe adverse outcomes of PND (Wisner et al., 2013). Recognition and evaluation of thoughts of self-harm and infant harm are therefore an important consideration during depression screening. Both the EPDS and the PHQ-9 have embedded questions related to self-harm or suicidal ideation (Cox et al., 1996; Spitzer et al., 1999). However, neither asks about risk of harm to the infant, and in a review of the literature, no tools to specifically screen for risk of harm to the infant were found (Fairbrother & Woody, 2008).

Summary recommendation: The EPDS and the PHQ-9 have the advantage of being brief, self-administered instruments that include assessment of suicidal ideation and are readily available in the public domain. The tools have been validated in several languages. The PHQ-9 is also useful for monitoring response to PND therapy. Two- or three-question tools, such as the PHQ-2 or NICE case-finding questions, can be administered even more rapidly and with high sensitivity but are subject to misclassification owing to high numbers of false positives. These brief tools must be followed by a more comprehensive tool for any woman with an elevated brief screening score. Screening tools for perinatal anxiety require further investigation prior to recommendations for widespread use.

When should screening occur?

The optimal timing for screening during pregnancy and the postpartum period remains undetermined (Gaynes et al., 2005). During pregnancy, the times available to screen for depression and anxiety depend to a significant extent on the woman's timing of seeking antenatal care and the timing of the delivery. Screening at the first visit may provide some information on prevalent depression and anxiety. Screening at 34–36 weeks has been found to have some value in predicting PND (Faisal-Cury & Menezes, 2012; Sutter-Dallay, Cosnefroy, Glatigny-Dallay, Verdoux, & Rascle, 2012).

Postpartum screening for depression has been done as early as 24–48 h postpartum, before women are discharged from the hospital postdelivery (Austin et al., 2013). However, the ability of screening completed within the first 48 h to predict continued depressive symptoms is limited. Women with prevalent (preexisting) depression may screen positive, but false-positive screens may result from unresolved "baby blues" or from the physical and emotional upheaval associated with a complex delivery or unexpected outcome. Early posthospital screening, at 5 days postpartum, lowered both the specificity and sensitivity (ability to identify all of the potential cases) when compared to screening at 6 weeks after delivery (Hannah, Adams, Lee, Glover, & Sandler, 1992). Screening at 6, 8, and 12 weeks postpartum has been shown to be equally effective in the identification of women at increased risk for prolonged PND (Wickberg & Hwang, 1997). Therefore, screening at a time when women may already be attending health-care visits (the routine 6–8-week postpartum visit or an early 4–8-week well-child visit) may provide adequate specificity and sensitivity while taking advantage of current health-care delivery patterns.

The AAP recommends rescreening women for PND at every visit for the infant (The Common Wealth Fund, 2007). When and how often to rescreen for PND have not been studied, and therefore, evidence-based recommendations cannot be made (Sheeder, Kabir, & Stafford, 2009).

Early data suggests that later screening at 6–12 months postpartum may identify additional women for further evaluation (Hannah et al., 1992; Wickberg & Hwang, 1997). However, due to lack of studies, no evidence-based recommendations for the timing of anxiety screening in the perinatal period can be made. However, from a practical perspective, it seems most efficient to screen for both depression and anxiety at the same time if both are to be included in a screening program.

Summary recommendation: Evidence supports PND screening at 4–12 weeks postpartum with early evidence suggesting rescreening at 6–12 months postpartum. No evidence exists for the timing of prenatal screening, but evaluation at the first prenatal visit may identify preexisting depression, and screening during late pregnancy may identify some women at risk for more severe PND. No evidence is available related to the optimal timing of anxiety screening, but if such screening becomes policy, timing similar to depression screening seems most practical until evidence is developed.

What is required if you do implement perinatal depression or anxiety screening?

Simply asking a few questions about PND, scoring and recording the results, and referring high-risk women for further evaluation or care are insufficient. The rest of this section will address those important and less studied next steps including the infrastructure, tools, and personnel required for evaluation and diagnosis, assisting women with selection of therapy, and management and follow-up of diagnosed depression and anxiety.

Evaluation of elevated screening scores

Women with elevated screening scores require further evaluation. Screening should not be confused with diagnostic evaluation. A small percentage of women who have high screening scores will have general medical conditions as the etiology of their symptoms. Hypothyroidism, hyperthyroidism, anemia, and other medical conditions as well as postnatal blues, problems with managing interpersonal difficulties or maladjustment to motherhood, substance use disorders, and postnatal grief reactions may present with symptoms similar to PND or postnatal anxiety (Bobo et al., 2014; Peiris, Oh, & Diaz, 2007). Therefore, in addition to evaluation of the woman's mental health, patients with positive PND screening results also require a thorough medical and psychosocial evaluation.

What constitutes an adequate diagnostic assessment for an elevated screening score remains controversial. Some health professionals report that all screened women require a standardized diagnostic interview by a trained mental health professional (Yonkers, Vigod, & Ross, 2011). However, this is likely to prove impractical since 15–25% of pregnant women would require lengthy evaluation from a mental health professional who are nationally and internationally in short supply (Gjerdingen et al., 2011).

Limited but growing evidence (Boyd, 2013; Dietrich et al., 2004; Frey & Sharma, 2013; Katon et al., 2010; Milgrom et al., 2011; Yawn et al., 2012a) shows that women can be evaluated by a primary care physician or perhaps another clinician with training in the diagnosis and management of depression. The evaluation must assess the severity and duration of the symptoms as well as their impact on the woman's ability to function in her usual roles. In addition, signs of other mood disorders (e.g. bipolar disorders), psychotic disorders (including postpartum psychosis), anxiety disorders, substance use disorders, or other serious mental health problems must be considered (Wisner et al., 2013). Referral to a mental health professional is then reserved for those women with unusual presentations, history of previous serious mental health problems, and depression resistant to therapies available in the primary setting (Yawn et al., 2012a, 2012b).

The results of the postscreening evaluation determine the next steps. If PND is diagnosed, the patient and, if possible, members of her support network should be engaged in a discussion that can begin by asking if they agree with concerns about the patient's depressed feeling or mood and if they feel that help would be desirable (Dietrich et al., 2004). This step is crucial. Patient engagement is necessary if they are to initiate and continue therapy and participate in follow-up and monitoring visits or phone calls (Katon et al., 2010; Yawn et al., 2012b).

Selecting therapeutic approach

Once the PND diagnosis has been established and engagement of the woman and her family begun, treatment is the next topic to approach. While the details of this are discussed in other chapters of this book (see chapter 7 and chapter 11), it is important to offer all reasonable types of treatment that are likely to result in remission of depressive symptoms and are available in the immediate region. For some sites, this may include cognitive behavioral therapy (CBT) or interpersonal therapy (IPT) delivered by telehealth (Segre et al., 2012) or perhaps even over the Internet (Baker, Kamke, O'Hara & Stuart, 2009; see also examples of online treatment in Chapter 15). When medication trials are being planned, breastfeeding status must be considered. The majority of antidepressant medications are considered to have an acceptable balance of risks and benefits especially in women with severe depression or depression that has failed nonpharmacologic therapy (Bobo et al., 2014; Patel & Wisner, 2011).

Guidelines have been developed for visits and interactions with adults with major depressive disorders (Gelenberg, 2010; Gyani, Pumphrey, Parker Shafran, & Rose, 2012). In general, each PND visit should monitor the woman's ability and desire to adhere to treatment and assess the functional status of the woman related to parenting, partner relationships, and work capacity. Reports of medication side effects are always important to acknowledge and address. Many early medication side effects can be minimized by beginning with low doses and moving to therapeutic levels. Pharmacotherapy for PND is dealt with further in Chapter 11 (O'Hara & McCabe, 2013)

Treatment of depression during pregnancy requires the same attention to evaluation, correct diagnosis, careful selection of therapy, follow-up, and monitoring as recommended and shown to be successful for PND (American Psychiatric Association, 2010; National Collaborating Center for Mental Health (UK), 2007; Patel & Wisner, 2011; Yonkers et al., 2009b).

Patient and family as partners in care

Patients and, when appropriate and willing, families need to be partners in the care of postnatal mood disorders. For some women, nonfamily members may be the most trusted, reliable, and willing supports. This should be explored with each woman to identify such supportive individuals and the willingness of the patient to engage with identified support individuals. For women with severe depression, initial participation in therapeutic decisions and therapy may be more limited than for women with less severe and incapacitating depression. Fathers may also suffer depression in the perinatal period and are more likely to do so if their partner has PND, further highlighting the need to engage and work with families (Fletcher, 2011).

Evaluating suicidal ideation

Many health-care professionals are concerned about the potential burden involved in screening for suicidal ideation. However, such screening is an important part of a PND program and required for women with severe depression (e.g., women with very high PND screening scores), women with history of suicidal ideation or attempts, women with a history of alcohol or other substance use disorders, and those for whom impulsive self-destructive behaviors may be frequent (Fairbrother & Woody, 2008; Wisner et al., 2013). In primary care practices, use of the tool depicted in Figure 2.1 was associated with increased comfort on the part of the clinic's staff and provided required information on suicidal thinking in a quick and easily used format (Yawn et al., 2009a). The reverse side of the form is not shown but includes the local numbers for emergency suicidal evaluation resources, the nearest emergency department, and local police. Chapter 4 provides further guidance to clinicians in conducting a risk assessment and supplementing procedures and forms with clinical judgment to ascertain the need for escalation of services.

Summary recommendation: Few programs have shown improvement in depression with PND screening, but those that have (including the TRIPPD trial) combined screening with follow-up care at the same site. The tools used in the TRIPPD trial (Yawn et al., 2012a) are freely available at http://www.aafp.org/patient-care/nrn/studies/all/trippd/ppd-toolkit.html.

Evidence gaps

The needs for basic, translational, implementation, and dissemination research in the fields of perinatal depression and anxiety remain vast. It is time to require that clinical studies in this field report meaningful patient outcomes, not simply process outcomes such as screening or therapy initiation rates. Previous failures and successes in PND screening should inform all future funded research (Hewitt et al., 2009). It is time to reorient the discussion of screening toward the steps needed to address elevated screening scores (Miller et al., 2012; Yawn et al., 2012a, 2012b).

For PND, the elements of effective screening and follow-up programs need to be tested in larger populations and in different settings such as pediatric, obstetric, and family or general medicine practices that provide on-site collaborative care for adults with PND (Hanbury, Farley, Thompson et al., 2012). Unique high-risk groups of women, for example, the mothers of infants receiving 3 weeks or more of care in the neonatal intensive care unit (NICU), should also be the subjects of future screening and follow-up studies for PND and postnatal anxiety (McCabe et al., 2012).

Screening for depression during pregnancy requires the same careful attention to process, evaluation, and follow-up that is required for PND (Reminick, Cohen, & Einarson, 2013) Preliminary evidence for improved outcomes exists for programs that provide screening

(a)

This form will be individualized to each site based on state laws and regulations and will be tailored to each practice.

IMMEDIATE ACTION PROTOCOL (IAP)

Use this action plan if any of the following:

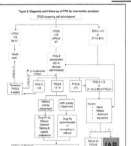

a. The EPDS score > 19.
b. The answer to EPDS Q #10 (The thought of harming myself has occurred to me) is "sometimes" or "yes, quite often".
c. The PHQ-9 score is ≥15.
d. The answer to PHQ-9 Q #9 (Thoughts that you would be better off dead or of hurting yourself in some way) is greater than "not at all".
e. Clinical judgment suggests concern about suicide.

First step: Assess suicidal risk:
 -This can be done by the primary care physician using the Suicide Risk Assessment Questions below.

Or

 -By immediate (same day) referral to a mental health professional who has access to an inpatient psychiatric facility or referral to an emergency department. Establish a verbal "No Suicide Contract" for at least 24 hours. (See reverse side for Immediate Referral Resources.)

Suicide Risk Assessment: Examples of questions.
a. Intent – *You have said that you think about killing or harming yourself. Have you made any plans?* (Use the answers on the EPDS or PHQ-9 to lead into the first question.)
b. Means – *Can you describe your plans?.* Or *How have you thought about killing yourself (your infant)? (You will want to assess access to weapons, drugs or other methods she has concerned)*
c. Likelihood – *Do you think you would actually harm or kill yourself?* (May be especially useful in those who state they think about but would never do it because it would leave their children without a mother or such reasons or those who report no social support.)
d. Impulsivity – *Have you tried before?* Factors such as alcoholism, drug use, or a history of previous attempts that suggest impulsive behavior or episodes of reduced control.

If the response to any of these is positive then referral to inpatient management is strongly recommended. Also establish a verbal "No Suicide Contract" for at least 24 hours. (See reverse side for Next Step Referral Resources.)

Patient not in the office:
If the clinician has a concern about active suicidal thought but the patient is not in the office:
 -Ask to speak with another adult in the house to alert them to the situation.
 -If no other person is available in the house and there is an immediate concern, keep the person on the phone and notify another staff member to dial 9-1-1.
 -Do not disconnect the phone.
 -Dispatch an ambulance/police and stay on the phone until someone arrives.
 -Establish a verbal "No Suicide Contract" for at least 24 hours.

> **Names, addresses and telephone numbers for referral and support are on the reverse side.**

Figure 2.1 (a) Example of Immediate Action Protocol (IAP) for suicidal ideation evaluation. (b) Diagnosis and follow-up of postpartum depression for intervention practices. (This is box inset of Figure 2.1a.).

and intervention services for patients with elevated depression or anxiety screening scores during pregnancy (Faisal-Cury & Menezes, 2012; Kozinszky et al., 2012; Kuo et al., 2013; Paul, Downs, Schaefer, Beiler, & Weisman, 2013; Smith & Kipnis, 2012). However, many of the studies are very small and focused on special groups of pregnant women such as adolescents or those experiencing interpersonal violence at home. Fundamental work is required

Immediate Referral Resources:

Referral for immediate (same day) assessment for suicidal risk:

Outpatient _____
                 Name of Clinic   Telephone #   Address

Inpatient _____
              Name of Clinic   Telephone #   Address

Mental Health Center_____
                Name of Center   Telephone #   Address

Crisis Facility _____
             Facility Name   Telephone #   Address

Emergency Department _____
                  Name of ED   Telephone #   Address

Other _____
           Name   Telephone #   Address

Next Step Referral Resources:

When the primary care physician has determined the woman is at risk for suicide (see Suicide Risk Assessment):

    Local Psychiatrist/Mental Health Professional _____
                         Name   Telephone #   Address

    Local Hospital _____
               Hospital Name   Telephone #   Address

    Local ED for Admission _____
                   Name of ED   Telephone #   Address

    Suicide Helpline_____
              Name   Telephone #   Address

    Distant Psychiatrist Consultation _____
                    Name   Telephone #   Address

    Other _____
           Name   Telephone #   Address

Transportation Resources:

If the woman/patient is resistant to inpatient management, transportation may better be accomplished by using non-family transportation.

    Police _____
            Telephone #

    Ambulance _____
               Telephone #

    Other _____
           Name   Telephone #

> *In most states physicians have the legal right and obligation to assure the suicidal patient is protected from self-harm. This usually includes the legal right to initiate a 24 to 72 hour involuntary "hold" for inpatient mental health assessment.*

Research Response:

Immediately notify central site of admission: 1-888-292-7164

Date Adverse Event Registry form completed: (Date) __/__/__

Date Adverse Event Form sent to Central Site: (Date) __/__/__

Figure 2.1   *(Continued)*

for each step of building a screening and follow-up program. Evidence is required for the appropriate timing of screening, the best tools to use, and frequency of repeat screenings. Research is required to identify additional treatment options for pregnant women with depression or anxiety.

Clinically significant anxiety during pregnancy and the postpartum period has become increasingly recognized as a significant public health problem (Matthey, Fisher, & Rowe, 2013; Reck, Noe, Gerstenlauer, & Stehle, 2012). However, development of screening and diagnostic tools for anxiety requires increased and immediate attention. Increased therapeutic approaches to anxiety also require study during the entire perinatal period.

(b)

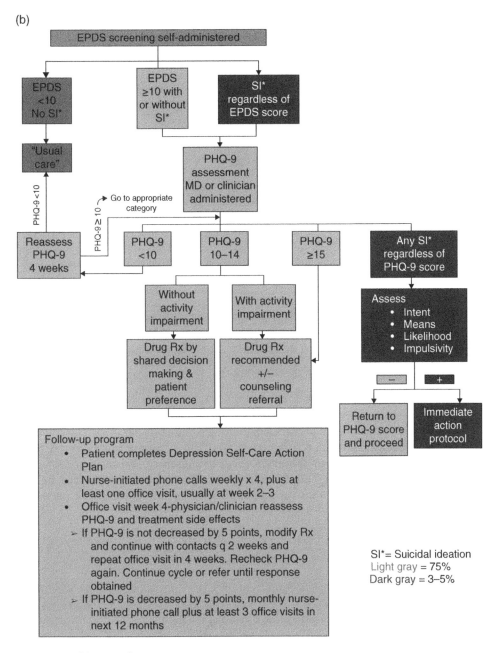

Figure 2.1 (*Continued*)

Finally, evidence needs to be gathered and shared on the impact of existing screening or "case-finding" policies such as those in the states of Illinois and New Jersey as well as the United Kingdom and Australia (Austin et al., 2010; Kozhimannil et al., 2011). We must demand rigorous evaluations and development of programs that are based not on what "sounds good" but rather on evidence of improved outcomes for women with PND and their families.

Table 2.3   Summary of evidence-based recommendations for PND screening

Why screen?	To improve the lives of the women, their infants, and families by reducing the burden of PND symptoms and associated adverse outcomes (Williams, 1968)
Who should screen?	Individuals or organizations that have the resources, infrastructure, and tools to assure further evaluation and follow-up (not just referral) of women with elevated screening scores (Yawn et al., 2012a, 2012b)
What screening tool?	The Edinburgh Postnatal Depression screening tool and the PHQ-9 have both been used in programs that improved outcomes, and the PHQ-9 can be used to follow the course of PND (Lowe et al., 2004; Yawn et al., 2009b, 2012a)
Where to screen?	A place that is convenient for women but also has the resources and infrastructure to go beyond the screening step and can support evaluation, treatment, follow-up, and monitoring (Leung, 2011; Morrell et al., 2011; Yawn et al., 2012a, 2012b)
When to screen?	4–12-week postpartum PND screening has been used in successful programs. Early data suggests that later screening at 6–12 months postpartum may identify additional women for further evaluation (Hannah et al., 1992; Wickberg & Hwang, 1997)
What is needed for screening program?	The infrastructure, tools, and procedures to evaluate, diagnose, treat/manage, and follow up PND should be imbedded in the site that begins the screening process (American Academy of Family Physicians, 2012; Gjerdingen et al., 2008, 2011; Lowe et al., 2004; Yawn et al., 2012a, 2012b)

Evidence-based recommendations when screening becomes policy

In the field of perinatal mood disorders, only screening for PND has sufficient evidence to make any "evidence-based" recommendations. These recommendations are now summarized as the answers to the basic question presented earlier in the chapter (Table 2.3). The research gaps identified earlier will need to be addressed before evidence-based recommendations can be made for prenatal depression or perinatal anxiety screening.

References

AHRQ Effective Health Care Program. (2012). *Efficacy and safety of screening for postpartum depression—research protocol.* Retrieved from http://www.effectivehealthcare.ahrq.gov/search-for-guides-reviews-and-reports/?pageaction=displayproduct&productID=997. Accessed December 16, 2014.

American Academy of Family Physicians. (2012). *Postpartum depression toolkit—National Research Network Studies.* Retrieved from http://www.aafp.org/patient-care/nrn/studies/all/trippd/ppd-toolkit.html. Accessed December 16, 2014.

American College of Obstetrics and Gynecology. (2012). *Screening for depression during and after pregnancy.* Retrieved from http://www.acog.org/Resources_And_Publications/Committee_Opinions/Committee_on_Obstetric_Practice/Screening_for_Depression_During_and_After_Pregnancy. Accessed December 16, 2014.

American Psychiatric Association. (2010). *Practice guideline for the treatment of patients with major depressive disorder*, (3rd ed.). Arlington, VA: American Psychiatric Association.

Apter-Levy, Y., Feldman, M., Vakart, A., Ebstein, R., & Feldman, R. (2013). Impact of maternal depression across the first 6 years of life on the child's mental health, social engagement, and empathy: The moderating role of oxytocin. *The American Journal of Psychiatry*, *170*(10), 1161–1168.

Augusto, A., Kumar, R., Calheiros, J., Matos, E., & Figueiredo, E. (1996). Post-natal depression in an urban area of Portugal: Comparison of childbearing women and matched cohorts. *Psychological Medicine*, *26*, 135–141.

Austin, M., Middelton, P., Reilly, N., & Highet, N. (2013). Detection and management of mood disorders in the maternity setting: The Australian Clinical Practice Guidelines. *Women and Birth*, *26*(1), 2–9.

Austin, M., Reilly, N., Milgrom, J., & Barnett, B. (2010). A national approach to perinatal mental health in Australia: Exercising caution in the roll-out of a public health initiative. *The Medical Journal of Australia*, *192*(2), 111.

Baker, C., Kamke, H., O'Hara, M., & Stuart, S. (2009). Web-based training for implementing evidence-based management of postpartum depression. *Journal of the American Board of Family Medicine*, *22*(5), 588–589.

Beck, C. (2002). Postpartum depression: A metasynthesis. *Qualitative Health Research*, *12*(4), 453–472.

Bertram, S., Graham, D., Kurland, M., Pace, W., Madison, S., & Yawn, B. (2013). Communication is the key to success in pragmatic clinical trials in Practice-based Research Networks (PBRNs). *Journal of the American Board of Family Medicine*, *26*, 571–578.

Bobo, W., Bertram, S., Wollan, P., Kurland, M., Lewis, G., Vore, K., … Yawn, B. (2014). Depressive symptoms and access to mental health care in women screened for post-partum depression and lose health insurance coverage after delivery: Findings from the TRIPPD effectiveness study. *Mayo Clinic Proceedings*, *89*(9), 1220–1228.

Boyd, R. (2013). Primary care-based screening, diagnosis and management of postpartum depression effective for improving symptoms. *Evidence-Based Medicine*, *18*(3), e27.

Boyd, R., Le, H., & Somberg, R. (2005). Review of screening instruments for postpartum depression. *Archives of Women's Mental Health*, *8*, 141–153.

Buist, A. (2006). Acceptability of routine screening for perinatal depression. *Journal of Affective Disorders*, *93*, 233–237.

Castle, D., Schweitzer, I., & Tiller, J. (2009). STAR*D: Has it taught us anything about the management of depression? *Australasian Psychiatry*, *17*(5), 360–364.

Chae, S., Chae, M., Tyndall, A., Ramirez, M., & Winter, R. (2012). Can we effectively use the two-item PHQ-2 to screen for postpartum depression? *Family Medicine*, *44*(10), 698–703.

Cox, J., Chapman, G., Murray, D., & Jones, P. (1996). Validation of the Edinburgh Postnatal Depression Scale (EPDS) in postnatal women. *Journal of Affective Disorders*, *39*(3), 185–189.

Davis, K., Pearlstein, T., Stuart, S., O'Hara, M., & Zlotnick, C. (2013). Analysis of brief screening tools for the detection of postpartum depression: Comparisons of the PRAMS 6-item instrument, PHQ-9, and structured interviews. *Archives of Women's Mental Health*, *16*(4), 271–277.

Dietrich, A. J., Oxman, T. E., & Williams, J. W. (2003a). Treatment of depression by mental health specialists and primary care physicians. *JAMA*, *290*(15), 1991–1996.

Dietrich, A., Oxman, T. E., Williams, J. W., Jr, Schulberg, H. C., Bruce, M. L., Lee, P. W., … Nutting, P. A. (2004). Re-engineering systems for the treatment of depression in primary care: Cluster randomized controlled trial. *BMJ (Clinical Research Edition)*, *329*(7466), 602.

Dietrich, A., William, J., Ciotti, M., Schulkin, J., Stotland, N., Rost, K., … Cornell, J. (2003b). Depression care attitudes and practices of newer obstetrician-gynecologists: A national survey. *American Journal of Obstetrics and Gynecology*, *189*, 267–273.

Fairbrother, N., & Woody, S. (2008). New mothers' thoughts of harm related to the newborn. *Archives of Women's Mental Health*, *11*(3), 221–229.

Faisal-Cury, A., & Menezes, P. (2012). Antenatal depression strongly predicts postnatal depression in primary health care. *Revista Brasileira de Psiquiatria*, *34*(4), 446–450.

Fletcher, R. (2011, December). Field testing of father-inclusive guidelines for web-based information and support aimed at families with perinatal depression. *Health Promotion Journal of Australia, 22*(3), 231–233

Frey, B., & Sharma, V. (2013). A primary care-based treatment programme improves postpartum depression at 12 months. *Evidence-Based Mental Health, 16*(1), 6.

Gaynes, B., Gavin, N., Meltzer-Brody, S., Lohr, K., Swinson, T., Gartlehner, G., … Miller, W. (2005). *Perinatal depression: Prevalence, screening accuracy, and screening outcomes* (Evidence Report 19). Rockville, MD: Agency for Healthcare Research and Quality. Retrieved from http://purl.access.gpo.gov/GPO/LPS58972. Accessed December 16, 2014.

Gelenberg, A. (2010). A review of the current guidelines for depression treatment. *Journal of Clinical Psychiatry, 7*, e15.

Georgiopoulos, A., Bryan, T., Wollan, P., & Yawn, B. (2001). Routine screening for postpartum depression. *The Journal of Family Practice, 50*(2), 117–122.

Gjerdingen, D., Katon, W., & Rich, D. (2008). Stepped care treatment of postpartum depression: A primary care-based management model. *Women's Health Issues, 18*(1), 44–52.

Gjerdingen, D., McGovern, P., & Center, B. (2011). Problems with a diagnostic depression interview in a postpartum depression trial. *Journal of the American Board of Family Medicine, 24*(2), 187–193.

Goodman, J., & Tyer-Viola, L. (2010). Detection, treatment, and referral of perinatal depression and anxiety by obstetrical providers. *Journal of Women's Health, 19*(3), 477–490.

Gyani, A., Pumphrey, N., Parker, H., Shafran, R., & Rose, S. (2012). Investigating the use of NICE guidelines and IAPT services in the treatment of depression. *Mental Health in Family Medicine, 9*(3), 149–160.

Hagan, J. F., Shaw, J. S., & Duncan, P. M. (2008). *Bright futures guidelines for health supervision of infants, children, and adolescents*. Elk Grove Village, IL: American Academy of Pediatrics.

Hanbury, A., Farley, K., Thompson, C., Wilson, P., & Chambers, D. (2012). Challenges in identifying barriers to adoption in a theory-based implementation study: Lessons for future implementation studies. *BMC Health Services Research, 12*, 422.

Hannah, P., Adams, D., Lee, A., Glover, V., & Sandler, M. (1992). Links between early post-partum mood and post-natal depression. *The British Journal of Psychiatry, 160*, 777–780.

Hewitt, C., Gilbody, S., Brealey, S., Paulden, M., Palmer, S., Mann, R., … Richards, D. (2009). Methods to identify postnatal depression in primary care: An integrated evidence synthesis and value of information analysis. *Health Technology Assessment, 13*(36), 1–229.

Horowitz, J., Murphy, C., Gregory, K., & Wojcik, J. (2009). Best practices: Community-based postpartum depression screening: Results from the CARE study. *Psychiatric Services, 60*(11), 1432–1434.

Hough, D. E. (2013). *Irrationality in health care what behavioral economics reveals about what we do and why*. Stanford, CA: Stanford Economics and Finance.

Illinois Chapter, American Academy of Pediatrics. (2008). *Perinatal mental health disorders including postpartum depression*. Retrieved from http://illinoisaap.org/wp-content/uploads/PostPartum-Depression-policy-brief-final-6-231.pdf. Accessed December 16, 2014.

Jadresic, E., Araya, R., & Jara, C. (1995). Validation of the Edinburgh Postnatal Scale (EPDS) in Chilean postpartum women. *Journal of Psychosomatic Obstetrics and Gynaecology, 16*, 187–191.

Janssen, P., Heaman, M., Urquia, M., O'Campo, P., & Thiessen, K. (2012). Risk factors for postpartum depression among abused and nonabused women. *American Journal of Obstetrics and Gynecology, 207*(6), 489.e1–489.e8.

Johanson, R., Chapman, G., Murray, D., Johnson, I., & Cox, J. (2000). The North Staffordshire Maternity Hospital prospective study on pregnancy-associated depression. *Journal of Psychosomatic Obstetrics and Gynecology, 21*, 93–97.

Jones, C., Creedy, D., & Gamble, J. (2013). Detection and management of perinatal depression by midwives. *Women and Birth, 26*(1), e66.

Katon, W., Lin, E., Von Korff, M., Ciechanowski, P., Ludman, E., Young, B., … McCulloch, D. (2010). Collaborative care for patients with depression and chronic illness. *The New England Journal of Medicine, 363*(27), 2611–2620.

Kelly, R., Zatzik, D., & Anders, T. (2001). The detection and treatment of psychiatric disorders and substance abuse among pregnant women cared for in obstetrics. *American Journal of Psychiatry, 158*, 213–219.

Kozhimannil, K., Adams, A., Soumerai, S., Busch, A., & Huskamp, H. (2011). New Jersey's efforts to improve postpartum depression care did not change treatment patterns for women on Medicaid. *Health Affairs, 30*(2), 293–301.

Kozinszky, Z., Dudas, R., Devosa, I., Csatordai, S., Tóth, E., Szabó, D., … Pál, A. (2012). Can a brief antepartum preventive group intervention help reduce postpartum depressive symptomatology? *Psychotherapy and Psychosomatics, 81*(2), 98–107.

Kroenke, K., Spitzer, R. L., Williams, J. B. (2001). The PHQ-9: Validity of a brief depression severity measure. *Journal of General Internal Medicine, 16*(9), 606–613.

Kuo, C., Schonbrun, Y., Zlotnick, C., Bates, N., Todorova, R., Kao, J., … Johnson, J. (2013). A qualitative stud of treatment needs among pregnant and postpartum women with substance use and depression. *Substance Use & Misuse, 48*(14), 1498–1508.

Letourneau, N., Dennis, C., Benzies, K., Duffett-Leger, L., Stewart, M., Tryphonopoulos, P., … Watson, W. (2012). Postpartum depression is a family affair: Addressing the impact on mothers, fathers, and children. *Mental Health Nursing, 33*(7), 445–457.

Leung, S., Lam, T. H., Hung, S. F., Chan, R., Yeung, T., Miao, M., … Lee, D. T. (2011). Outcome of a postnatal depression screening programme using the Edinburgh Postnatal Depression Scale: A randomized controlled trial. *Journal of Public Health (Oxford, England), 33*(2), 292–301.

Liberto, T. (2012). Screening for depression and help-seeking in postpartum women during well-baby pediatric visits: An integrated review. *Journal of Pediatric Health Care, 26*(2), 109–117.

Liu, C., & Tronick, E. (2013). Rates and predictors of postpartum depression by race and ethnicity: Results from the 2004 to 2007 New York City PRAMS survey (Pregnancy Risk Assessment Monitoring System). *Maternal and Child Health Journal, 17*(9), 1599–1610.

Lowe, B., Kroenke, K., Herzog, W., & Grafe, K. (2004). Measuring depression outcome with a brief self-report instrument: Sensitivity to change of the Patient Health Questionnaire (PHG-9). *Journal of Affective Disorders, 81*(1), 61–66.

Mann, R., Adamson, J., & Gilbody, S. (2012). Diagnostic accuracy of case-finding questions to identify perinatal depression. *CMAJ, 184*(8), E424–E430.

Matthey, S., Fisher, J., & Rowe, H. (2013). Using the Edinburgh postnatal depression scale to screening for anxiety disorders: Conceptual and methodological considerations. *Journal of Affective Disorders, 146*(2), 224–230.

McCabe, K., Blucker, R., Gillaspy, J., Cherry, A., Mignogna, M., Roddenbery, A., … Gillaspy, S. (2012). Reliability of the postpartum depression screening scale in the neonatal intensive care unit. *Nursing Research, 61*(6), 441–445.

McDonald, S., Wall, J., Forbes, K., Kingston, D., Kehler, H., Vekved, M., & Tough, S. (2012). Development of a prenatal psychosocial screening tool for post-partum depression and anxiety. *Paediatric and Perinatal Epidemiology, 26*(4), 316–327.

McGill, H., Burrows, V., Holland, L., Langer, H., & Sweet, M. (1995). Postnatal depression: A Christchurch study. *The New Zealand Medical Journal, 108*(999), 162–165.

Mercier, R., Garrett, J., Thorp, J., & Siega-Riz, A. (2013). Pregnancy intention and postpartum depression: Secondary data analysis from a prospective cohort. *BJOG: An International Journal of Obstetrics & Gynaecology, 120*(9), 1116–1122.

Milgrom, J., Holt, C., Gemmill, A., Ericksen, J., Leigh, B., Buist, A., & Schembri, C. (2011). Treating postnatal depressive symptoms in primary care: A randomised controlled trial of GP management, with and without adjunctive counselling. *BMC Psychiatry, 11*, 95.

Miller, L., McGlynn, A., Suberlak, K., Rubin, L., Miller, M., & Pirec, V. (2012). Now what? Effects of on-site assessment on treatment entry after perinatal depression screening. *Journal of Women's Health, 10*, 1046–1052.

Morrell, C. J., Ricketts, T., Tudor, K., Williams, C., Curran, J., & Barkham, M. (2011, January). Training health visitors in cognitive behavioural and person-centred approaches for depression in postnatal women as part of a cluster randomised trial and economic evaluation in primary care: The PoNDER trial. *Primary Health Care Research & Development, 12*(1), 11–20.

National Collaborating Center for Mental Health (UK). (2007). *Antenatal and postnatal mental health: The NICE guideline on clinical management and services* (Report no. 45). Retrieved from http://www.nice.org.uk/nicemedia/live/11004/30433/30433.pdf. Accessed December 16, 2014.

Nelson, D., Freeman, M., Johnson, N., McIntire, D., & Leveno, K. (2013). A prospective study of post-partum depression in 17 648 parturients. *The Journal of Maternal-Fetal & Neonatal Medicine, 26*(12), 1155–1161.

Nhiwatiwa, S., Patel, V., & Acuda, W. (1998). Predicting postnatal mental disorder with a screening questionnaire: A prospective cohort study from Zimbabwe. *Journal of Epidemiology & Community Health, 59*, 262–266.

O'Hara, M., & McCabe, J. (2013). Postpartum depression: Current status and future directions. *Annual Review of Clinical Psychology, 9*, 379–407.

O'Hara, M., Stuart, S., Watson, D., Dietz, P., Farr, S., & D'Angelo, D. (2012). Brief scales to detect post-partum depression and anxiety symptoms. *Journal of Women's Health (2002), 21*(12), 1237–1243.

O'Higgins, M., Roberts, I., Glover, V., & Taylor, A. (2013). Mother-child bonding at 1 year; associations with symptoms of postnatal depression and bonding in the first few weeks. *Archives of Women's Mental Health, 16*(5), 381–389.

Olson, A., Dietrich, A., Prazar, G., & Hurley, J. (2006). Brief maternal depression screening at well-child visits. *Pediatrics, 118*(1), 207–219.

Patel, S., & Wisner, K. (2011). Decision making for depression treatment during pregnancy and the postpartum period. *Depression and Anxiety, 28*(7), 589–595.

Paul, I., Downs, D., Schaefer, E., Beiler, J., & Weisman, C. (2013). Postpartum anxiety and maternal-infant health outcomes. *Pediatrics, 131*(4), e1218–e1224.

Peindl, K., Wisner, K., & Hanusa, B. (2004). Identifying depression in the first postpartum year: Guidelines for office-based screening and referral. *Journal of Affective Disorders, 80*(1), 37–44.

Peiris, A., Oh, E., & Diaz, S. (2007). Psychiatric manifestations of thyroid disease. *Southern Medical Journal, 100*(8), 773–774.

Petrozzi, A., & Gagliardi, L. (2013). Anxious and depressive components of Edinburgh Postnatal Depression Scale in maternal postpartum psychological problems. *Journal of Perinatal Medicine, 41*(4), 343–348.

Price, S., Corder-Mabe, J., & Austin, K. (2012). Perinatal depression screening and intervention: Enhancing health provider involvement. *Journal of Women's Health (2002), 21*(4), 447–455.

Quevedo, L., Silva, R., Godoy, R., Jansen, K., Matos, M., Tavares Pinheiro, K., & Pinheiro, R. (2012). The impact of maternal post-partum depression on the language development of children at 12 months. *Child: Care, Health and Development, 38*(3), 420–424.

Reck, C., Noe, D., Gerstenlauer, H., & Stehle, E. (2012). Effects of postpartum anxiety disorder and depression on maternal self-confidence. *Infant Behavior & Development, 35*(2), 264–272.

Reminick, A., Cohen, S., & Einarson, A. (2013). Managing depression during pregnancy. *Women's Health, 9*(6), 527–535.

Rhodes, A., & Segre, L. (2013). Perinatal depression: A review of US legislation and law. *Archives of Women's Mental Health, 16*(4), 259–270.

Rollans, M., Schmied, V., Kemp, L., & Meade, T. (2013). Digging over that old ground: An Australian perspective of women's experience of psychosocial assessment and depression screening in pregnancy and following birth. *BMC Women's Health, 13*, 18.

Rosenfield, A. I. (Ed.). (2007). Barriers to postpartum depression screening, diagnosis and treatment. In *New research on postpartum depression* (pp. 59–68). New York, NY: Nova Science Publishers.

Rowan, P., Greisinger, A., Brehm, B., Smith, F., & McReynolds, E. (2012). Outcomes from implementing systematic antepartum depression screening obstetrics. *Archives of Women's Mental Health, 15*(2), 115–120.

Segre, L., O'Hara, M., Brock, R., & Taylor, D. (2012). Depression screening of perinatal women by the Des Moines Healthy Start Project: Program description and evaluation. *Psychiatric Services, 63*(3), 250–255.

Shapiro, G., Fraser, W., & Seguin, J. (2012). Emerging risk factors for postpartum depression: Serotonin transporter genotype and omega-3 fatty acid status. *Canadian Journal of Psychiatry*, *57*(11), 704–712.

Sharp, L., & Lipsky, M. (2002). Screening for depression across the lifespan: A review of measures for use in primary care settings. *American Family Physician*, *66*, 1001–1008.

Sheeder, J., Kabir, K., & Stafford, B. (2009). Screening for postpartum depression at well-child visits: Is once enough during the first 6 months of life? *Pediatrics*, *123*(6), e982–e988.

Sit, D., Flint, C., Svidergol, D., White, J., Wimer, M., Bish, B., & Wisner, K. (2009). Best practices: An emerging best practice model for perinatal depression care. *Psychiatric Services*, *60*(11), 1429–1431.

Smith, T., & Kipnis, G. (2012). Implementing a perinatal mood and anxiety disorders program. *MCN: The American Journal of Maternal/Child Nursing*, *37*(2), 80–85.

Smith, M., Shao, L., Howell, H., Wang, H., Pschman, K., & Yonkers, K. (2009). Success of mental health referral among pregnant and postpartum women with psychiatric distress. *General Hospital Psychiatry*, *31*(2), 155–162.

Spitzer, R., Kroenke, K., & Williams, J. (1999). Validation and utility of a self-report version of PRIME-MD: The PHQ primary care study. Primary Care Evaluation of Mental Disorders. Patient Health Questionnaire. *JAMA*, *282*, 1737–1744.

Sutter-Dallay, A., Cosnefroy, O., Glatigny-Dallay, E., Verdoux, H., & Rascle, N. (2012). Evolution of perinatal depressive symptoms from pregnancy to two years postpartum in a low-risk sample: The MATQUID cohort. *Journal of Affective Disorders*, *139*(1), 23–29.

Sword, W., Clark, A., Hegadoren, K., Brooks, S., & Kingston, D. (2012). The complexity of postpartum mental health and illness: A critical realist study. *Nursing Inquiry*, *19*(1), 51–62.

The Common Wealth Fund, Olson, A., & Gaffney, C. (2007). *Parental depression screening for pediatric clinicians: An implementation manual*. Retrieved from http://www.commonwealthfund.org/Publications/Fund-Manuals/2007/Apr/Parental-Depression-Screening-for-Pediatric-Clinicians--An-Implementation-Manual.aspx. Accessed December 16, 2014.

Truitt, F., Pina, B., Person-Rennell, N., & Angstman, K. (2013). Outcomes for collaborative care versus routine care in the management of postpartum depression. *Quality in Primary Care*, *21*(3), 171–177.

U.K. National Screening Committee. (2011). *The UK NSC policy on postnatal depression screening in pregnancy*. Retrieved from http://www.screening.nhs.uk/postnataldepression. Accessed December 16, 2014.

United States Preventive Services Task Force. (2009). Depression screening in adults. Retrieved from http://www.uspreventiveservicestaskforce.org/uspstf09/adultdepression/addeprrs.htm. Accessed December 16, 2014.

University of Minnesota. (2012). *Need to improve state screening policies*. Retrieved from http://sph.umn.edu/postpartum-depression-screening-policies/. Accessed December 16, 2014.

Whooley, M. A., Avins, A. L., Miranda, J., & Browner, W. S. (1997). Case-finding instruments for depression: Two questions are as good as many. *Journal of General Internal Medicine*, *12*, 439–445.

Wickberg, B., & Hwang, C. (1996). The Edinburgh Postnatal Depression Scale: Validation on a Swedish community sample. *Acta Psychiatrica Scandinavica*, *94*, 181–184.

Wickberg, B., & Hwang, C. (1997). Screening for postnatal depression in a population-based Swedish sample. *Acta Psychiatrica Scandinavica*, *95*(1), 62–66.

Williams, B. (1968). 48-hour maternity discharge—Good or bad? *Nursing Mirror and Midwives Journal*, *127*(15), 33–35.

Wisner, K., Sit, D. K., McShea, M. C., Rizzo, D. M., Zoretich, R. A., Hughes, C. L., … Hanusa, B. H. (2013). Onset timing, thoughts of self-harm, and diagnoses in postpartum women with screen-positive depression findings. *JAMA*, *70*(5), 490–498.

Wu, Q., Chen, H., & Xu, X. (2012). Violence as a risk factor for postpartum depression in mothers: A meta-analysis. *Archives of Women's Mental Health*, *15*(2), 107–114.

Yawn, B., Dietrich, A., Wollan, P., Bertram, S., Graham, D., Huff, J., … Pace, W. (2012a). TRIPPD: A practice-based network effectiveness study of postpartum depression screening and management. *Annals of Family Medicine*, *10*(4), 320–329.

Yawn, B., Dietrich, A., Wollan, P., Bertram, S., Kurland, M., Pace, W., … Huff, J. (2009a). The IAP: A simple tool to guide assessment and immediate action for suicidal ideation. *Family Practice Management, 16*(5), 17–20.

Yawn, B., Olson, A., Bertram, S., Pace, W., Wollan, P., & Dietrich, A. (2012b). *Postpartum depression: Screening, Diagnosis, and Management Programs 2000 through 2010.* Depression Research and Treatment. doi:2012:363964.

Yawn, B., Pace, W., Wollan, P., Bertram, S., Kurland, M., Graham, D., & Dietrich, A. (2009b). Concordance of Edinburgh Postnatal Depression Scale (EPDS) and Patient Health Questionnaire (PHQ-9) to assess increased risk of depression among postpartum women. *Journal of the American Board of Family Medicine, 22*(5), 483–491.

Yonkers, K., Smith, M., Lin, H., Howell, H., Shao, L., & Rosenheck, R. (2009a). Depression screening of perinatal women: An evaluation of the healthy start depression initiative. *Psychiatric Services, 60*(3), 322–328.

Yonkers, K., Vigod, S., & Ross, L. (2011). Diagnosis, pathophysiology, and management of mood disorders in pregnant and postpartum women. *Obstetrics & Gynecology, 117*(4), 961–977.

Yonkers, K., Wisner, K., Stewart, D., Oberlander, T., Dell, D., Stotland, N., … Lockwood, C. (2009b). The management of depression during pregnancy: A report from the American Psychiatric Association and the American College of Obstetricians and Gynecologists. *Obstetrics & Gynecology, 114*(3), 703–713.

3

Acceptability, Attitudes, and Overcoming Stigma

Anne Buist, Heather O'Mahen, and Rosanna Rooney

Introduction

While there is evidence that a number of screening measures can detect perinatal depression with very good sensitivity and adequate specificity, there remains debate about the merits of universal screening, particularly if not integrated into care pathways (as discussed in the previous chapters). There is also limited evidence regarding the validity of screening measures across ethnic and cultural groups (King, 2012). Further, treatment engagement rates remain low, with studies reporting that only 12–30% of women with perinatal depression receive any kind of treatment (Bowen, Bowen, & Butt, 2012; Flynn et al., 2006; see Chapter 1 of this book).

Implementation difficulties exist at each stage of the identification, referral, and treatment processes. These difficulties have been characterized in both the broader and perinatal-specific depression literature as practical (accessibility, linkage between screening and treatment, cost, child care) and attitudinal barriers (stigma, beliefs about screening and treatment). This chapter seeks to review literature that can inform strategies aimed at overcoming barriers.

A growing body of literature has examined the reciprocal roles of both provider and patient barriers on the provision and uptake of screening, depression referral, and treatment engagement (Brealey, Hewitt, Green, Morrell, & Gilbody, 2010), and these are detailed in the following text.

Acceptability of Screening

Historically, there has been a lack of consensus on the acceptability of screening as an identification strategy (Shakespeare, Blake, & Garcia 2003). Increasingly, it has been found that women themselves find screening both simple and acceptable (Bilszta, Ericksen, Buist, &

Identifying Perinatal Depression and Anxiety: Evidence-Based Practice in Screening, Psychosocial Assessment, and Management, First Edition. Edited by Jeannette Milgrom and Alan W. Gemmill.
© 2015 John Wiley & Sons, Ltd. Published 2015 by John Wiley & Sons, Ltd.

Milgrom, 2007a, 2010; Brealey et al., 2010). The percentage of women who are approached to be screened and agree to do so in both empirical studies and clinical practice is high (85–90%; Evins, Theofrastous, & Galvin, 2000; Georgiopoulos, Bryan, Wollan, & Yawn, 2001). However, rates of screening are lower among cultural minorities and women with lower incomes (Gjerdingen & Yawn, 2007; Morris-Rush, Freda, & Bernstein 2003), suggesting there may be unique barriers to screening among these women. This is of particular concern given the higher prevalence of depression among these populations. There have been a number of studies that directly examine women's views of screening (Brealey et al., 2010).

Antenatal acceptability of screening

In a telephone interview study of 407 women who had been screened for depression during pregnancy, 100% indicated that they found the process acceptable, with an additional 50% of women stating that the process raised their awareness of perinatal depression (Leigh & Milgrom, 2006). Reports of stigma or distress did not spontaneously emerge in any of the interviews. Notably, all women had received immediate feedback about their screen from their midwives, and they described finding this feedback reassuring.

In another Australian study, 202 women were interviewed about the acceptability of screening antenatally, 98 of whom were Arabic- or Vietnamese-speaking women (Matthey et al., 2005). There were high rates of reported acceptability of the screening process throughout the perinatal period. Notably, Arabic- and Vietnamese-speaking women also reported finding screening acceptable and recommended only a few culture-specific changes to the screening processes such as partner being referred to as "husband."

Postnatal acceptability of screening

In the postnatal period, findings about acceptability have been mixed. In one study, Gemmill and colleagues (2006) sent surveys asking women about a screening program and whether they had found the process "comfortable" and "a good idea." Acceptability was high. Of the 472 respondents, only 18.8% found it less than comfortable, and 97% thought it was a "good idea" to screen. In another survey of 860 women in Australia, all of whom had been screened for postnatal depression (PND) in the previous year, high rates of acceptability were found, with 93% reporting that the Edinburgh Postnatal Depression Scale (EPDS; Cox, Holden, & Sagovsky, 1987; Cox & Holden, 2003) was easy to use and 83% reporting that they did not find it uncomfortable (Buist et al., 2006). Reports of discomfort in filling out the EPDS screen were associated with having an EPDS score of 13 or greater. A total of 25% of women in the study were advised they were at risk. Of these women, 16% ignored the assessment, 29% experienced some level of upset, 27% were unsure of the results, and 23% were somewhat relieved. These latter findings are important, as they highlight the distinction between the acceptability of being asked screening questions and how women manage the feedback they receive.

By contrast, in a qualitative study of the acceptability of screening for depression by health visitors in the postnatal period in the United Kingdom, 46% of the 39 women interviewed reported low rates of acceptability of depression screening (Shakespeare et al., 2003). Although all but two of the women had completed the EPDS, those who found the process difficult reported the reasons underlying their ratings of low acceptability: they did not like having the screen administered in the clinic setting, preferring the privacy and comfort of their own home; were sensitive to the health visitor's reaction to the screen (e.g., sense that health visitor was feeling "rushed"); and preferred to talk about their mood symptoms in a more conversational fashion versus on a questionnaire. A number of women commented that they worried about factors associated with stigma and so were either reluctant to respond to the screen or responded untruthfully. In another small Australian qualitative study, women reported mixed experiences of the screening process. Although some found the process helpful, others reported low levels of acceptability. The authors noted that women who had a caring relationship with the health provider conducting the screening and were subsequently appropriately referred to available treatment resources reported positive experiences of screening (Armstrong & Small, 2010).

The results of Shakespeare and colleagues highlight the critical role health-care providers play in the screening process (Shakespeare et al., 2003). The interaction of stigma and women's perceptions of the health visitor's lack of time or interest in their problems reduced women's willingness to disclose their symptoms or left them uncomfortable with the process. Although health visitors in the United Kingdom, where the study took place, had received training in administering and responding to the depression screen, it may be that other practical, logistical, and provider attitudinal barriers affected how health visitors administered and implemented the screening.

In different cultural groups, there may be additional shortcomings of screening instruments. For example, the EPDS appears to be an excellent screening instrument in certain Western samples, but it does not include somatic symptoms. Many groups such as Iraqi, Ethiopian, and Sudanese migrant women focus on somatic symptoms if depressed in the year following the birth of their baby (Di Ciano, Rooney, Wright, Hay, & Robinson, 2010), and so screening with a measure such as the EPDS is likely to miss cases at risk when used universally. Although King (2012) was able to replicate Tuohy and McVey's (2008) three-factor model within a sample of low socioeconomic status African American women, the three-factor model of the EPDS needs to be fully investigated via confirmatory factor analysis among a diverse range of groups before it can be used across cultures as there is limited evidence for the stability of the factor structure across diverse cultural groups (King, 2012). The implication here is that both the factor structure of the EPDS and the relevance of symptoms such as somatic symptoms appear to vary across cultures. A single version of the EPDS is neither likely to be acceptable universally nor culturally appropriate for all groups.

In summary, these studies suggest that screening is broadly acceptable to women, especially during pregnancy, although the findings in the postnatal period are mixed. Quantitative studies with large samples have largely found that screening is acceptable to most women. Smaller qualitative studies have demonstrated nuances in the acceptability of screening to specific women. In Brealey et al.'s systematic review (2010), women raised some concerns in two smaller UK studies and one Australian study in a culturally diverse sample, but a majority of women were positive about being screened. The Australian *beyondblue* initiative has involved implementing systematic screening on a national basis, with large numbers of health-care providers participating nationally (Buist et al., 2007). Clear guidelines around how and when to screen and refer women have been produced in Australia (*beyondblue*, 2011), and the emphasis is on using the screening tool as a point of discussion, which may overcome some of the issues identified by Armstrong and Small (2010) and Shakespeare et al. (2003). In Australia, this has occurred alongside public health campaigns aimed at improving knowledge about depression. As a consequence, women may be more accustomed to screening as a part of normal perinatal care and may therefore find the process of screening generally more acceptable, particularly where health professional training is available. Finally, given the interactional nature of depression screening, referral, and treatment engagement, it is also important to understand the systemic and attitudinal factors affecting health-care providers in this process.

Health-Care Provider Attitudes

In surveys of health-care provider attitudes about depression in the perinatal period, providers stated that they believe perinatal depression is common, serious, and treatable (Gjerdingen & Yawn, 2007). However, providers in areas with high proportions of low-income and/or minority groups underestimated depression rates in these populations. While estimates of depression point prevalence in these groups is up to 35%, health-care providers estimate depression prevalence at 15% (Morris-Rush et al., 2003), rates that are consistent with white, higher-income groups. Further, despite their general awareness of the prevalence and seriousness of perinatal depression, provider implementation of regular screening is low, ranging between 0% and 50% (Seehausen, Baldwin, Runkle, & Clark, 2005). Many practices that aim to implement screening often use unvalidated tools or informal assessments and fail to systematically implement screening procedures, instead relying on clinical judgment alone (Seehausen et al., 2005). This is problematic given that informal screening has been demonstrated to be ineffective and potentially harmful, detecting fewer than half of women potentially suffering from depression (Evins et al., 2000; Georgiopoulos et al., 2001).

Health-care providers report a number of reasons why implementing screening is difficult, including lack of time, competing demands, limited knowledge of available resources, perceived reluctance of patients to engage in depression treatment, poor availability of treatment, lack of patient resources to pay for treatment, fear of legal repercussions, and inadequate training around depression screening (Brealey et al., 2010; Byatt, Moore Simas, Lundquist, Johnson, & Ziedonis, 2012; Gjerdingen & Yawn, 2007). Interestingly, some provider-level barriers are consistent with patient-perceived barriers. Where providers reported a lack of time and competing demands, patients reported a sense that providers are "ticking a box" without time to follow-up appropriately. Qualitative studies on patients suggest that provider unease in asking depression questions is also quickly detected by patients who are sensitive to their discomfort. This reciprocal process may create an overall sense of interactional unease in both the provider and patient. Training programs in screening, when regularly and systematically used, may improve the comfort providers have in administering screening. However, this process of training needs follow-up and continuing supervisor support to ensure ongoing revision around acceptable and effective screening implementation (Rollans, Schmied, Kemp, & Meade, 2013a, 2013b).

Notably, the results of a number of studies strongly suggest that screening programs alone do not improve mental health outcomes in women (Gjerdingen & Yawn, 2007). For screening to be effective, programs must be implemented within a system of referral and support (Myers et al., 2013; Yawn et al., 2012). These findings are reflected in health-care providers' concerns that discussing depression with a patient opens up areas of vulnerability for both the provider and patient. This is especially the case when the provider does not feel skilled and is without the time to assist the patient in treating the depression or where there is a lack of available resources and support for referral. This needs addressing if screening is to work effectively at a population level. This is further compounded by providers' accurate perception that treatment engagement rates among patients who screen positive for depression are low, with between 12% and 30% of depressed perinatal patients engaging in treatment (Bowen et al., 2012; Flynn et al., 2006).

Barriers to Seeking Treatment

Effective linkage between screening and treatment is critical in order to positively impact on women's mental health. Further, if depression goes unidentified, it is likely to go untreated (Thio, Oakley Browne, Coverdale, & Argyle, 2006). Providing accessible and acceptable treatment is needed to successfully engage women. Integral to this is screening women at appropriate time periods. For example, in Bowen et al.'s (2012) sample, there was no follow-up after four weeks' postpartum, even though symptoms are likely to persist for many up to six months (Vliegen et al., 2010).

Studies have shown that awareness of sources of assistance for PND is variable and influenced by education. Use of a psychoeducational emotional health booklet in the Australian *beyondblue* study showed, in an evaluated subset of 1309 women, that the booklet was associated with better ability to recognize a hypothetical case of depression and better assess personal mental health. This was most effective for women with lower scores on the EPDS (Buist et al., 2007). Depression itself, or risk factors for depression (such as being younger, drug use, lower education, or cultural factors), may increase risk for both nondetection and nonrecognition of personal symptoms, making women less likely to present for treatment (Bowen et al., 2012; McGarry, Kim, Sheng, Egger, & Baksh, 2009; Sealy, Fraser, Simpson, & Evans, 2009). With increased awareness, there is still a relatively low recognition of anxiety and antenatal depression as found in a later Australian study (Highet, Gemmill, & Milgrom, 2011).

A number of additional factors are likely to influence women's attitudes to treatment uptake: risks to the infant/fetus, past experience with treatments (either their own, friends, or family members), partner support, and personality and cultural attitudes to illness and treatment (Bilszta et al., 2010; Di Ciano et al., 2010; Misri et al., 2010).

Other barriers have been noted once treatment is sought. Availability, accessibility, and affordability are all critical for new mothers who must juggle the practicalities of bringing a child to an appointment or arranging child care, changes in family finances, and locating the type of therapy they prefer (Goodman 2004; O'Mahen et al., 2012).

Barriers to seeking psychological treatment for mood symptoms

A number of studies have identified women's preference for psychological treatments over medication. Dennis and Chung-Lee (2006) identified a strong desire among women to talk about their feelings, but that the listener needed to be nonjudgmental and understand their problem. Reactions against accepting treatment included women "normalizing" their own symptoms or being offered unacceptable/unwanted treatments (Sword, Busser, Ganann, McMillan, & Swinton, 2008). The relationship with the health professional is seen as critical (Shakespeare et al., 2003), and the reactions of nurses, and more so time-pressured doctors, who may first turn to a prescription pad, act as a barrier to both accepting diagnosis and treatment (Bilszta et al., 2010; Sword et al., 2008; Webster et al., 2001).

While work has been limited, there have been reports by women from a range of culturally and linguistically diverse (CALD) groups of stigma in the year following the birth of their baby. Being from a migrant background in general, particularly having a baby aged

0–12 months has been shown to act as a barrier to identification of mental health problems and seeking treatment. For example, in Australia, it has been found that there is a high degree of stigma surrounding mental illness among people from culturally diverse backgrounds. Bakshi and colleagues (1999) reported that being a migrant, being unemployed, and being diagnosed with a mental illness are associated with the underlying psychological issue being harder to identify, which in turn reduces the likelihood of seeking help. Perceived stigma of mental illness is increased as motherhood is often a time where society expects women to cope well and appear happy. While work has been limited, there have been qualitative reports of stigma reported by women in the year following the birth of their baby from a range of groups including African American (O'Mahen et al., 2012), Iraqi (Di Ciano et al., 2010), Ethiopian, and Sudanese women (Down, Palacios, & Wright, 2005).

When planning interventions for CALD women in the postnatal period, an emerging theme in the literature is the critical importance and centrality of a mother's explanatory models of motherhood and PND. For example, one of the key things that women from Iraqi, Sudanese, and Ethiopian backgrounds wanted in the year following the birth of their baby was support and help from their mother whose input was reportedly greatly missed (Di Ciano et al., 2010; Down et al., 2005). Consistent with this, de Castro, Hinojosa-Ayala, and Hernandex-Prado (2011) found that for Mexican mothers, support protected against the risk of developing PND and this effect was even stronger for adolescents than for adults. Buist et al. (2007) also found that lack of support was associated with an increase in PND in CALD women in Australia. Similarly, Barnett, Matthey, and Karatas (2005) concluded in their review that practical support such as being able to access traditional rituals and emotional support were associated with a decrease in risk for PND in Arabic and Vietnamese women.

Although there are very few studies of interventions that are culturally specific or sensitive for PND, there is some information about women's preferences. Group support may be beneficial with Arabic women, who express that it would be useful to be able to sit with other Arabic mothers to talk about their experience of parenting in Australia and relevant issues (Matthey et al., 2005; Nahas, Hillege, & Amasheh, 1999). Barnett et al. (2005) compared preference for individual counseling, group therapy, phone support, antenatal classes, and home visits among Arabic and Vietnamese women. While phone support was the most popular option, all options were found to be helpful although it was unclear which had the best effects or how much the content was culturally specific or sensitive.

Incorporating support and their explanatory models of motherhood and PND into an intervention for Iraqi women, Gent and colleagues (2014) found that, on average, the Iraqi participant's EPDS scores decreased. From a high risk of depression with mean scores over 12, they fell to a low level of depression (mean scores under 9) at posttest and 5 weeks after delivery of the intervention. The researchers also reported that women reported between 4/5 and 5/5 ratings of enjoyment for each session and the numbers wanting to join the group increased each week as word of the groups spread. Other factors which improved engagement included running the group in the participant's language with a "motherly" Iraqi facilitator who was able to bring their cultural songs alive through singing and was able to generally be a "mother figure" to the women which was a critical factor in their explanatory models of motherhood that was missing after migrating to Australia. The absence of a mother figure in support and intervention has been commonly reported by a range of migrant women when arriving in Australia (Di Ciano et al., 2010; Down et al., 2005). However, randomized controlled trials need to be carried out among a range of CALD groups to see if support groups incorporating CALD mother's explanatory models are effective. Similarly, studies comparing patient preferences and outcomes are lacking in non-CALD groups.

Barriers to seeking treatments for mother–infant difficulties

For some women, practical issues with the infant bring them to support services, looking for an explanation for their child's sleep or eating issues and not necessarily identifying issues within themselves or in their relationship with their infant as a cause of concern (Bilszta et al., 2010). As research has shown that treating maternal depression will not necessarily improve compromised interactions and longer-term negative child outcomes (Forman et al., 2007; Milgrom, Ericksen, McCarthy, & Gemmill, 2006), there has been an increased focus on designing interventions targeting the mother–infant relationship in PND treatment. As yet there is limited evidence of efficacy for better outcomes for the child (Milgrom & Gemmil, 2013; Milgrom et al., 2006) as well as limited availability. For women who may feel like a failure as a mother, referral for intervention in the mother–infant relationship runs the risk of confirming their beliefs. The challenge for the health professional is to make such a referral in a sensitive manner that allows women to feel empowered as a mother rather than criticized.

Conversely, the perinatal period is the one time many women are more likely to seek treatment as they are motivated to be a good mother (e.g., decreased alcohol use) and to see the period a chance to improve their lives and their child's life.

Barriers to seeking biological treatment

In Dennis and Chung-Lee's qualitative systematic review (2006), women were reluctant to take medication, even after education, citing fear of addiction and beliefs that the symptoms would resolve without medication. Acceptance was particularly low in breastfeeding mothers, and noncompliance or intermittent compliance was also an issue (Boath, Bradley, & Henshaw, 2004).

This contrasts somewhat with doctors' attitudes. In Buist et al.'s (2006) study of attitudes and knowledge, general practitioners had a significantly higher propensity to recommend antidepressants than other health professionals. This was at odds with the preferences of the women themselves for natural remedies. Antenatally, women were particularly concerned about medication, but this concern was also reflected among surveyed doctors in Canada and Australia (Bilszta, Han, Tsuchiya, Einarson, & Buist, 2007b).

For some women, particularly those with past positive experiences of antidepressants and those with severe disabling symptoms, antidepressants are considered the best treatment option by the women themselves. However, anxiety can persist regarding the potential harmful effects on the infant, either in utero or via breast milk (Turner, Sharp, Folkes, & Chew-Graham, 2008). Pregnant mothers in Bowen et al.'s sample (2012) were significantly less likely to use antidepressants. Those that did use antidepressants had higher depression scores, suggesting higher use in moderate to severe depression and that severity of symptomatology may be one of the factors that influence women's attitudes.

Misri et al. (2010) followed 50 depressed women recruited in pregnancy to 1 month postpartum, 30 of whom adhered to medication and 20 who did not. Besides finding better outcomes for the adherers, they examined differences between the two groups and found adherers to be more accepting of their illness, whereas the decliners had less insight. The main reasons for declining were fear of fetal exposure and that their symptoms did not warrant the medication. No differences were found between the exposed and unexposed infants, but the sample was small and not followed up.

Stepanuk, Fisher, Wittmann-Price, Posmontier, and Bhattacharya (2013) investigated the decision-making process in postpartum women with respect to taking medication and subsequent satisfaction. This study broke the process of emancipated decision-making (EDM) into three subsections: personal knowledge, awareness of social norms, and flexible environment. Those with higher levels of EDM, particularly personal knowledge, were more likely to be satisfied with their decision regarding medication.

Steps Forward

In order to overcome barriers to identification, referral, and treatment, it is critical that we address underlying attitudes as well as systemic issues. The interaction of patient and pro- vider's attitudes in the screening, referral, and treatment engagement process suggests that there is a need to address factors impacting attitudes from both perspectives (Armstrong & Small, 2010; Bilszta et al., 2010; Dennis & Chung-Lee, 2006; Webster et al., 2001). A number of studies have reported facilitation aimed at improving depression treatment. Firstly, there is a need to recognize that depression is a stigmatized condition and many women are not motivated to seek treatment. During the perinatal period, evidence suggests that the stigma of depression is compounded with notions of being a "bad mother" (Bilszta et al., 2007a; Buultjens & Liamputtong, 2007; O'Mahen et al., 2012). As a result, there is a need for health providers to approach the screening, referral, and treatment process both sensitively and actively. Women have reported it is helpful to have encouragement from referrers to attend treatment, flexible referrals that are tailored to patient needs, and active facilitation of the referral process by providers. Another issue to consider for pregnant and breastfeeding women is the potential risk or fear of risk to the infant regarding medication options. Although absolute certainty regarding the safety of medications is lacking, with increasing research in the field (Sie et al., 2012), clear, concise, best current evidence-based information can be provided. A second opinion from an alternative expert may also be considered. Women's preferences for treatment should be considered however, as many women prefer nonpharmaceutical treatment options.

Once screened, the evidence suggests that there is a critical window of opportunity in which women are more likely to act on referrals and commence treatment. As such, women prefer referral processes that have minimal steps involved and mental health referrals and appointments that are timely (Byatt et al., 2012; Flynn, Henshaw, O'Mahen, & Forman, 2010). Further, a number of studies have found that women prefer to have treatment colo- cated in familiar health-care settings or in the home setting (Flynn et al., 2010; O'Mahen et al., 2012). In Myers et al.'s (2013) comparative effectiveness review, there was substantially higher referral where identification, diagnosis, and treatment were in the same setting.

The interpersonal style of the health-care provider is another area of central importance. Women respond positively to providers who are genuine, warm, and optimistic and who take time to listen in a fashion that is not judgmental. Women reported benefiting from providers contextualizing their problems without downplaying their seriousness (Henshaw, Flynn, Himle, O'Mahen, & Forman, 2010; Jesse, Dolbier, & Blanchard, 2008). Psycho- education about depression is useful in helping women understand both their symptoms and their options. However, symptom knowledge may not be enough. In a recent qualitative study on treatment-seeking delays in general major depression, participants avoided labeling their symptoms as depression, even when they recognized their problems as impactful, because of beliefs that "being a depressed person" damaged their identity and their ability to achieve in valued domains (Farmer, Farrand, & O'Mahen, 2012). To that end, open discussions about the stigmatizing nature of depression may be helpful in assisting women to find a path toward accepting "mood difficulties" or depression and to take on change through treatment while also recognizing they remain a valuable and capable person.

Research suggests that adequate training in assessment measures for depression specifically, and mental health problems more generally, improves the depression treatment process (Byatt et al., 2012). However, providers also indicate that they are more satisfied when they have additional support and feedback from mental health providers. Attitudinal barriers can often be improved by making positive systemic changes as well. A health culture that routinely and effectively screens, refers, and engages depressed women in treatment can reciprocally impact on provider views (Kim et al., 2009). Processes such as establishing office prompts for screening, identifying a person who can "champion" depression care processes in the healthcare setting, and setting reasonable provider expectations can all impact positively on perceptions of perinatal depression care (Kim et al., 2009). Lastly, giving providers the requisite time to carry out tasks related to depression care is critical. Limited provider time is endemic to many health-care systems internationally. Failure to spend appropriate time on important and disabling conditions such as depression can generate a false economy.

In one study, midwives who were trained to screen and refer for depression during pregnancy found that the screening process helped them to more efficiently determine who needed extra time. Thus, they were able to allocate their time more effectively (Brugha, Morrell, Slade, & Walters, 2011). It is still important, however, to recognize that referring women to treatment is often not enough; successful depression care often requires considerable outreach from providers. In a recent randomized controlled trial of depression screening and coordinated follow-up of depression care in primary settings, nurses reported that they made three or more attempts before reaching women on the phone. Further, nurses reported they struggled to find time in their own workload to reach women, many of whom had returned to work or were difficult to engage (Yawn et al., 2012). Such reallocations of time and resources require a shifting of attitudes in services away from the expectation that patients require a single referral or input around care for chronic and disabling conditions. Ongoing support and outreach is a critical investment in the well-being of women in the perinatal period.

References

Armstrong, S. J., & Small, R. E. (2010). The paradox of screening: Rural women's views on screening of postnatal depression. *BMC Public Health, 10*(744).

Bakshi, L., Rooney, R., & O'Neil, K. (1999). Reducing stigma about mental illness in transcultural mental settings. In *Australian Transcultural Mental Health Network: National Mental Health Strategy*. Melbourne: Australian Transcultural Mental Health Network.

Barnett, B., Matthey, S., & Karatas, J. (2005). In beyondblue (Ed.) *New South Wales Intervention Initiative: Clinical Interventions for and Preferences of, Women from Vietnamese and Arabic-Speaking Backgrounds* (National PND Program Final Report). Melbourne, Australia: Beyondblue: The National Depression Initiative.

Beyondblue. (2011). *Clinical Practice Guidelines for Depression and Related Disorders—Anxiety, Bipolar Disorder and Puerperal Psychosis—In the Perinatal Period. A Guideline for Primary Care Health Professionals.* Melbourne, Australia: Beyondblue: The National Depression Initiative.

Bilszta, J., Ericksen, J., Buist, A., & Milgrom, J. (2007a). Exploring the lived experiences of women with postnatal depression: A qualitative study. *Journal of Midwifery & Women's Health, 27*(3), 44–54.

Bilszta, J., Ericksen, J., Buist, A., & Milgrom, J. (2010). Women's experience of postnatal depression— Beliefs and attitudes as barriers to care. *Australian Journal of Advanced Nursing, 27*(3), 44–54.

Bilszta, J. L. C., Han, K., Tsuchiya, S., Einarson, A., & Buist, A. E. (2007b). *Determinants of general practitioner's attitudes and practices regarding antidepressant use during pregnancy.* Paper presented at the International Women's Mental Health, Melbourne, Australia.

Boath, E., Bradley, E., & Henshaw, C. (2004). Women's views of antidepressants in the treatment of postnatal depression. *Journal of Psychosomatic Obstetrics and Gynaecology, 25*(3–4), 221–233.

Bowen, A., Bowen, R., & Butt, P. (2012, March). Patterns of depression and treatment in pregnant and postpartum women. *Canadian Journal of Psychiatry, 57*(3), 161–167.

Brealey, S. D., Hewitt, C., Green, J. M., Morrell, J., & Gilbody, S. (2010). Screening for postnatal depression—Is it acceptable to women and healthcare professionals? A systematic review and meta-synthesis. *Journal of Reproductive & Infant Psychology, 28*, 328–344.

Bronwyn, L., & Milgrom, J. (2006). Acceptability of antenatal screening for depression in routine antenatal care. *Australian Journal of Advanced Nursing, 24*(3), 14–18.

Brugha, T. S., Morrell, C. H., Slade, P., & Walters, S. J. (2011). Universal prevention of depression in women postnatally: Cluster randomized trial evidence in primary care. *Psychological Medicine, 41*, 739–748.

Buist, A. E., Condon, J., Brooks, J., Speelman, C., Milgrom, J., Hayes, B., … Bilszta, J. (2006). Acceptability of routine screening for postnatal depression. *Journal of Affective Disorders, 93*, 233–237.

Buist, A., Ellwood, D., Brooks, J., Milgrom, J., Hayes, B., Sved-Williams, A., … Bilszta, J. (2007). National Program for Depression Associated with Childbirth: The Australian Experience. In edited by Guest Editor: T. K. H. Chung. Editor in Chief: S. Arulkumaran, *Clinical Obstetrics & Gynaecology.* (pp. P193–P206). London, UK: Best Practice & Research.

Buultjens, M., & Liamputtong, P. (2007). When giving life starts to take the life out of you: Women's experiences of depression after childbirth. *Midwifery, 23*, 77–91.

Byatt, N., Moore Simas, T. A., Lundquist, R. S., Johnson, J. V., & Ziedonis, D. M. (2012). Strategies for improving perinatal depression treatment in North American outpatients obstetric settings. *Journal of Psychosomatic Obstetrics & Gynecology, 33*, 143–161.

Cox, J., & Holden, J. (2003). Using the EPDS in clinical settings: Research evidence. In J. Cox, J. Holden, & C. Hensaw (Eds.), *Perinatal mental health—A guide to the EPDS* (pp. 26–33). Glasgow, UK: Royal College of Psychiatrists, no. Bell & Bain Ltd.

Cox, J. L., Holden, J. M., & Sagovsky, R. (1987). Detection of postnatal depression: Development of the 10-item Edinburgh Postnatal Depression Scale. *British Journal of Psychiatry, 150*, 782–786.

de Castro, F., Hinojosa-Ayala, N., & Hernandex-Prado, B. (2011). Risk and protective factors associated with postnatal depression in Mexican adolescents. *Journal of Psychosomatic Obstetrics and Gynecology, 32*, 210–217.

Dennis, C.-L., & Chung-Lee, L. (2006). Postpartum depression help-seeking barriers and maternal treatment preferences: A qualitative systematic review. *Birth, 33*(4), 323–331.

Di Ciano, T., Rooney, R., Wright, B., Hay, D., & Robinson, L. (2010). Postnatal social support group needs and explanatory models of Iraqi Arabic speaking mothers in Perth, Western Australia. *Advances in Mental Health, 9*, 162–176.

Down, C., Palacios, V., & Wright, B. (2005). *Investigation into childbirth, families and emotional well being in Three Culturally and Linguistically Diverse (CALD) communities.* Perth, Australia: WA Perinatal Mental Health.

Evins, G., Theofrastous, J., & Galvin, S. (2000). Postpartum depression: A comparison of screening and routine clinical evaluation. *American Journal of Obstetrics and Gynecology, 182*, 1080–1082.

Farmer, C., Farrand, P., & O'Mahen, H. A. (2012). Understanding help-seeking rates for major depressive disorder: The role of identify conflict. *BMC Psychiatry, 2*, 164.

Flynn, H. A., Henshaw, E., O'Mahen, H., & Forman, J. (2010). Patient perspectives on improving the depression referral processes in obstetrics settings: A qualitative study. *General Hospital Psychiatry, 32*, 9–16.

Flynn, H. A., O'Mahen, H. A., Massey, L., & Marcus, S. (2006). The impact of a brief obstetrics clinic-based intervention on treatment use for perinatal depression. *Journal of Women's Health, 15*(10), 1195–1204.

Forman, D. R., O'Hara, M. W., Stuart, S., Gorman, L. L., Larsen, K. E., & Coy, K. C. (2007). Effective treatment for postpartum depression is not sufficient to improve the developing mother-child relationship. *Development & Psychopathology, 19*(2, Spring), 585–602.

Gemmill, A. W., Leigh, B., Ericksen, J., & Milgrom, J. (2006). A survey of the clinical acceptability of screening for postnatal depression in depressed and non-depressed women. *BMC Public Health, 6*(211), 1–8.

Gent, V., DiCiano, T., Rooney, R., Wright, B., & Kane, R. (2014). The pilot and evaluation of a post-natal support group for Iraqi women in the year following the birth of their baby. *Frontiers in Psychology, 5*, 16.

Georgiopoulos, A. M., Bryan, T. L., Wollan, P., & Yawn, B. P. (2001). Routine screening for postpartum depression. *Journal of Family Health Practice, 50*, 117–122.

Gjerdingen, D. K., & Yawn, B. P. (2007). Postpartum depression screening: Importance, methods, barriers and recommendations for practice. *Journal of American Board Family Medicine, 20*, 280–288.

Goodman, J. H. (2004). Postpartum depression beyond the early postpartum period. *Journal of Obstetric, Gynecologic, & Neonatal Nursing, 33*(4), 410–420.

Henshaw, E., Flynn, H. A., Himle, J., O'Mahen, H., & Forman, J. (2010). Patient preferences for clinical interactional style in treatment of perinatal depression: A qualitative study. *Qualitative Health Research, 721*, 936–951.

Highet, N. J., Gemmill, A. W., & Milgrom, J. (2011). Depression in the perinatal period: Awareness, attitudes and knowledge in the Australian population. *Australian & New Zealand Journal of Psychiatry, 45*, 223–231.

Jesse, D. E., Dolbier, C. L., & Blanchard, A. (2008). Barriers to seeking help and treatment suggestions for prenatal depressive symptoms: Focus groups with rural low-income women. *Issues in Mental Health Nursing, 29*, 3–19.

Kim, J. J., La Porte, L. M., Adams, M. G., Gordon, T. E., Kuendig, J. M., & Silver, R. K. (2009). Obstetric care provider engagement in a perinatal depression screening program. *Archives of Women's Mental Health, 1*, 167–172.

King, L. (2012). Replicability of structural models of the Edinburgh Postnatal Depression Scale (EPDS) in a community sample of postpartum African American women with low socio-economic status. *Archives of Women's Mental Health, 15*, 77–86.

Matthey, S., White, T., Phillips, J., Taouk, R., Chee, T., & Barnett, B. (2005). Acceptability of routine antenatal psychosocial assessments to women from English and non-English speaking backgrounds. *Archives of Women's Mental Health, 8*, 171–180.

McGarry, J., Kim, H., Sheng, X., Egger, M., & Baksh, L. (2009, January/February). Postpartum depression and help-seeking behaviour. *Journal of Midwifery & Women's Health, 54*(1), 50–56.

Milgrom, J., Ericksen, J., McCarthy, R. M., & Gemmill, A. W. (2006). Stressful impact of depression on early mother-infant relations. *Stress and Health, 22*, 229–238.

Milgrom, J., & Gemmil, A. W. (2013). Identification and treatment of depression in the perinatal period. In M. Caltabiano & L. Ricciardelli (Eds.), *Applied Topics in Health Psychology* (pp. 212–227). Chichester, UK: John Wiley & Sons, Ltd.

Misri, S., Kendrick, K., Oberlander, T. F., Norris, S., Tomfohr, L., Zhang, H., & Grunau, R. E. (2010). Antenatal depression and anxiety affect postpartum parenting stress: A longitudinal, prospective study. *Canadian Journal of Psychiatry, 55*(4), 222–228.

Morris-Rush, J. K., Freda, M. C., & Bernstein, P. S. (2003, May). Screening for postpartum depression in an inner-city population. *American Journal of Obstetrics and Gynecology, 188*, 1217–1219.

Myers, E. R., Aubuchon-Endsley, N., Bastian, L. A., Gierisch, J. M., Kemper, A. R., Swamy, G. K., … Sanders, G. D. (2013). *Efficacy and safety of screening for postpartum depression* (Comparative Effectiveness Review 106). Rockville, MD: Agency for Healthcare Research and Quality.

Nahas, V. L., Hillege, S., & Amasheh, N. (1999, January/February). Postpartum depression: The lived experiences of Middle Eastern migrant women in Australia. *Journal of Nurse Midwifery, 44*(1), 65–74.

O'Mahen, H. A., Henshaw, E., Fedock, G., Himle, J., Forman, J., & Flynn, H. (2012). Modifying CBT for perinatal depression: What do women want a qualitative study. *Cognitive & Behavioural Psychotherapy, 19*(2), 359–371.

Rollans, M., Schmied, V., Kemp, L., & Meade, T. (2013a). Negotiating policy in practice: Child and family health nurses' approach to the process of postnatal psychosocial assessment. *BMC Health Services Research, 13*, 133.

Rollans, M., Schmied, V., Kemp, L., & Meade, T. (2013b). Digging over that old ground: An Australian perspective of women's experience of psychosocial assessment AMD depression screening in pregnancy and following birth. *BMC Women's Health, 13*, 18.

Sealy, P. A., Fraser, J., Joanne, P., Simpson, M. E., & Hartford, A. (2009). Community awareness of postpartum depression. *Journal of Obstetric, Gynecologic, & Neonatal Nursing, 38*, 121–133.

Seehausen, D. A., Baldwin, L. M., Runkle, H. P., & Clark, G. (2005). Are family physicians appropriately screening for postnatal depression? *Journal of the American Board of Family Medicine, 18*, 104–112.

Shakespeare, J., Blake, F., & Garcia, J. (2003). A qualitative study of the acceptability of routine screening of postnatal women using the Edinburgh postnatal depression scale. *British Journal of General Practice, 53*(493), 614–619.

Sie, S. D., Wennink, J. M. B., van Driel, J. J., te Winkel, A. G. W., Castleelen, G., & van Weissenbruch, M. M. (2012). Maternal use of SSRIs, SNRIs and NaSSAs: Practical recommendations during pregnancy and lactation. *Archives of Disease in Childhood. Fetal and Neonatal Edition, 97*, F462–F476 .

Stepanuk, K. M., Fisher, K. M., Wittmann-Price, R., Posmontier, B., & Bhattacharya, A. (2013). Women's decision-making regarding medication use in pregnancy for anxiety and/or depression. *Journal of Advanced Nursing, 69*(11), 2470–2480.

Sword, W., Busser, D., Ganann, R., McMillan, T., & Swinton, M. (2008). Women's care-seeking experiences after referral for postpartum depression. *Qualitative Health Research, 18*(9), 1161–1173.

Thio, I. M., Oakley Browne, M. A., Coverdale, J. H., & Argyle, N. (2006). Postnatal depressive symptoms go largely untreated: A probability study in urban New Zealand. *Social Psychiatry and Psychiatric Epidemiology, 41*, 814–818.

Tuohy, A., & McVey, C. (2008). Subscales measuring symptoms of non-specific depression, anhedonia, and anxiety in the Edinburgh Postnatal Depression Scale. *British Journal of Clinical Psychology, 47*(2), 153–169.

Turner, K. M., Sharp, D., Folkes, L., & Chew-Graham, C. (2008). Women's views and experiences of antidepressants as a treatment for postnatal depression: A qualitative study. *Family Practice, 25*, 450–455.

Vliegen, N., Luyten, P., Besser, A., Casalin, S., Kempke, S., & Tang, E. (2010). Stability and change in levels of depression and personality: A follow-up study of postpartum depressed mothers that were hospitalized in a mother–infant unit. *Journal of Nervous and Mental Disease, 198*, 45–51.

Webster, J., Pritchard, M. A., Linnare, S. W. L., Roberts, J. A., Hinson, J. K., & Starrenburg, S. E. (2001). Postnatal depression: Use of health services and satisfaction with health-care providers. *Journal of Quality in Clinical Practice, 21*, 144–148.

Yawn, B. P., Dietrich, A. J., Wollan, P., Bertram, S., Graham, D., Huff, J., … Pace, W. D. (2012). TRIPPD: A practice-based network effectiveness study of postpartum depression screening and management. *Annals of Family Medicine, 10*, 320–329.

4

How to Use the EPDS and Maximize Its Usefulness in the Consultation Process
A Clinician's Guide

Carol Henshaw and Jennifer Ericksen

Rationale for the Use of Screening Tools to Identify Perinatal Depression and Anxiety

Perinatal depression and anxiety are common, with around 13–15% of pregnant women or new mothers becoming depressed (Leahy-Warren & McCarthy, 2007; O'Hara & Swain, 1996). Consequences can be serious and long lasting for the woman and her family, particularly if left untreated (Beyondblue, 2014; Milgrom, Ericksen, McCarthy, & Gemmill, 2006; Milgrom, Gemmill, & Westley, 2004; Murray & Cooper, 1997). Although most women with depression and anxiety can be treated successfully, many will not spontaneously seek help for their symptoms. A number of barriers have been identified (Bilszta, Ericksen, Buist, & Milgrom, 2010), and thus, primary care needs to be proactive in identifying parents who may be in need of additional support and assistance. In universal services, this involves routinely asking women and their partners (if present) about their mental health, often with the use of a screening tool. Early identification of mental health concerns increases referral for management (Reilly et al., 2013) and should avoid some of the negative impacts on mother and infant (Austin & Priest, 2005).

The mental health and adjustment of partners are also important to consider. Wee, Skouteris, Pier, Richardson, and Milgrom (2011) reviewed the literature and identified correlates associated with perinatal depression in men. Having a depressed partner, a poor-quality relationship with her, as well as low social support was most commonly reported by men. Paternal depression can also impact on the amount of support he can provide, affecting mothers' well-being as well as infant development (Ramchandani & Psychogiou, 2009; Ramchandani et al., 2008). Identification of emotional difficulties in new fathers is covered in detail in Chapter 10.

In this chapter, we discuss the use of the Edinburgh Postnatal Depression Scale (EPDS) (Cox, Holden, & Henshaw, 2014; Cox, Holden, & Sagovsky, 1987) in clinical

Identifying Perinatal Depression and Anxiety: Evidence-Based Practice in Screening, Psychosocial Assessment, and Management, First Edition. Edited by Jeannette Milgrom and Alan W. Gemmill.
© 2015 John Wiley & Sons, Ltd. Published 2015 by John Wiley & Sons, Ltd.

practice. Its main use is in routine screening in a population of perinatal women for likelihood of depression, but it has also been used to monitor progress, as it is sensitive to change over time (Matthey, 2004). Identifying women in need of further assessment and possible support for depression through screening gives women the opportunity to discuss their situation and the option to take up treatment in line with their individual health beliefs.

The EPDS

The EPDS is a simple, short, and free 10-item self-rated screening questionnaire (Cox et al., 1987). Women read statements and choose one of four responses related to their mood as they have experienced it in the last week. It allows health professionals to identify most of the women who might need help and require a referral for a full diagnostic assessment.

Who Can Use the EPDS?

Internationally, the EPDS is the most widely applied perinatal depression screening instrument and can be used by any health professional or researcher trained in its use and in how to carry out a clinical assessment (Cox et al., 1987, 2014). In addition, it has been validated as a screening tool for antenatal women and is recommended nationally for use in the antenatal population in Australia (Beyondblue, 2014; Gibson, McKenzie-McHarg, Shakespeare, Price, & Gray, 2009).

Well-coordinated and well-resourced universal screening can increase the detection of depression (Milgrom, Mendelsohn, & Gemmill, 2011) and other postnatal mood disorders and distress. Discussions with primary care health professionals about the benefits of universal screening often highlight their experience that some women appear to be coping well but return surprisingly elevated EPDS scores. Up to 60% of cases can be missed if screening is targeted only at those who the health professional thinks might be depressed rather than universally undertaken (Cox & Holden, 2003). Barriers to help seeking such as stigma, denial, lack of knowledge, unrealistic expectations, and a need to keep up appearances and not to ask for help until the "time is right" make detection more difficult without a screening tool such as the EPDS (Bilszta et al., 2010).

In a recent survey (Ericksen, Rallis, Cox, & Holt, 2014) of 1053 Australian primary health-care professionals' main concerns about implementing universal screening, the most often noted concerns were inadequate referral pathways and consultation time, lack of confidence in their skills to communicate results effectively, and concerns about not screening properly (missing women). Training health professionals to address some of these concerns is covered in Chapter 13.

How to Administer the EPDS

The EPDS is usually administered as a pencil and paper test. Although it is free to use, the copyright is held by the Royal College of Psychiatrists, and this means the scale must be reproduced in the original, validated format (including the validation reference) unless the college has granted specific permission. Nonetheless, some unvalidated versions are in circulation.

Underlining the required response for each item was how the EPDS was originally designed. However, a number of versions (including electronic versions: Glaze & Cox, 1991) have developed other means of identifying response (tick boxes, circles). Some versions have the score next to the response for easier totaling of the scale. We are not aware of any validation of this practice, and anecdotal evidence from health professionals using such versions suggests that women underreport if the scores are visible.

Any woman completing the EPDS should do this by herself without discussion with others unless she has literacy difficulties or an intellectual disability (Gaskin & James, 2006). In these cases, it can be administered verbally by reading out, explaining, and simplifying the questions. The EPDS is ideally completed in the presence of a health professional, but there are circumstances where this might not be possible, for example, in rural areas or if a woman is unable to travel or be visited at home.

Glaze and Cox (1991) introduced a computerized version of the EPDS reporting that women had no difficulty completing it in this way. The benefits are it can be done privately in a woman's own time, but there must be clear instructions and guidance regarding the clinical assessment of high scorers and referral pathways. A small study in the United States explored the feasibility and acceptability of online screening with the EPDS (Drake, Howard, & Kinsey, 2014). The women entered their demographic data into a laptop while in the maternity hospital and, 3 months later, were sent a reminder e-mail asking them to complete the online EPDS. Having done this, they received an individualized score with referral information, guidance, and links to available resources. However, none of the women in the study accessed these.

The Internet and a growing number of websites providing information and resources for perinatal women have made the EPDS readily available for women to self-screen. There is little literature on this practice but it does raise issues with respect to risk management, interpretation of results, and access to pathways to care. Responsible sites/resources include information about appropriate pathways to care and action to be taken related to EPDS scores. While this manner of screening may not be optimal, it may be argued that it helps to increase access and detection.

When to Screen with the EPDS

When originally developed and validated, the EPDS was used to screen for depression 6 weeks after delivery, when women in the United Kingdom are offered a postnatal check by their GP or health visitor. However, it can be used at any point postpartum. Most guidelines recommend screening between 4 and 6 weeks after delivery as completing the EPDS too soon after delivery, for example, in the first week, may be measuring postpartum blues rather than depression.

The beyondblue Clinical Practice Guidelines Good Practice Point 11 (Beyondblue, 2011) advises that all women should complete the EPDS at least once, preferably twice, in both the antenatal period and the postnatal period (ideally 6–12 weeks after the birth) using a cutoff score of 13 or above. Good Practice Point 13 recommends for women who score 10, 11, and 12 to readminister the EPDS after 2–4 weeks. Some depressive episodes will onset later so a second screening could take place 3–6 months after delivery. The EPDS can be administered at the discretion of the health professional and can be administered multiple times as indicated.

Screening should only be carried out when the woman is in a situation conducive to the process, where she has privacy and time to concentrate on the scale (help may be needed with children) and is free of unhelpful or intrusive family support that may interfere with her screening.

Explaining Screening to Women

Woman-centered care is a model of perinatal service delivery that seeks to embrace the concept of providing a holistic approach to care. The key characteristics of the model are:

- Treating the woman as an individual
- Understanding her context
- Honoring her preferences and individual needs
- Involving her in making decisions about her care

Screening can be conducted within this model by introducing the process with a full explanation and gaining consent. Using effective communication skills to ask psychosocial questions based on known risk factors for postnatal depression, gaining an understanding about her context, and involving the woman in discussions about her preferences for support and intervention are all steps in providing a woman-centered perinatal care.

Although reference is made to "woman-centered" care and to mothers as the primary carer, the same issues and principles apply to partners and other carers (e.g., same-sex couples, grandparents, foster parents, etc.). As always, practice needs to be modified and delivered in a way that is appropriate to the individual and acknowledges the various family constellations and care arrangements.

It is important to explain fully why screening is taking place before a woman is asked to complete the EPDS and to gain her consent. Ideally, a clinician she knows and can trust should administer it as part of routine care. It is suggested that screening is introduced as a conversation about how the woman is coping. It is also a good idea to provide women with an explanation regarding the purpose of the screening and some psychoeducation about early parenthood being a challenging time followed by comments about offering screening routinely to everyone at this point and that some women may need some extra support. Here are some examples of how to explain screening as part of routine practice and how to integrate consent:

> *"This appointment is focused a little more on you and how you are coping with all the changes and challenges since your baby has arrived. Routine care here at … (YOUR AGENCY) involves asking you to complete a short scale about how you have been feeling over the last week. It will help me to understand a bit more about you and your situation and, if necessary, assist me to help you and your baby. Is that alright with you? All the information we discuss today will remain confidential, and you will not have to follow up anything you don't want to."*
>
> *"I routinely ask all women some questions about how they have been feeling since the birth of their baby. I prefer to do this using this EPDS screening scale. Would you mind reading the instructions and filling it out? Then we can talk about it."*

It is important to explain to her that she is to choose the response which comes closest to how she has felt in the last 7 days, not just how she is feeling at the time of completing the scale. She should complete all 10 questions and take as long as she needs to do this (usually 5–10 min).

If a woman declines to undertake the assessment, she should not be coerced to do so. Document that she has declined, and offer a further assessment at subsequent consultations. It may also be prudent to inquire as to why consent has been declined. Feedback from nurses would suggest that women who are already aware of their depression may feel further screening is unnecessary and women in denial may also refuse.

There is still considerable stigma attached to depression, and women may also be concerned about the treatment they might be offered (e.g., antidepressants) or be under the misapprehension that their children may be removed by child protection services.

Generally, screening is acceptable to perinatal women, both depressed and nondepressed (Gemmill, Leigh, Ericksen, & Milgrom, 2006; Leigh & Milgrom, 2007). In the Australian setting, the vast majority of women believe universal screening is a good thing. One thousand and two hundred Australians were surveyed, and 83% agreed with a universal screening policy (Highet, Gemmill, & Milgrom, 2011). Ninety percent of women thought the EPDS questions were reasonable ones to be asked (Matthey et al., 2005).

Conducting Screening with Women from Culturally and Linguistically Diverse Backgrounds

All health professionals must ensure that their services are delivered in a culturally sensitive manner. When working with perinatal populations, it is important to remember that increasing numbers of women who give birth are born in other countries. Often, these women may have higher rates of mental health problems because of their background, the circumstances that surrounded their migration, and possible history of trauma and loss. Refugee, asylum-seeking, and immigrant women may have higher postnatal depression rates (24–42%) compared to other women (10–15%) (Collins, Zimmerman, & Howard, 2011).

Women from different backgrounds have been found to experience perinatal depression and anxiety, but there may be differences in the understanding and attitudes about mental health among women, their families, and communities (Dennis & Chung-Lee, 2006). Sensitivity to possible differences in cultural norms and a woman-centered approach are therefore essential. For example, some women may be accompanied to all appointments by their partner or a family member so the opportunity for confidentiality is greatly diminished. Clifford, Day, Cox, and Werrett (1999) noted that some Punjabi women accompanied by their mother-in-law felt uncomfortable completing the EPDS because being identified as depressed would be seen as bringing negative consequences on the family.

Some key challenges (Henshaw & Elliott, 2005) for health professionals working with culturally and linguistically diverse (CALD) families may include:

1 Language and barriers
2 Understanding the diversity of cultural norms
3 Considering health professional's own prejudices, preconception, and attitudes
4 Understanding women's concepts of "health" or "illness"
5 Appropriate modes of communication—for example, the use of interpreters and link workers
6 Arranging suitable access

The EPDS has now been translated into at least 60 difference languages, but is not validated in all of these (see Cox et al., 2014). Merely translating the scale however accurately does not ensure that it is culturally appropriate or that the same cutoffs will operate as in an English-speaking population. Meanings and idiom may be quite different. The process of developing and validating a translation has been described by Clifford and colleagues (1999). Clinicians should therefore check before using a translation to ensure that is has been validated.

In Australia, resources have been developed for primary health-care professionals to assist in dealing with women from CALD backgrounds (Beyondblue, 2011). They recommend, however, that "Care should be provided in a woman-centred way based on her individual needs and her preferences not the assumed needs of her ethnic or religious background." It should be noted that women from different cultures may experience and understand emotional distress in different ways, may not have an equivalent word for depression, and may describe physical rather than emotional symptoms.

It is important to undertake a cultural assessment with a woman to determine what culture she identifies with, what language she prefers to use, and what cultural and religious practices she is accustomed to and wishes to continue to practice. These things need to be discussed and not be taken at face value.

An example of opening up this conversation:

> *"I don't know a lot about you and the country and culture that you come from. Can you tell me a bit about this to help me to understand you, so I can be aware and respectful of your beliefs and wishes?"*

There is benefit in involving others with cultural expertise including ethnic and bilingual health workers, with the woman's permission.

How to Score and Interpret EPDS Results

Each of the 10 items of the EPDS is scored 0–3 with 0 indicating no change from normal functioning and 3 indicating most change from normal functioning. Some items are reverse scored. The scores should not appear on the copy that the woman fills out. The scores on all ten items are totaled, giving a maximum score of 30. Care should be taken when scoring the EPDS as errors do occur. One study identified scoring errors in 16.9% of completed cases in four clinical services in a major city in Australia (Matthey, Lee, Crnec, & Trapolini, 2013). They recommended the use of overlaying a scoring template and adding the scores twice, once from item 1 to 10 and the second from item 10 to 1.

The EPDS measures the presence of symptoms that can indicate current depression or possible symptoms of anxiety but does not predict who will become depressed (Austin & Lumley, 2003).

Generally, a score greater than or equal to 13 is considered a positive screen, indicating that follow-up assessment is required. Scores of 10, 11, or 12 need a follow-up readministration in 2–4 weeks. Figueredo et al. (2012) carried out a telephone study of women in the last trimester of pregnancy or postpartum. They reported that a cutoff of greater than 10 offered the best sensitivity and specificity and should be used when screening by telephone. The first pregnancy validation advised a cutoff of greater than 14 (Murray & Cox, 1990).

Hewitt et al. (2009) found an optimal cutoff of 12 for detecting major depression and 10 for detecting major and minor depression after reviewing 40 studies using the EPDS. A comparative review found the sensitivity (% of actual cases identified) and specificity

(% of negative cases identified as negative) of the EPDS ranges from 80 to 90% at the most commonly applied cutoffs.

The positive predictive value of the EPDS has been estimated as 50–60%, which means 6 out of 10 women who score positive on the EPDS will meet the diagnostic criteria for major depression. Others may meet the criteria for minor depression, adjustment, or other mental disorders, and many will experience significant postnatal distress (Matthey, 2009; Milgrom, Holt, Gemmill et al., 2011).

Like any screening tool, the EPDS will produce both false positives (women identified as "at risk" when they are not) and false negatives (women not identified when they are "at risk"); however, the EPDS' performance is favorable compared to other tests. Always be aware that a low score may not mean a woman is not depressed. That is, some depressed women will underreport their symptoms and score below the threshold (a **false-negative** result), so you must always follow your own clinical judgment and discuss the results with her. If a score on one item seems to be at variance with the remainder or with her presentation, then discuss this with the woman. **The EPDS result must not replace your clinical judgment.**

Some women may not feel ready to fill out the EPDS honestly and will mark all answers as if they are coping well. Health professionals who use the EPDS regularly comment that very low overall scores or scores of zero raise their suspicion and their clinical judgment suggests following up with some additional questioning about coping. Anecdotally, the common range of scores for postnatal women would appear to be between 3 and 8 points.

As the EPDS is not a diagnostic instrument, the Community Practitioners' and Health Visitors' Association (CPHVA) stress: "The EPDS should never be used in isolation, it should form part of a full and systematic mood assessment of the mother, supporting professional judgement and a clinical interview" (CPHVA, 2003). Nevertheless, screening with the EPDS appears "numerically worthwhile at a population level, with the potential to facilitate substantial increases in identification" (Milgrom, Mendelsohn, & Gemmill, 2011).

It takes professional judgment to determine whether the score is an honest indication of how the woman is feeling versus what she may be trying to portray:

> *"It looks like things are going well for you at present; remember you can always come and talk to me or another health professional if you feel that you need to. It is not uncommon for women to need a bit of extra support as they make the transition to parenthood, and this can make a huge difference to how you feel and manage. Let's have a look at each of your answers."*

Although a woman might not be willing to answer the EPDS honestly on this occasion, it does give her some appreciation of the symptoms that are associated with depression. It also opens up the conversation about depression and lets her know that this health professional would be interested in her mood should she wish to discuss it at a later date. She may wish to follow her own management pathway independently.

The EPDS can also be used to monitor progress in treatment. Matthey (2004) calculated that a clinically significant change was four points on the scale.

In summary, a score of 13 or greater generally indicates the woman is likely to be depressed, but there are other mental health disorders (anxiety, bipolar disorder, etc.) that may be prevalent in this group (Milgrom, Ericksen, Negri, & Gemmill, 2005). Life events and stressors may indicate that the symptoms constitute an adjustment disorder. Similarly, a recently bereaved woman might have a high score, but this would clearly be related to her grief rather than a depressive illness. Physical health problems can have symptoms similar to those of depression and are common in the postpartum period, for example, anemia or thyroid dysfunction. These need to be investigated and treated rather than assuming the symptoms are depression.

How to Interpret the Anxiety Subscale

The EPDS purposely excludes some symptoms of depression that are commonly experienced by women in the perinatal period (fatigue, sleep, and appetite disturbance) and includes three questions (questions 3–5) that may tap into symptoms of anxiety as well as depression (Matthey, 2008, Matthey, Fisher, & Rowe, 2013). These three items in the EPDS are known to have a correlation with clinical anxiety:

Q3: "I have blamed myself unnecessarily when things went wrong."
Q4: "I have been anxious or worried for no good reason."
Q5: "I have felt scared or panicky for no very good reason."

It is worth noting a woman's response on these questions for all women including those who score below the overall threshold of 13 for the EPDS. However, note that the validity of these items for screening for anxiety has not been formally established. Currently, there is no strong evidence that any one tool (including the EPDS) is reliable enough for screening for anxiety in perinatal women (see Chapter 6).

How to Explain Screening Results to Women

For all women, acknowledging and discussing their responses and offering further assessment and/or support in line with their wishes form the basis of screening in the context of woman-centered care.

Some ways to open the conversation about the meaning of a **positive screening result**:

"Thanks for completing the EPDS scale which is quite sensitive and can pick up lots of different things including symptoms of depression, anxiety and other distress."
"Looking at your responses, you have indicated that you have been feeling … (discuss her responses)."
"What do you think is influencing your responses on the scale just now?" (Use clinical judgment to decide whether to monitor and readminister or refer.)
"What do you think you would like to do about how you are feeling and coping?"

Suggestions for discussing the meaning of a **negative screening result**:

"Thanks for completing the EPDS scale; you seem to be coping quite well. Is that how you feel too? Remember that I am happy to talk with you about further support you think you might need at any stage should things change."

How to Respond to Question 10: Risk Assessment

An advantage of the EPDS is that it allows for rapid identification of women who are experiencing suicidal ideation. This is often anxiety provoking for the health professional, especially those with minimal mental health training and experience and limited time to manage the situation. It should be remembered that the majority of new mothers are unlikely to act on such suicidal feelings and that asking about these thoughts will not exacerbate them or induce an act of self-harm.

Question 10 focuses on thoughts of self-harm/suicidal ideation. Any score other than 0 requires following up with a more detailed risk assessment. Howard, Flach, Mehay, Sharp, and Tylee (2011) reported that 9% of women screened with the EPDS answered question 10 positively. On the basis of her answer, you will be able to know what the next step is. Careful exploration to discriminate between accidental misinterpretation of the question, thoughts of self-harm, and true suicidal intent will need to be undertaken. Each organization undertaking screening will need to develop some clear guidelines and referral pathways for managing women who are experiencing thoughts of self-harm or suicidal ideation (see also Chapter 2).

Many women who indicate "hardly ever" on question 10 go on to describe thoughts of wishful thinking "not wanting to be in their current situation," "wanting to escape," or "return to previous life" with no plan or suicidal intent. Further questioning elicits resounding denial of suicidality and embarrassment that they have triggered further assessment. Others will deny those thoughts in the past week but report on other times when they have felt this way. While this is not what the EPDS was asking about, it does provide relevant history for their management.

The wording of "self-harm" can also be interpreted as cutting, burning, or other methods of self-harm. For some, suicidal thoughts are present and need to be asked about directly:

"I notice you have indicated that you have sometimes thought about harming yourself. Can you tell me a bit more about these feelings?"
  "Have you had thoughts that life isn't worth living?"
  "Have you thought about suicide?"
  "What exactly have you been thinking you might do?"

This should include precisely what thoughts she has been having, the frequency and severity of thoughts, and whether she can resist them or has made any plans (has she the means?) or attempts to harm herself or others. Are there factors and supports that are preventing her from acting out her thoughts? Ask if she self-harmed in the past, as this increases the risk of further self-harm postpartum (Healey et al., 2013). An urgent psychiatric opinion and/or crisis management support must be sought if she is actively suicidal. It is important for clinicians to remember that discussing suicidal ideation is not going to make her more likely to harm herself.

A woman's thoughts about suicide usually involve one method she has been thinking about (overdose of medication, hanging, etc.), so removing the means (the medication or rope) and increasing family and social supports to assist with monitoring can increase safety in the short term until other treatment can be arranged.

If a woman is experiencing suicidal thoughts, it is also important to ascertain whether she is also experiencing any thoughts of harming her baby and/or any other children she has. If she is profoundly depressed, her baby/children may be at risk of neglect.

Also, ask about thoughts of harm toward the baby:

"Have you had thoughts of harming your baby?"
  "Have you felt irritated or scared by your reaction to your baby's behavior?"
  "Have you wanted to shake or slap your baby?"
  "Have you ever harmed your baby?"
  "What did you do?"
  "Thank you for being so honest today about … I know it has been a difficult conversation for us to have. Together, we can put some things in place that can support you to keep yourself and your baby safe."

Developing a management plan

Having spent some time with the woman introducing and completing the EPDS, discussing her responses, and summarizing the content, then a plan for management is made. Usually, this is best done by supplementing the EPDS with broader psychosocial questions (see Chapter 8). For many, this is all too much to undertake on one occasion, and the offer needs to be made to return for a further conversation or to connect with another mental health professional for further assessment and management, for example, if a positive EPDS requires further diagnostic assessment (see Chapter 7). Women are not always of a mind to take action about their mental health. Low levels of engagement with appropriate services after screening have been consistently reported at around 20% (Milgrom, Holt, Gemmill et al., 2011) and 30–40% (Austin et al., 2008), so we need to be working with women to help them to resolve their ambivalence and to explore what actions they would like to take and options that fit with their health beliefs. Motivational interviewing techniques successful in other areas of health (Rubik, Sandbaek, Lauritzen, & Christensen, 2005) are being used to help women to explore their motivation to take action about their mental health issues. Grote and Bledsoe (2007) found 60% more depressed women attended an initial treatment session after receiving an engagement interview involving these techniques. Involving women in making decisions about their management, listening to them, and encouraging them to talk about their ambivalence about engaging with support, rather than giving advice about what they should do, have improved uptake/compliance. If consultation time is limited, you are better off asking women why they would want to and how they would go about get help rather than that they should (Rollnick, Miller, & Butler, 2008):

> *"Considering the issues we have discussed today, it seems like you are having some difficulties with…* (e.g., lowered mood and lack of social support).*"*
>
> *"What are your reasons for wanting to deal with some of these issues?"*
> *"What do you think would be most helpful for you?"*
> *"How important is it to you to…?"*
> *"If you did decide to … How would you go about it?"*
> *"I have some information about things that have been helpful for others. Would it be ok if I shared it with you?"*

Document the results of this assessment and the actions you have taken. Referral is a process rather than a one-off event, so it may take some time. Refer to an appropriate health professional, document, and most importantly follow up to make sure referral is acted on and review progress at subsequent visits. Women report they are concerned about losing the relationship they have with you by being referred on to someone else (Bilszta et al., 2010).

Conclusions

Around the world, the EPDS is used in many different settings in various formats and translations. In practice, there are several key points to ensuring acceptable, worthwhile screening:

- Universal screening is recommended to increase detection of postnatal mental health disorders as:
  - Significant barriers exist preventing women from self referring.
  - Undiagnosed and untreated postnatal depression may have deleterious effects on the woman and her partner, infant, and other children.

- A woman-centered approach provides the context to screening and discussion of results.
- The EPDS should be used for its intended purpose and in a validated format by trained health professionals:
  - Paper and pencil administration.
  - Ensuring privacy and environment conducive to the task.
  - Cutoff score of 13 or above.
  - Four to six weeks postnatal and able to be repeated as required.
  - Care needs to be taken to ensure scoring accuracy.
  - EPDS items should be discussed with women paying attention to the items associated with anxiety questions 3–5 and 10 risk of self-harm.
- Detailed risk assessment to be done with anyone scoring 1, 2, or 3 on question 10 including risk to baby/other children.
- Screening should pay attention to the woman's broader psychosocial context:
  - Psychosocial factors impacting on the woman.
  - The needs of CALD families.
- Developing a management plan with the woman is important and may take time but ensures that positive screens are considered in the context of a woman's history.
- Motivational interviewing techniques increase engagement with help seeking.

References

Austin, M.-P., Frilingos, M., Lumley, J., Hadzi-Pavlovic, D., Roncolato, W., Acland, S., … Parker, G. (2008). Brief antenatal cognitive behaviour therapy group intervention for the prevention of postnatal depression and anxiety: A randomised controlled trial. *Journal of Affective Disorders, 105*, 35–44. doi:10.1016/j.jad.2007.04.001.

Austin, M.-P., & Lumley, J. (2003). Antenatal screening for postnatal depression: A systematic review. *Acta Psychiatrica Scandinavica, 107*, 10–17. doi:10.1034/j.1600-0447.2003.02024.x.

Austin, M.-P., & Priest, S. (2005). Clinical issues in perinatal mental health: New developments in the detection and treatment of perinatal mental mood and anxiety disorders. *Acta Psychiatrica Scandinavica, 112*, 97–104. doi:10.1111/j.1600-0447.2005.00549.x.

Beyondblue. (2011). *Perinatal clinical practice guidelines*. Retrieved from http://www.beyondblue.org.au/resources/health-professionals/perinatal-mental-health. Accessed February 3, 2014.

Beyondblue. (2014). *Fact Sheet. Perinatal Depression and Anxiety: Evidence related to infant cognitive and emotional development*. Retrieved from www.beyondblue.org.au/resources. Accessed February 3, 2014.

Bilszta, J., Ericksen, J., Buist, A., & Milgrom, J. (2010). Women's experience of postnatal depression-beliefs and attitudes as barriers to care. *Australian Journal of Advanced Nursing, 2*, 44–54.

Clifford, C., Day, A., Cox, J., & Werrett, J. (1999). A cross-cultural analysis of the use of the Edinburgh Post-Natal Depression Scale (EPDS) in health visiting practice. *Journal of Advanced Nursing, 30*, 655–664. doi:10.1046/j.1365-2648.1999.01115.x.

Collins, C., Zimmerman, C., & Howard, L. (2011). Refugee, asylum seeker, immigrant women and postnatal depression: Rates and risk factors. *Archives of Women's Mental Health, 14*, 3–11. doi: 10.1007/s00737-010-0198-7.

Cox, J., & Holden, J. (2003). Perinatal Mental Health. A Guide to the Edinburgh Postnatal Depression Scale (EPDS). London, UK: Gaskell.

Cox, J., Holden, J., & Henshaw, C. (2014). *Perinatal Mental Health: The EPDS Manual* (2nd ed.). London, UK: RCPsych Publications.

Cox, J., Holden, J., & Sagovsky, R. (1987). Detection of postnatal depression: The development of the 10-item Edinburgh Postnatal Depression Scale. *British Journal of Psychiatry, 150*, 782–786.

Community Practitioners and Health Visitors Association. (2003). *Postnatal depression and maternal mental health in a multicultural society: Challenges and solutions*. London, UK: CPHVA.

Dennis, C. L., & Chung-Lee, L. (2006). Postpartum depression help-seeking barriers and maternal treatment preferences: A qualitative systematic review. *Birth*, *33*(4), 323–331.

Drake, E., Howard, E., & Kinsey, E. (2014). Online screening and referral for postpartum depression: An exploratory study. *Community Mental Health Journal*, *50*(3), 305–311. doi:10.1007/s10597-012-9573-3.

Ericksen, J., Rallis, S., Cox, P., & Holt, C. (2014). *Depression and Psychosocial Assessment: A report on Maternal and Child Heath knowledge, comfort and confidence* (Report to Department of Education and Early Child Hood Development). Melbourne, Australia: Parent Infant Research Institute.

Figueredo, F. P., Balarini, F. B., Silva, A. P. C., Cavalli, R. C., Silva, A. A. M., Bettiol, H., … Del-Ben, C. M. (2012). EPDS by telephone—What cut off point use. *European Psychiatry*, *1*(Suppl), 1. doi:10.1016/S0924-9338(12)75632-8.

Gaskin, K., & James, H. (2006). Using the Edinburgh Postnatal Depression Scale with learning disabled mothers. *Community Practitioner*, *79*, 392–396.

Gemmill, A. W., Leigh, B., Ericksen, J., & Milgrom, J. (2006). A survey of the clinical acceptability of screening for postnatal depression in depressed and non-depressed women. *BMC Public Health*, *6*, 211.

Gibson, J., McKenzie-McHarg, K., Shakespeare, J., Price, J., & Gray, R. (2009). A systematic review of studies validating the Edinburgh Postnatal Depression Scale in antepartum and postpartum women. *Acta Psychiatrica Scandinavica*, *119*(5), 350–364.

Glaze, R., & Cox, J. (1991). Validation of a computerised version of the 10-item (self-rating) Edinburgh Postnatal Depression Scale. *Journal of Affective Disorders*, *22*, 73–77.

Grote, N., & Bledsoe, S. (2007). Predicting postpartum depressive symptoms in new mothers: The role of optimism and stress frequency during pregnancy. *Health & Social Work*, *32*, 107. doi:10.1093/hsw/32.2.10.

Healey, C., Morriss, R., Henshaw, C., Wadoo, O., Sajjad, A., & Scholefield, H. (2013). Self-harm in postpartum depression: An audit of referrals to a perinatal mental health team. *Archives of Women's Mental Health*, *16*, 237–245. doi:10.1007/s00737-013-0335-1.

Henshaw, C., & Elliott, S. (Eds.). (2005). *Screening for perinatal depression*. London, UK: Jessica Kingsley.

Hewitt, C., Gilbody, S., Brealey, S., Paulden, M., Palmer, S., Mann, R., … Richards, D. (2009). Methods to identify postnatal depression in primary care: An integrated evidence synthesis and value of information analysis. *Health Technology Assessment*, *13*: 36. doi:10.3310/hta13360.

Highet, N. J., Gemmill, A. W., & Milgrom, J. (2011). Depression in the perinatal period: Awareness, attitudes and knowledge in the Australian population. *Australian & New Zealand Journal of Psychiatry*, *45*, 223–231.

Howard, L. M., Flach, C., Mehay, A., Sharp, D., & Tylee, A. (2011). The prevalence of suicidal ideation identified by the Edinburgh Postnatal Depression Scale in postpartum women in primary care: Findings from the RESPOND trial. *BMC Pregnancy and Childbirth*, *11*, 57. doi:10.1186/1471-2393-11-57.

Leahy-Warren, P., & McCarthy, G. (2007). Postnatal depression: Prevalence, mother's perspectives and treatments. *Archives of Psychiatric Nursing*, *21*(2), 91–100.

Leigh, B., & Milgrom, J. (2007). Acceptability of antenatal screening for depression in routine antenatal care. *The Australian Journal of Advanced Nursing*, *24*(3), 14–18.

Matthey, S. (2004). Calculating clinically significant change in postnatal depression studies using the Edinburgh Postnatal Depression Scale. *Journal of Affective Disorders*, *78*, 269–272. doi:10.1016/S0165-0327(02)003130.

Matthey, S. (2008). Using the Edinburgh Postnatal Depression Scale to screen for anxiety disorders. *Depression and Anxiety*, *25*, 926–931. doi:10.1002/da.20415.

Matthey, S. (2009). Are we overpathologising motherhood? *Journal of Affective Disorders*, *120*, 263–266. doi:10.1016.j.jad.2009.05.004.

Matthey, S., Fisher, J., & Rowe, H. (2013). Using the Edinburgh postnatal depression scale to screen for anxiety disorders: Conceptual and methodological considerations. *Journal of Affective Disorders*, *146*, 224–230. doi:10.1016.j.jad.2012.09.009.

Matthey, S., Lee, C., Crnec, R., & Trapolini, T. (2013). Errors in scoring the Edinburgh Postnatal Depression Scale. *Archives of Women's Mental Health*, *16*, 117–122. doi:10.1007/s00737-012-0324-9.

Matthey, S., White, T., Phillips, J., Taouk, R., Chee, T. T., & Barnett, B. (2005). Acceptability of routine antenatal psychosocial assessments to women from English and non-English speaking backgrounds. *Archives of Women's Mental Health*, *8*, 171–180.

Milgrom, J., Ericksen, J., McCarthy, R., & Gemmill, A. W. (2006). Stressful impact of depression on early mother-infant relations. *Stress and Health*, *22*(4), 229–238.

Milgrom, J., Ericksen, J., Negri, L., & Gemmill, A. W. (2005). Screening for perinatal depression in routine primary care: Properties of the Edinburgh Postnatal Depression Scale in an Australian sample. *Australian and New Zealand Journal of Psychiatry*, *39*, 833–839.

Milgrom, J., Gemmill, A. W., & Westley, D. (2004). The mediating role of maternal responsiveness in some longer term effects of postnatal depression on infant development. *Infant Behaviour and Development*, *27*(4), 443–454.

Milgrom, J., Holt, C., Gemmill, A. W., Ericksen, J., Leigh, B., Buist, A., & Schembri, C. (2011). Treating postnatal depressive symptoms in primary care: A randomised controlled trial of GP management, with and without adjunctive counselling. *BMC Psychiatry*, *11*, 95–103. doi:10.1186/1471-244X-11-95.

Milgrom, J., Mendelsohn, J., & Gemmill, A. W. (2011). Does postnatal depression screening work? Throwing out the bathwater, keeping the baby. *Journal of Affective Disorders*, *132*, 301–310. doi:10.1016/j/jad.2010.09.031.

Murray, L. D., & Cooper, P. (1997). Postpartum depression and child development. *Psychological Medicine*, *27*, 253–260.

Murray, L. D., & Cox, J. L. (1990). Screening for depression during pregnancy with the Edinburgh Depression Scale (EPDS). *Journal of Reproductive and Infant Psychology*, *8*, 99–107.

O'Hara, M., & Swain, A. (1996). Rates and risk of postpartum depression—A meta-analysis. *International Review of Psychiatry*, *8*, 37–54.

Ramchandani, P. G., & Psychogiou, L. (2009). Paternal psychiatric disorders and children's psychosocial development. *Lancet*, *374*, 646–653. doi:10.1016/S0140-6736(09)60238-5.

Ramchandani, P. G., Stein, A., O'Connor, T. G., Heron, J., Murray, L., & Evans, J. (2008). Depression in men in the postnatal period and later child psychopathology: A population cohort study. *Journal of American Academy of Child and Adolescent Psychiatry*, *47*, 390–398. doi:10.1097. CHI.0b013e31816429c2.

Reilly, N., Harris, S., Loxton, D., Chojenta, C., Forder, P., Milgrom, J., & Austin, M.-P. (2013). Referral for management of emotional health issues during the perinatal period: Does mental health assessment make a difference? *Birth*, *40*(4), 297–306. doi:10.1111/birt.12067.

Rollnick, S., Miller, W. R., & Butler, C. C. (2008). *Motivational Interviewing in Healthcare*. New York, NY: Guilford Press.

Rubik, S., Sandbaek, A., Lauritzen, T., & Christensen, B. (2005). Motivational interviewing: A systematic review and meta-analysis. *British Journal of General Practice*, *55*, 305–312.

Wee, K. Y., Skouteris, H., Pier, C., Richardson, B., & Milgrom, J. (2011). Correlates of ante- and postnatal depression in fathers: A systematic review. *Journal of Affective Disorders*, *130*, 358–377.

5

Screening Tools and Methods of Identifying Perinatal Depression

Rachel Mann and Jonathan Evans

Introduction

The Edinburgh Postnatal Depression Scale (EPDS) (Cox, Holden, & Sagovsky, 1987) is the most widely used method to screen for perinatal depression (Hewitt, Gilbody, Mann, & Brealey, 2010). A number of other instruments have also been used; these include generic and perinatal-specific self-report questionnaires. Alternative methods include the use of clinician-rated scales and case-finding questions.

Choosing the best screening instrument depends on the context in which it is being used. It is important to consider who is going to be administering the instrument and interpreting the results and what action is planned in the event of a positive screen. Self-report scales which include somatic items such as disturbance in sleep and appetite are likely to lead to high false-positive rates in pregnancy and postnatally, so those instruments which exclude somatic questions are preferable at this time. As screening for depression during pregnancy is becoming more commonplace in routine practice, the length of the screen in terms of time taken to use and number of items is important. The first assessment with midwives can be lengthy, and so the shortest depression screens are more likely to be favored in practice.

This chapter describes the EPDS and a number of alternative self-report questionnaires and clinician-rated measures that have been used in the perinatal period and then discusses the use of a brief case-finding instrument to identify perinatal depression.

EPDS

The EPDS, as its name suggests, was developed specifically for use in the postnatal period to screen for depression. It is a 10-item self-report instrument which requires women to respond to 10 statements relating to symptoms of depressed mood, anhedonia, anxiety, and

Identifying Perinatal Depression and Anxiety: Evidence-Based Practice in Screening, Psychosocial Assessment, and Management, First Edition. Edited by Jeannette Milgrom and Alan W. Gemmill.
© 2015 John Wiley & Sons, Ltd. Published 2015 by John Wiley & Sons, Ltd.

self-harm in the previous week. For each item, there are four possible responses rated from 0 to 3 according to severity or frequency. It is deliberately brief and has been in wide use internationally for both antenatal and postnatal populations (Cox & Holden, 2003). The EPDS deliberately excludes somatic symptoms (changes in appetite, energy levels, and sleeping patterns) that are common to women in the perinatal period. Responses for the 10 items are summed to yield a maximum score of 30. Three items in the EPDS load on an anxiety factor in both antenatal and postnatal populations (Jomeen & Martin, 2005; Matthey, 2008; Matthey, Fisher, & Rowe, 2012; Tuohy, McVey, Tuohy, & McVey, 2008), and the last item concerns thoughts of self-harm. The EPDS has also been validated for antenatal use (Bergink et al., 2011; Gibson, Mckenzie-Mcharg, Shakespeare, Price, & Gray, 2009) and is available in several non-English language translations. As there are no items which are specific to the perinatal period, items included are similar to those used in generic depression measures, and it has also been used and validated outside the perinatal period and in men (Edmondson, Psychogiou, Vlachos, Netsi, & Ramchandani, 2010). The most commonly used cutoff score for indicating possible depression is greater than or equal to 13. A synthesis of more than 40 studies located an optimal EPDS cutoff point of greater than or equal to 13 for major depression and 10 for major and minor depression combined (Hewitt et al., 2009). A recent comparative effectiveness review found moderate strength of evidence that the sensitivity and specificity of the EPDS both range from 80 to 90% at commonly applied cutoffs (Myers et al., 2013). However, there is considerable variation among studies in terms of setting, population, screening threshold used, etc. The EPDS, like any other screening tool for depression, yields both false-positive and false-negative results and should inform, not replace, clinical judgment. Compared to other instruments that have been used to screen for perinatal depression, the test performance of the EPDS appears favorable (Myers et al., 2013).

The average positive predictive value of the English language version of the EPDS in postnatal populations has been estimated at around 50–60% (Matthey, 2009; Milgrom, Mendelsohn, & Gemmill, 2011). This means that 40–50% of those screening positive will not have depression when assessed clinically. However, given the close relationship between anxiety and depression, some of those who are false positive for depression may have generalized anxiety disorder or mixed anxiety and depression. Therefore, further assessment may have some value even in those who do not reach criteria for a specific diagnosis of depression. This is not usually taken into account in studies of the utility of the EPDS or other scales. This last point emphasizes the importance of being clear why screening is being conducted in the first place, what kind of assessment will be made following a positive screen, and what management options are available. Screening with the EPDS is usually aimed at identifying those who would benefit from further assessment as it is not sufficient to use the scale alone as a diagnostic instrument.

The EPDS has been judged, according to the UK National Screening Committee's screening criteria, to be a "simple, safe, precise and validated screening test" for which suitable cutoffs can be defined (Hewitt et al., 2009; Hill, 2010). However, further research is required to compare the performance of the EPDS with other measures to identify depression and evaluate the clinical and cost-effectiveness of perinatal screening (Hill, 2010). Currently, a population mass screening program, which meets all of the UK Screening Committee criteria (which includes evidence for clinical and cost-effectiveness of a screening program) to identify perinatal depression, is not recommended in the United Kingdom at this time (screening is recommended in some other countries however; see Chapter 12).

Generic Self-Report Instruments

There are many different generic self-report instruments available to identify depressive disorders and with potential value as a screen for depression; some are global measures that contain a depression-specific category, and others are depression-specific measures; some examples are shown in Table 5.1 although not all tools have been used in perinatal populations.

Self-report generic instruments that have been used in the perinatal period include the General Health Questionnaire (GHQ), Beck Depression Inventory (BDI), and Patient Health Questionnaire (PHQ).

The GHQ has been validated against gold-standard diagnostic criteria in perinatal populations in various countries (Abiodun, 1994; Aguado et al., 2012; Kadir, Nordin, Ismail, Yaacob, & Mustapha, 2004; Kitamura, Shima, Sugawara, & Toda, 1994; Lee, Yip, Chiu, Leung, & Chung, 2001; Lee et al., 2003; Navarro et al., 2007). For example, the GHQ-12 has been validated against standardized *Diagnostic and Statistical Manual of Mental Disorders, Fourth Edition* (DSM-IV) diagnostic criteria (American Psychiatric Association, 1994) with modest sensitivity and specificity of 89 and 80.4%, respectively, to identify postnatal depression (PND) (Navarro et al., 2007). The GHQ has also been used in a large longitudinal cohort study in the United Kingdom to examine the impact of a range of genetic, socioeconomic, environmental, and health-related factors such as psychological well-being on maternal, family, and child health and on child development (Raynor & the Born in Bradford Collaborative Group, 2008). An analysis of the GHQ-28 subscales to examine psychological well-being in a large, ethnically diverse subsample of pregnant women within the cohort found that the meaning of the underlying concepts for some items differed according to language of administration and between ethnic groups. Therefore, the GHQ-28 may have limitations when used to screen for depression in ethnically diverse populations (Prady et al., 2013).

The original BDI (Beck, Ward, Mendelson, Mock, & Erbaugh, 1961) has been through multiple revisions: the BDI-1A (Beck, Rush, Shaw, & Emery, 1979) is an amended version of the original BDI, is commonly referred to in the literature as the BDI, and has 21 items, and the time frame considers symptoms "over one week, including today" (Beck & Steer, 1987); the BDI-II (Beck, Steer, & Brown, 1996) includes addition of symptoms related to worthlessness, concentration difficulty, agitation, and loss of energy, and the time frame considers symptoms "over two weeks, including today"; and the seven-item BDI-Fast Screen (BDI-FS) (Beck, Steer, & Brown, 2000), formerly known as the BDI-Primary Care (Beck, Guth, Steer, & Ball, 1997), comprises nonsomatic items derived from the BDI-II covering sadness, loss of pleasure, suicidal thoughts, pessimism, past failure, self-dislike, and self-criticalness.

The BDI-1A and BDI-II have been validated against gold-standard diagnostic criteria in the perinatal period (Adewuya, Adekunle, & Adejare, 2005; Beattie-Clarke, 2003; Beck & Gable, 2001; Holcomb, Stone, Lustman, Gavard, & Mostello, 1996; Lee et al., 2003; Milgrom, Ericksen, Negri, & Gemmill, 2005; Teng et al., 2005; Whiffen, 1988).

While the BDI is commonly regarded as a gold-standard depression assessment instrument, it has been criticized for low sensitivity (Whiffen, 1988). Further, for pregnant populations, a higher cutoff score is recommended than the cutoff used in nonpregnant populations (Holcomb et al., 1996). The BDI-II has been found to have moderate correlation with a PND-specific instrument (the Postpartum Depression Screening Scale (PDSS); Beck & Gable, 2001). However, limitations of the BDI-II relate to the

Table 5.1 Generic self-report instruments

Instrument	Items[a]	Scope	Time frame	Score range	Approximate administration time (min)
BDI (Beck et al., 1961)	21, 7	Depression specific	1–2 weeks/today	0–63	5
PHQ (Kroenke et al., 2001; Kroenke et al., 2003)	9, 2	Depression specific	Past 2 weeks	0–27	5
GHQ (Goldberg, 1972)	30, 28, 12	Global psychological symptoms	Past few weeks	0–28	2–10
HADS (Zigmond & Snaith, 1983)	14	Depression and anxiety	Past week	0–21	≤2
CES-D (Radloff, 1977)	20, 10	Depression specific	Past week	0–60	5–10
Zung SDS (Zung, Richards, & Short, 1965)	20	Depression specific	Recently	25–100	2–5
HSCL (Derogatis, Lipman, Rickels, Uhlenhuth, & Covi, 1974)	25, 13	Global with depression-specific category	Past week	25–100	2–5
SCL-90-R (Derogatis, 1992)	90	Global with depression-specific category	Past week	0–360	Up to 15

BDI, Beck Depression Inventory; CES-D, Center for Epidemiologic Studies Depression Scale; GHQ, General Health Questionnaire; HADS, Hospital Anxiety and Depression Scale; HSCL, Hopkins Symptom Checklist; PHQ, Patient Health Questionnaire; SCL-90-R, Symptom Checklist-90-Revised; Zung SRDS, Zung Self-Rating Depression Scale.

[a]Numbers refer to different versions.

items concerned with somatic symptoms, which potentially impact on the accuracy of depression assessment during the perinatal period as endorsement of items is difficult to differentiate from common postnatal sequelae (Manian, Schmidt, Bornstein, & Martinez, 2013). As described, the BDI-II is a modification of the BDI-1A, a key aspect of this revision being the extension of the reporting time frame to 2 weeks in order to correspond with the time frame for a DSM-IV diagnosis of major depression (Beck et al., 1996). Pooled estimates of sensitivity and specificity for the BDI and BDI-II using a cutoff score of 10 postnatally (validated with DSM-IV criteria) are 72 and 91%, respectively (Hewitt et al., 2009). The BDI-II has shown modest sensitivity and specificity when validated against DSM-IV diagnostic criteria in pregnancy of 74 and 83%, respectively, and head-to-head comparison with the EPDS found the psychometric properties of the EPDS superior as BDI-II psychometric properties were potentially affected by the somatic items and poor validity (Su et al., 2007). Another head-to-head comparison of EPDS and BDI-II found that the scales performed similarly (Milgrom et al., 2005), but in some studies, traditional cutoff points did not perform at expected levels of sensitivity and specificity with optimum cutoff points for the scales being lower than currently recommended (Chaudron et al., 2010). This makes it difficult to judge the relative merits of one scale over another in comparison studies, and it is therefore difficult to draw conclusions about optimum instruments. Caution in the use of the BDI-II has been specifically advocated in postnatal populations as the total score may overrepresent depressive symptoms, and "screeners" are advised to pay particular attention to cognitive and affective items endorsed on the scale (Conradt, Manian, & Bornstein, 2012). There appears to be a lack of evidence for use of the BDI-FS in perinatal populations, which is surprising given the brevity of the scale.

The Patient Health Questionnaire-9 (PHQ-9) (Kroenke, Spitzer, & Williams, 2001) is a commonly used generic self-report instrument used in primary care, but there are relatively few studies of its use in the perinatal period (Davis, Pearlstein, Stuart, O'Hara, & Zlotnick, 2013; Flynn, Sexton, Ratliff, Porter, & Zivin, 2011; Hanusa, Scholle, Haskett, Spadaro, & Wisner, 2008; Sidebottom, Harrison, Godecker, & Kim, 2012; Weobong et al., 2009; Yawn et al., 2009). The PHQ-9 contains somatic items including questions on sleep, appetite, and energy and also includes a question on thoughts of self-harm. The PHQ-2 (Kroenke, Spitzer, & Williams, 2003) consists of the first two PHQ-9 items; there is a stem question: "Over the last 2 weeks, how often have you been bothered by any of the following problems?" Respondents are required to answer the following two statements: (1) "little interest or pleasure in doing things" and (2) "feeling down, depressed, or hopeless." Responses are scored according to a four-point Likert-type scale as per the PHQ-9, with a score range of 0–6. The purpose of the PHQ-2 was to develop an extremely brief measure for screening depression in large patient-volume, US primary care clinics, whereby the measure would minimize false-positive responses (Kroenke et al., 2003).

In one US study, the PHQ-9 and PHQ-2 were validated against standardized diagnostic criteria for depressive disorder in the postnatal period (Gjerdingen, Crow, McGovern, Miner, & Center, 2009). Sensitivity and specificity of the PHQ-9 using the simple summary scoring method were 82 and 84%, respectively, and using the complex diagnostic algorithm scoring were 67 and 92%, respectively. The sensitivity and specificity of the PHQ-2 were 84 and 79%, respectively. The PHQ-9 has also been validated in one study against DSM diagnostic criteria in pregnancy; using the summative scoring method, the sensitivity and specificity of the instrument at a cutoff of 10 were 85 and 84%, respectively (Sidebottom et al., 2012).

The Hospital Anxiety and Depression Scale (HADS) (Zigmond & Snaith, 1983) was designed for use in medical settings and so specifically excluded somatic items. There is a seven-item depression subscale. Despite its potential value as a screen for depression during pregnancy, there have been few studies to evaluate this scale (Tsai et al., 2013).

There has been some interest in use of the Kessler-10 (K-10) to identify antenatal depression and PND in African countries (Baggaley et al., 2007; Spies et al., 2009). The K-10 is a generic 10-item self-report measure designed to identify psychological distress. It is comprised of five response categories ranked on a five-point scale, and individual items are summed to give a total score. In a study of 129 pregnant women (Spies et al., 2009), the K-10 was validated against the Structured Clinical Interview for DSM-IV (SCID DSM-IV) (First & Gibbon, 1997). At a cutoff of greater than or equal to 21.5, the sensitivity and specificity were 73 and 54%, respectively. In a study of 61 postnatal women (Baggaley et al., 2007), the K-10 and K-6 were validated against ICD-10 criteria for depression (World Health Organisation, 2005). At a cutoff of greater than or equal to 14 for the K-10, sensitivity and specificity were 59 and 91%, respectively. The K-10 has been proposed as a standard screening instrument for primary care especially in the context of depression identification in developing countries such as South Africa rather than use of multiple types of generic or perinatal-specific instruments such as the EPDS. The generic nature of the K-10, simplified scoring system, and desirability of one tool to standardize depression assessment in primary care populations (including perinatal populations) are cited as reasons why use of this instrument appeals in countries with resource constraints.

Not all generic instruments have been validated for use against a gold-standard diagnostic interview, for example, Duke Anxiety-Depression Scale, Index of Depression, and Inventory of Depressive Symptomatology (Parkerson, Broadhead, & Tse, 1996; Popoff, 1969; Rush, Giles, & Schlesser, 1986). This suggests that selection of a generic tool to assess perinatal depression should be undertaken with careful consideration with regard to the type of items contained within an instrument and the psychometric properties of the instrument. Furthermore, it is suggested that generic instruments may be more useful in the latter part of the postnatal period when somatic symptoms associated with the first few weeks after delivery are less likely to impact on the assessment of perinatal depression (Boyd, Le, & Somberg, 2005); use of generic instruments with somatic items is likely to falsely identify women as depressed (Manian et al., 2013).

Evidence synthesized from a detailed report for the Agency for Healthcare Research and Quality in the United States (Gaynes, Gavin, Meltzer-Brody, & Lohr, 2005) found limited evidence of high-quality studies to assess any screening instruments in the perinatal period. There were only 10 studies meeting the review inclusion criteria; these criteria were restricted to screening instruments in English. The most widely studied screening instrument was the EPDS. Only three other instruments were included in these studies: two generic instruments, the Beck Depression Inventory (BDI-I and BDI-II) and the CES-D (Radloff, 1977), and one perinatal-specific instrument, the PDSS (Beck & Gable, 2000) (described in the following section). Specificity of both the generic instruments was relatively high, indicating that a positive screen was relatively accurate in ruling in the presence of depression. However, in a condition where missing depression cases (false negatives) could be worse than falsely identifying the condition, sensitivity of the instrument may be more important. Indications were that the sensitivity of the BDI was lower than the other instruments although confidence intervals were wide, and therefore, it was not possible to be certain about the relative merits of the different scales.

A review and evidence synthesis by Hewitt et al. (2009) of strategies to identify PND identified use of both perinatal-specific instruments (e.g., the EPDS) and generic measures in the antenatal and postnatal period. The review applied stringent criteria, and only studies that validated identification instruments against a recognized gold-standard diagnostic interview for depression were included. Generic measures identified for inclusion in the review were the GHQ, BDI, BDI-II, Zung SDS, HADS, HSCL, and SCL-90-R. However, data synthesis of studies conducted in the antenatal period could not be undertaken due to insufficient numbers of studies that had validated generic instruments against gold-standard criteria during pregnancy. Evidence synthesis of the BDI for diagnosis of minor or major depression indicated that compared to the EPDS, the BDI was less sensitive but more specific. However, a limitation of this data synthesis was that only four studies contained data suitable for statistical pooling, and therefore, conclusions regarding the psychometric properties of the BDI to identify PND warrant caution.

As concluded by Hewitt et al. (2009), a relatively limited amount of validation work has been conducted with generic instruments in perinatal depression, as opposed to validation work with the EPDS, for example, making it difficult to draw robust conclusions as to the utility of their psychometric properties in the perinatal period or indeed make a firm recommendation with regard to the merits of one generic instrument over another.

In conclusion, regarding generic tools, a review of screening instruments to identify PND by Boyd et al. (2005) suggested that use of generic instruments to identify perinatal depression was promising. However, evidence from subsequent systematic reviews (Gaynes et al., 2005; Gibson et al., 2009; Hewitt et al., 2009) demonstrates that little research has been attempted in recent years to capitalize on this promise and there is a paucity of research to support the use of generic instruments in the perinatal period compared to the EPDS.

Other Perinatal-Specific Self-Report Instruments

In addition to the EPDS, several other perinatal-specific instruments have been developed.

Pregnancy Risk Assessment Monitoring System

The Pregnancy Risk Assessment Monitoring System (PRAMS) was originally developed in the United States by the Centers for Disease Control (CDC) to assess prevalence and provide statewide surveillance of health-related issues in pregnancy. Further validation of PRAMS items with the highest prediction of postnatal depressive symptoms has been undertaken to develop PRAMS as a screening tool for PND resulting in PRAMS-6 (O'Hara et al., 2012). PRAMS-6 is intended to be an ultrabrief screening tool that assesses PND symptoms since the woman delivered. It comprises six items: three items assess depressive symptoms (depressed mood, hopelessness, feeling slowed down physically), and three items assess anxiety symptoms (feeling fearful, panic, and feeling restless or fidgety). Items are rated on a Likert scale from 1 (never) to 5 (always). A study by the developers of PRAMS-6 administered a diagnostic interview using the SCID DSM-IV (First & Gibbon, 1997) to women suspected of having PND based on a PHQ-9 score greater than or equal to 10. Use of 80% sensitivity was chosen by the authors as the optimum level of sensitivity in terms of false-negative and false-positive cases, which determined an optimum cutoff score for PRAMS-6 of 15. A study limitation was that women were selected for inclusion in the study based on the presence of depressive symptoms (Coronado-Montoya, Kwakkenbos, Levis, & Thombs, 2013); therefore, PRAMS-6 requires further validation work in a well-designed diagnostic test accuracy study in a consecutive sample of women presenting for maternity care in routine practice (Knottnerus & Muris, 2002).

PDSS

The PDSS was developed by Beck and Gable (2000). The instrument is a 35-item Likert-type self-report measure created specifically for new mothers and consists of seven dimensions including sleeping/eating disturbances, anxiety/insecurity, emotional lability, cognitive impairment, loss of self, guilt/shame, and thoughts of self-harm. Respondents are asked to indicate their agreement or disagreement on a five-point scale ranging from "strongly agree" to "strongly disagree" regarding how they have felt in the last 2 weeks. The screening measure yields an overall severity score falling into one of three ranges: normal adjustment, significant symptoms of PND, and positive screen for major PND. A study by Beck and Gable of 150 mothers at 12 weeks' postdelivery who completed the PDSS, the BDI, and the EPDS found that the PDSS was strongly correlated to the BDI ($r=0.81$) and EPDS ($r=0.79$) (Beck & Gable, 2001). A PDSS cutoff score of 80 was recommended for identification of major PND with a sensitivity and specificity of 91 and 72%, respectively. There is also a PDSS short form consisting of the first 7 items of the 35-item version (Beck & Gable, 2001). The PDSS-7 and PDSS-35 have been subsequently validated against DSM diagnostic criteria in a sample of indigenous women in Canada (Beattie-Clarke, 2003) and Spanish-speaking women (Beck & Gable, 2005). In another study, the PDSS-7 and EPDS were found to be more accurate than the PHQ-9 (Hanusa et al., 2008).

Bromley Postnatal Depression Scale

The Bromley Postnatal Depression Scale (BPDS) was specifically developed as a screening tool to identify the presence of both current and previous episodes of PND and consists of 10 items with yes/no and open-ended responses. One study has validated the BPDS against the Dunedin Scale (Stein & Van Den Akker, 1992), a questionnaire which examines feeling within the first year of childbirth which was validated against the DSM-III (American Psychiatric Association, 1980) criteria for major depression. Assuming a positive response to the Dunedin Scale was equal to a DSM-III diagnosis, the sensitivity and specificity of the BPDS were 62 and 94%, respectively.

The Pitt Depression Scale

The Pitt Depression Scale (PDS) (Pitt, 1968) is a 24-item screening questionnaire based on clinical experience and measures maternal anxiety and depression before and after childbirth. The items are listed as questions, for example, "Do you worry a lot about the baby?" and "Are you as happy as you ought to be?" Respondents indicate whether each symptom was present "today or over the past few days" and respond yes, no, or don't know. The total scores range from between 0 and 48. The PDS correlates highly with the EPDS; however, it has not been validated and is used infrequently.

Clinician-Rated Scales

An alternative method to identify perinatal depression is the use of clinician-rated scales. These are measures of depression used to standardize clinical judgments and provide ratings of duration and severity of symptoms. Several clinician-rated scales are available and include the seven-item Pregnancy Depression Scale (PDS) (Altschuler et al., 2008). This is a brief clinician-administered screening tool developed for specific use in identifying depression in pregnancy. Others are the Raskin Depression Rating Scale (Raskin, Schulterbrandt, Reatig, & McKeon, 1969), the Hamilton Depression Rating Scale (HAM-D) (Hamilton, 1960), and the Montgomery–Asberg Depression Rating Scale (MADRS) (Montgomery & Asberg, 1979). Scores on the MADRS in women 6–12 weeks postnatally have been found to be highly correlated with the BDI, EPDS, and HADS (Berle, Aarre, Mykletun, Dahl, & Holsten, 2003). However, there are limiting factors for the use of these instruments. First, they are designed for use during a clinical consultation and not for large-scale population-based screening. Second, they do not replace the need for clinical assessment to confirm the diagnosis. Third, they include somatic items which present problems of interpretation in perinatal populations. The HAM-D and MADRS were developed to measure severity and to be sensitive to change particularly for use during clinical trials. The MADRS has since been developed as a self-report questionnaire (Fantino & Moore, 2009) to identify major depressive disorder, and therefore, this generic nine-item self-report screening tool has the potential to be validated in a perinatal population alongside other perinatal-specific tools.

Case-Finding Perinatal Depression

An alternative method to identify perinatal depression, rather than multi-item self-report screening questionnaires, is the use of ultrabrief case finding. In practice, this would often be the first stage in a two-stage screening process with a more detailed tool used as a second stage.

Case finding for conditions is not concerned with large-scale population screening, as is the case with mass screening programs such as cervical and breast cancer screening programs. Case finding has been variously defined as

> "the identification of cases within routine systems of health care delivery for example during a visit to the doctor's office for some related or unrelated cause" (Kirch, 2008) and " the search for additional illness in those with medical problems." (Henshaw, Cox, & Barton, 2009)

Case-finding questions

In recent years, a move away from the "traditional" multi-item paper and pencil tests has been advocated. Instead, case-finding questions have been advocated due to their ability to identify depression with acceptable accuracy without the burden of long, complex questionnaires that require scoring and interpretation (Mitchell & Coyne, 2007).

The concept of using case-finding questions in mental health prior to subsequent in-depth assessment evolved from the development of the Primary Care Evaluation of Mental Disorders (PRIME-MD) procedure (Spitzer et al., 1994). The PRIME-MD was designed to identify five groups of mental disorders commonly encountered in primary care. The patient questionnaire of the PRIME-MD contains two initial questions regarding mood and loss of interest:

> *During the past month, have you often been bothered by feeling down, depressed, or hopeless?* and
> *During the past month, have you often been bothered by little interest or pleasure in doing things?*

These questions address the essential features that are necessary (but not sufficient) for a diagnosis of depression according to DSM criteria. To demonstrate the potential advantage of these two brief case-finding questions compared to traditional "paper and pencil" measures, Whooley, Avins, Miranda, and Browner (1997) validated the two case-finding questions, which require only a simple yes or no response, alongside several measures including the BDI (Beck & Steer, 1987) and Diagnostic Interview Schedule (DIS) (Robins, Helzer, Croughan, & Ratcliff, 1981) against diagnostic criteria in 536 consecutive male patients attending a Veterans Affairs Medical Center.

In the study, Whooley et al. (1997) found that a positive response to either of the two case-finding questions had a sensitivity and specificity of 96% (95% CI 90%, 99%) and 57% (95% CI 53%, 62%), respectively.

Arroll, Smith, Kerse, Fishman, and Gunn (2005) examined the utility of an additional question to inquire if a respondent needed help: *Is this something you feel you need or want help with?* triggered by a positive response to either or both of the case-finding questions.

A positive response to either question plus the "help" question had a sensitivity and specificity of 96% (95% CI 86%, 99%) and 89% (95% CI 87%, 91%), respectively.

In 2007, clinical guidance issued by the UK National Institute for Health and Clinical Excellence (NICE, 2007) strongly advocated asking perinatal women the two case-finding questions and an additional question to inquire if help is needed or wanted. A positive response to either question triggers the use of the additional help question. Use of the case-finding questions were presumed as more compatible with routine practice than the EPDS or other generic self-report measures, despite the absence of evidence in the perinatal context at the time the guidance was issued.

Case-finding questions were cited as a less elaborate but equally effective method to identify perinatal depression. Use of the case-finding questions should potentially be considered in the context of a triage strategy, rather than viewed as a replacement strategy to existing methods of assessment (Mann & Gilbody, 2011). Use of case-finding questions could be considered in a two-step strategy. The potential benefit of a brief case-finding triage approach within clinical settings where routine perinatal care takes place is to reduce the numbers of those who need further evaluation; therefore, initial case finding with these two questions narrows the number of women that would require further assessment with longer instruments.

There has been limited work validating these case-finding questions in the perinatal period. While the addition of the help question had little effect on sensitivity in nonperinatal populations, studies that have investigated the validity of this method in perinatal women showed a substantial fall in sensitivity with the inclusion of the help question. Gjerdingen et al. (2009) investigated the first two case-finding questions postnatally against a diagnostic interview and reported a sensitivity of 100% and a specificity of 44%. Mann, Adamson, and Gilbody (2012) found similar results both postnatally and when used in the third trimester of pregnancy (sensitivity 100%, specificity 65%, sensitivity 100%, and specificity 68%, respectively). For the positive "screens," specificity of the additional "help"

question antenatally and postnatally was 91 and 100%, respectively. With posttest probability of antenatal and PND of 65 and 95%, respectively, women who answer "yes" to the
help question warrant further clinical evaluation for depressive disorder. However, the
additional "help" question was found to decrease the sensitivity to 39% postnatally and to
58% in the third trimester.

This casts some doubt on the use of the help question in the perinatal context when
women decline help. It may be unclear what "help" means to pregnant women who may
consider that this implies antidepressants or are concerned this may result in scrutiny of
their parenting. Elliot and Henshaw (2005) suggest deliberate concealment of feelings
might be viewed as an ethical issue of a woman's choice arising from their feeling the need
to do so, rather than a fault with a questionnaire. Despite the concern regarding false-negative cases, some suggest that the help question remains clinically relevant—even if some
patients decline help, it highlights those willing to accept additional support (Baker-Glen,
Park, Granger, Symonds, & Mitchell, 2011; Lombardo et al., 2011).

An additional consideration is who will administer the case-finding questions and how
will they be asked. This will vary, for example, in the United Kingdom, screening during
pregnancy is undertaken by midwives and postnatally by health visitors. One limitation is
the timely availability of appropriate further assessment and treatment. In the United
Kingdom, there has been a considerable expansion in psychological treatment services, but
provision remains limited with delays in receiving treatment for women in the perinatal
period. This has an impact on the confidence health professionals have in screening for
depression during the perinatal period, when they may be left to try to manage depression
themselves. This is an important point for use of screening self-report scales, as all positive
screens need to be followed up with further assessment/treatment. Knowledge in how to
administer screening questions and the need for health professionals such as midwives and
health visitors to receive training to improve skills in developing a management plan is an
important consideration for perinatal health policy.

Screening Tools for Culturally Diverse Populations

Instruments specifically for use in ethnic minority groups of women have been developed.
These include the Punjabi Postnatal Depression Scale (Bhatti-Ali & Hussain, 2000) and the
Doop Chaon©. Use of these instruments was examined in a sample of South Asian women
living in the United Kingdom to screen for depressed mood in the postnatal period (Downe,
Butler, & Hinder, 2007). Quality criterion applied to the instruments was not met, and the
study concluded that at present none of the instruments were sufficiently evaluated for
clinical use and could not be recommended for use in these groups. The study found that,
in similarity with findings from qualitative work undertaken with the EPDS (Shakespeare,
Blake, & Garcia, 2003), women preferred to talk face-to-face rather than complete paper
and pencil questionnaires. The EPDS has been translated into various languages, but further
work is required to evaluate their use (Hewitt et al., 2010).

Conclusion

There is limited evidence to support the use of any self-report screening measures apart
from the EPDS in perinatal populations.

Studies that examine the diagnostic test accuracy (validity) of screening tools for perinatal depression are often conducted in populations with a higher prevalence of depression than the general perinatal population which limits generalizability.

The two-question case-finding screen may be useful due to the brevity of the questions; they may be administered, for example, in the course of a discussion with a woman during perinatal assessment and preclude the need for "pencil and paper" questionnaires, which have been shown as less preferable than face-to-face discussion. However, there is a danger that screening may not be followed by a further longer screen or more detailed diagnostic assessment in routine clinical practice. The help question may lead to particular problems in the perinatal period especially if women choose to decline additional support. More detailed validation studies of the two-question case-finding approach are needed before it can be recommended strongly.

At time of writing, very few studies have assessed validity of screening tools to identify depression during pregnancy. This may be a particularly valuable opportunity for screening as early mental health contact combined with the opportunity to intervene early may prevent adverse effects on the fetus either directly or through reducing harmful health-related behaviors. Finally, the availability of treatment programs may affect the willingness of health professionals to screen perinatal women for depression. Managed referral and treatment programs, while desirable, may not be the only benefits from screening or case-finding approaches. In cases where perinatal depression is identified, there is also the potential for other constructive outcomes, for example, awareness and knowledge of the condition may lead to self-help, family involvement, and additional links to supportive services.

References

Abiodun, O. A. (1994). A validity study of the Hospital Anxiety and Depression Scale in general hospital units and a community sample in Nigeria. *The British Journal of Psychiatry, 165,* 669–672.

Adewuya, A., Adekunle, A., & Adejare, L. (2005). Prevalence of postnatal depression in Western Nigerian women: A controlled study. *International Journal of Psychiatry in Clinical Practice, 9,* 60–64.

Aguado, J., Campbell, A., Ascaso, C., Navarro, P., Garcia-Esteve, L., & Luciano, J. V. (2012). Examining the factor structure and discriminant validity of the 12-item General Health Questionnaire (GHQ-12) among Spanish postpartum women. *Assessment, 19,* 517–525.

Altschuler, L., Cohen, L., Vitonis, A., Faraone, S., Harlow, B., Suri, R., ... Stowe, Z. (2008). The Pregnancy Depression Scale (PDS): A screening tool for depression in pregnancy. *Archives of Women's Mental Health, 11,* 277–285.

American Psychiatric Association. (1980). *Diagnostic and statistical manual of mental disorders (DSM-III)* (3rd ed.). Washington, DC.

American Psychiatric Association. (1994). *Diagnostic and statistical manual of mental disorders (DSM-IV)* (4th ed.). Washington, DC.

Arroll, B., Smith, F. G., Kerse, N., Fishman, T., & Gunn, J. (2005). Effect of the addition of a "help" question to two screening questions on specificity for diagnosis of depression in general practice: Diagnostic validity study. *British Medical Journal, 331,* 884.

Baggaley, R. F., Ganaba, R., Filippi, V., Kere, M., Marshall, T., Sombié, I., ... Patel, V. (2007). Short communication: Detecting depression after pregnancy: The validity of the K10 and K6 in Burkina Faso. *Tropical Medicine & International Health, 12,* 1225–1229.

Baker-Glen, E. A., Park, B., Granger, L., Symonds, P., & Mitchell, A. J. (2011). Desire for psychological support in cancer patients with depression or distress: Validation of a simple help question. *Psycho-Oncology, 20,* 525–531.

Beattie-Clarke, P. (2003). Validation of two postpartum screening scales in a sample of Saskatchewan First Nations and Metis women. (Master's thesis). University of Regina, Regina, Canada.

Beck, A. T., Guth, D., Steer, R. A., & Ball, R. (1997). Screening for major depression disorders in medical inpatients with the Beck Depression Inventory for primary care. *Behaviour Research & Therapy, 35,* 785–791.

Beck, A. T., Rush, A. J., Shaw, B. F., & Emery, G. (1979). *Cognitive therapy of depression.* New York, NY: Guilford Press.

Beck, A. T., & Steer, R. A. (1987). *Manual for the Beck Depression Inventory.* San Antonio, TX: Psychological Corporation.

Beck, A. T., Steer, R. A., & Brown, G. K. (1996). *Manual for Beck Depression Inventory-II.* San Antonio, TX: Psychological Corporation.

Beck, A. T., Steer, R. A., & Brown, G. K. (2000). *BDI: Fast screen for medical patients manual.* San Antonio, TX: Psychological Corporation.

Beck, A. T., Ward, C. H., Mendelson, M. M., Mock, J. J., & Erbaugh, J. (1961). An inventory for measuring depression. *Archives of General Psychiatry, 4,* 561–571.

Beck, C. T, & Gable, R. K. (2000). Postpartum depression screening scale: Development and psychometric testing. *Nursing Research, 49,* 272–282.

Beck, C. T, & Gable, R. K. (2001). Further validation of the Postpartum Depression Screening Scale. *Nursing Research, 50,* 150–164.

Beck, C. T, & Gable, R. K. (2005). Screening performance of the postpartum depression screening scale—Spanish version. *Journal of Transcultural Nursing, 16,* 331–338.

Bergink, V., Kooistra, L., Lambregtse-van den Berg, M. P., Wijnen, H., Bunevicius, R., van Baar, A., & Pop, V. (2011). Validation of the Edinburgh Depression Scale during pregnancy. *Journal of Psychosomatic Research, 70*(4), 385–389.

Berle, J. Ø., Aarre, T. F., Mykletun, A., Dahl, A. A., & Holsten, F. (2003). Screening for postnatal depression. *Journal of Affective Disorders, 76*(1), 151–156.

Bhatti-Ali, R., & Hussain, A. (2000). The development and evaluation of a Punjabi Postnatal Depression Scale. Report available from Bradford Community Healthcare Trust, Shipley, UK.

Boyd, R. C., Le, H. N., & Somberg, R. (2005). Review of screening instruments for postpartum depression. *Archives of Women's Mental Health, 8,* 141–153.

Chaudron, L. H., Szilagyi, P. G., Tang, W., Anson, E., Talbot, N. L., Wadkins, H. I., … Wisner, K. L. (2010). Accuracy of depression screening tools for identifying postpartum depression among Urban mothers. *Pediatrics, 125,* e609-e617.

Conradt, E., Manian, N., & Bornstein, M. H. (2012). Screening for depression in the postpartum using the Beck Depression Inventory-II: What logistic regression reveals. *Journal of Reproductive & Infant Psychology, 30,* 427–435.

Coronado-Montoya, S., Kwakkenbos, L., Levis, B., & Thombs, B. (2013). Reassessing the clinical utility of the Patient Health Questionnaire (PHQ)-9 for depression screening in prenatal women: A commentary on Sidebottom et al. *Archives of Women's Mental Health, 16,* 253–254.

Cox, J., & Holden, J. (2003). *Perinatal mental health. A guide to the Edinburgh Postnatal Depression Scale (EPDS).* London, UK: Gaskell.

Cox, J. L., Holden, J. M., & Sagovsky, R. (1987). Detection of postnatal depression: Development of the 10-item Edinburgh Postnatal Depression Scale. *British Journal of Psychiatry, 150,* 782–786.

Davis, K., Pearlstein, T., Stuart, S., O'Hara, M., & Zlotnick, C. (2013). Analysis of brief screening tools for the detection of postpartum depression: Comparisons of the PRAMS 6-item instrument, PHQ-9, and structured interviews. *Archives of Women's Mental Health, 16,* 1–7.

Derogatis, L. R. (1992). *SCL-90-R: Administration, scoring and procedures manual-II for the (R)evised version and other instruments of the psychopathology rating scale service.* Towson, MD: Clinical Psychometric Research.

Derogatis, L. R., Lipman, R. S., Rickels, K., Uhlenhuth, E. H., & Covi, L. (1974). The Hopkins Symptom Checklist (HSCL): A self-report symptom inventory. *Behavioural Science, 19*, 1–15.

Downe, S. M., Butler, E., & Hinder, S. (2007). Screening tools for depressed mood after childbirth in UK-based South Asian women: A systematic review. *Journal of Advanced Nursing, 57*, 565–583.

Edmondson, O. J., Psychogiou, L., Vlachos, H., Netsi, E., & Ramchandani, P. G. (2010). Depression in fathers in the postnatal period: Assessment of the Edinburgh Postnatal Depression Scale as a screening measure. *Journal of Affective Disorders, 125*(1–3), 365–368.

Elliot, S., & Henshaw, C. (2005). Conclusions. In C. Henshaw & S. Elliot (Eds.), *Screening for perinatal depression*. London, UK: Jessica Kingsley.

Fantino, B., & Moore, N. (2009). The self-reported Montgomery-Asberg depression rating scale is a useful evaluative tool in major depressive disorder. *BMC Psychiatry, 9*, 26.

First, M. B., & Gibbon, M. (1997). *User's guide for the structured clinical interview for DSM-IV axis I disorders SCID-I: Clinician version*. Arlington, VA: American Psychiatric Press.

Flynn, H. A., Sexton, M., Ratliff, S., Porter, K., & Zivin, K. (2011). Comparative performance of the Edinburgh Postnatal Depression Scale and the Patient Health Questionnaire-9 in pregnant and postpartum women seeking psychiatric services. *Psychiatry Research, 187*, 130–134.

Gaynes, B. N., Gavin, N., Meltzer-Brody, S., & Lohr, K. N. (2005). *Perinatal depression: Prevalence, screening accuracy and screening outcomes*. Rockville, MD: Agency for Healthcare Research and Quality.

Gibson, J., Mckenzie-Mcharg, K., Shakespeare, J., Price, J., & Gray, R. (2009). A systematic review of studies validating the Edinburgh Postnatal Depression Scale in antepartum and postpartum women. *Acta Psychiatrica Scandinavica, 119*, 350–364.

Gjerdingen, D., Crow, S., McGovern, P., Miner, M., & Center, B. (2009). Postpartum depression screening at well-child visits: Validity of a 2-question screen and the PHQ-9. *The Annals of Family Medicine, 7*, 63–70.

Goldberg, D. (1972). *The detection of psychiatric illness by questionnaire*. London, UK: Oxford University Press.

Hamilton, M. (1960). A rating scale for depression. *Journal of Neurology, Neurosurgery and Psychiatry, 26*, 56–62.

Hanusa, B., Scholle, S., Haskett, R., Spadaro, K., & Wisner, K. L. (2008). Screening for depression in the postpartum period: A comparison of three instruments. *Journal of Women's Health, 17*, 585–596.

Henshaw, C., Cox, J., & Barton, J. (2009). *Modern management of perinatal psychiatric disorder*. London, UK: Royal College of Psychiatrists.

Hewitt, C. E., Gilbody, S. M., Brealey, S., Paulden, M., Palmer, S., Mann, R., … Richards, D. (2009). Methods to identify postnatal depression in primary care: An integrated evidence synthesis and value of information analysis. *Heath Technology Assessment, 13*(36), 147–230.

Hewitt, C. E., Gilbody, S. M., Mann, R., & Brealey, S. (2010). Instruments to identify post-natal depression: Which methods have been the most extensively validated, in what setting and in which language? *International Journal of Psychiatry in Clinical Practice, 14*:72–76.

Hill, C. (2010). *An evaluation of screening for postnatal depression against NSC criteria*. London, UK: National Screening Committee.

Holcomb, W., Stone, L., Lustman, P., Gavard, J., & Mostello, D. (1996). Screening for depression in pregnancy: Characteristics of the Beck Depression Inventory. *Obstetrics & Gynecology, 88*, 1021–1025.

Jomeen, J., & Martin, C. R. (2005). Confirmation of an occluded anxiety component within the Edinburgh Postnatal Depression Scale (EPDS) during early pregnancy. *Journal of Reproductive and Infant Psychology, 23*(2), 143–154. doi:10.1080/02646830500129297.

Kadir, A., Nordin, R., Ismail, S., Yaacob, M., & Mustapha, W. (2004). Validation of the Malay version of the Edinburgh Postnatal Depression Scale for postnatal women in Kelantan, Malaysia. *Asia Pacific Family Medicine, 3*, 9–18.

Kirch, W. (2008). *Encyclopaedia of public health*. New York, NY: Springer.

Kitamura, T., Shima, S., Sugawara M., & Toda, M. A. (1994). Temporal variation of validity of self-rating questionnaires: Repeated use of the General Health Questionnaire and Zung's Self-rating Depression Scale among women during antenatal and postnatal periods. *Acta Psychiatrica Scandinavica, 90*, 446–450.

Knottnerus, J., & Muris, J. (2002). Assessment of the accuracy of diagnostic tests: The cross-sectional study. In J. Knottnerus (Ed.), *The evidence base of clinical diagnosis* (p. 39). London, UK: BMJ Publishing Group.

Kroenke, K., Spitzer, R. L., & Williams, J. B. (2001). The PHQ-9: Validity of a brief depression severity measure. *Journal of General Internal Medicine, 16*, 606–613.

Kroenke, K., Spitzer, R. L., & Williams, J. B. (2003). The Patient Health Questionnaire-2: Validity of a two-item depression screener. *Medical Care, 41*, 1284–1292.

Lee, D., Yi, A., Chan, S., Tsui, M., Wong, W., & Chung, T. (2003). Postdelivery screening for postpartum depression. *Psychosomatic Medicine, 65*, 357–361.

Lee, D., Yip, A., Chiu, H., Leung, T., & Chung, T. (2001). Screening for postnatal depression: Are specific instruments mandatory? *Journal of Affective Disorders, 63*, 233–238.

Lombardo, P., Vaucher, P., Haftgoli, N., Burnand, B., Favrat, B., Verdon, F., ... Herzig, L. (2011). The "help" question doesn't help when screening for major depression: External validation of the three-question screening test for primary care patients managed for physical complaints. *BMC Medicine, 9*, 114.

Manian, N., Schmidt, E., Bornstein, M. H., & Martinez, P. (2013). Factor structure and clinical utility of BDI-II factor scores in postpartum women. *Journal of Affective Disorders, 149*, 259–268.

Mann, R., Adamson, J., & Gilbody, S. M. (2012). Diagnostic accuracy of case-finding questions to identify perinatal depression. *Canadian Medical Association Journal, 184*, E424–E430.

Mann, R., & Gilbody, S. M. (2011). Validity of two case finding questions to detect postnatal depression: A review of diagnostic test accuracy. *Journal of Affective Disorders, 133*, 388–397.

Matthey, S. (2008). Using the Edinburgh Postnatal Depression Scale to screen for anxiety disorders. *Depression & Anxiety, 25*(11), 926–931.

Matthey, S. (2009). Are we overpathologising motherhood? *Journal of Affective Disorders, 120*(1–3), 263–266.

Matthey, S., Fisher, J., & Rowe, H. (2012). Using the Edinburgh Postnatal Depression Scale to screen for anxiety disorders: Conceptual and methodological considerations. *Journal of Affective Disorders, 146*(2), 224–230. doi:10.1016/j.jad.2012.09.009.

Milgrom, J., Ericksen, J., Negri, L., & Gemmill, A. W. (2005) Screening for postnatal depression in routine primary care: Properties of the Edinburgh Postnatal Depression Scale in an Australian sample. *Australian and New Zealand Journal of Psychiatry, 39*, 833–839.

Milgrom, J., Mendelsohn, J., & Gemmill, A. W. (2011). Does postnatal depression screening work? Throwing out the bathwater, keeping the baby. *Journal of Affective Disorders, 132*(3), 301–310.

Mitchell, A., & Coyne, J. (2007). Do ultra-short screening instruments accurately detect depression in primary care? A pooled analysis and meta-analysis of 22 studies. *British Journal of General Practice, 57*, 144–151.

Montgomery, S. A., & Asberg, M. (1979). A new depression scale designed to be sensitive to change. *The British Journal of Psychiatry, 134*, 382–389.

Myers, E. R., Aubuchon-Endsley, N., Bastian, L. A., Gierisch, J. M., Kemper, A. R., Swamy, G. K., ... Sanders, G. D. (2013). *Efficacy and safety of screening for postpartum depression. Comparative effectiveness review 106*. Rockville, MD: Agency for Healthcare Research and Quality.

National Institute for Health & Clinical Excellence [NICE]. (2007). *Ante-natal and post-natal mental health. The NICE guideline on clinical management and service guidance*. London, UK: The British Psychological Society & The Royal College of Psychiatrists.

Navarro, P., Ascaso, C., Garcia-Esteve, L., Aguado, J., Torres, A., & Martin-Santos, R. (2007). Postnatal psychiatric morbidity: A validation study of the GHQ-12 and the EPDS as screening tools. *General Hospital Psychiatry, 29*, 1–7.

O'Hara, M., Stuart, S., Watson, D., Dietz, P., Farr, S., & D'Angelo, D. (2012). Brief scales to detect postpartum depression and anxiety symptoms. *Journal of Women's Health, 21,* 1237–1243.

Parkerson, G. R., Broadhead, W. E., & Tse, C. K. (1996). Anxiety and depressive symptom identification using the Duke Health Profile. *Journal of Clinical Epidemiology, 49,* 85–93.

Pitt, B. (1968). "Atypical" depression following childbirth. *The British Journal of Psychiatry, 114,* 1325–1335.

Popoff, L. M. (1969). A simple method for diagnosis of depression by the family physician. *Clinical Medicine, 76,* 24–27.

Prady, S., Miles, J., Pickett, K., Fairley, L., Bloor, K., Gilbody, S., … Wright, J. (2013). The psychometric properties of the subscales of the GHQ-28 in a multi-ethnic maternal sample: Results from the Born in Bradford cohort. *BMC Psychiatry, 13,* 55.

Radloff, L. S. (1977). The CES-D scale: A self-report depression scale for research in the general population. *Applied Psychological Measurement, 1,* 385–401.

Raskin, A., Schulterbrandt, J., Reatig, N., & McKeon, J. J. (1969). Replication of factors of psychopathology in interview, ward behavior and self-report ratings of hospitalized depressives. *The Journal of Nervous and Mental Disease, 148,* 87–98.

Raynor, P., & the Born in Bradford Collaborative Group. (2008). Born in Bradford, a cohort study of babies born in Bradford, and their parents: Protocol for the recruitment phase. *BMC Public Health, 8,* 327.

Robins, L., Helzer, J., Croughan, J., & Ratcliff, K. (1981). The NIMH Diagnostic Interview Schedule, its history, characteristics and validity. *Archives of General Psychiatry, 38,* 381–389.

Rush, A. J., Giles, D. E., & Schlesser, M. A. (1986). The inventory for depressive symptomatology (IDS): Preliminary findings. *Psychiatry Research, 18,* 65–87.

Shakespeare, J., Blake, F., & Garcia, J. (2003). A qualitative study of the acceptability of routine screening of postnatal women using the Edinburgh Postnatal Depression Scale. *British Journal of General Practice, 53,* 614–619.

Sidebottom, A., Harrison, P., Godecker, A., & Kim, H. (2012). Validation of the Patient Health Questionnaire (PHQ)-9 for prenatal depression screening. *Archives of Women's Mental Health, 15,* 367–374.

Spies, G., Stein, D. J., Roos, A., Faure, S. C., Mostertr, J., Seedat, S., & Vythilingum, B. (2009). Validity of the Kessler 10 (K-10) in detecting DSM-IV defined mood and anxiety disorders among pregnant women. *Archives of Women's Mental Health, 12,* 69–74.

Spitzer, R. L., Williams, J. B., Kroenke, K., Linzer, M., Degruy, F. V. I., Hahn, S. R., … Johnson, J. G. (1994). Utility of a new procedure for diagnosing mental disorders in primary care: The PRIME-MD 1000 study. *Journal of the American Medical Association, 272,* 1749–1756.

Stein, G., & Van Den Akker, O. (1992). The retrospective diagnosis of postnatal depression by questionnaire. *Journal of Psychosomatic Research, 36,* 67–75.

Su, K.-P., Chiu, T.-H., Huang, C.-L., Ho, M., Lee, C.-C., Wu, P.-L., … Pariante, C. M. (2007). Different cutoff points for different trimesters? The use of Edinburgh Postnatal Depression Scale and Beck Depression Inventory to screen for depression in pregnant Taiwanese women. *General Hospital Psychiatry, 29,* 436–441.

Teng, H.-W., Hsu, C.-S., Shih, S.-M., Lu, M.-L., Pan, J.-J., & Shen, W. W. (2005). Screening postpartum depression with the Taiwanese version of the Edinburgh Postnatal Depression Scale. *Comprehensive Psychiatry, 46,* 261–265.

Tsai, A. C., Scott, J. A., Hung, K. J., Zhu, J. Q., Matthews, L. T., Psaros, C., & Tomlinson, M. (2013). Reliability and validity of instruments for assessing perinatal depression in African settings: Systematic review and meta-analysis. *PloS One, 8*(12), e82521.

Tuohy, A., McVey, C., Tuohy, A., & McVey, C. (2008). Subscales measuring symptoms of non-specific depression, anhedonia, and anxiety in the Edinburgh Postnatal Depression Scale. *British Journal of Clinical Psychology, 47*(Pt 2), 153–169.

Weobong, B., Akpalu, B., Doku, V., Owusu-Agyei, S., Hurt, L., Kirkwood, B., & Prince, M. (2009). The comparative validity of screening scales for postnatal common mental disorder in Kintampo, Ghana. *Journal of Affective Disorders, 113,* 109–117.

Whiffen, V. (1988). Screening for postpartum depression: A methodological note. *Journal of Clinical Psychology, 44*, 367–371.

Whooley, M., Avins, A., Miranda, J., & Browner, W. (1997). Case-finding instruments for depression: Two questions are as good as many. *Journal of General Internal Medicine, 12*, 439–445.

World Health Organisation. (2005). *ICD-10: International Statistical Classification of Diseases and Related Health Problems: Tenth revision* (2nd ed.). Geneva, Switzerland: Author.

Yawn, B. P., Pace, W., Wollan, P. C., Bertram, S., Kurland, M., Graham, D., & Dietrich, A. (2009). Concordance of Edinburgh Postnatal Depression Scale (EPDS) and Patient Health Questionnaire (PHQ-9) to assess increased risk of depression among postpartum women. *The Journal of the American Board of Family Medicine, 22*, 483–491.

Zigmond, A. S., & Snaith, R. P. (1983). The hospital anxiety and depression scale. *Acta Psychiatrica Scandinavica, 67*, 361–370.

Zung, W. K., Richards, C., & Short, M. J. (1965). Self-rating depression scale in an outpatient clinic: Further validation of the SDS. *Archives of General Psychiatry, 13*, 508–515.

6

Identifying Perinatal Anxiety

Susan Ayers, Rose Coates, and Stephen Matthey

The importance of anxiety in the health of women and their children means that the issue of how we measure anxiety during pregnancy and after birth is critical, although not without controversy. Anxiety is broadly defined as "an emotion characterized by feelings of tension, worried thoughts and physical changes like increased blood pressure" (American Psychiatric Association, 2013). Symptoms include affective, cognitive, and behavioral components. Diagnostic categories for anxiety disorders are varied and encompass generalized anxiety disorder (GAD), phobias, panic disorder, agoraphobia, social anxiety disorder, separation anxiety disorder, selective mutism, and posttraumatic stress disorder prior to its reclassification as a trauma and stressor-related disorder (DSM-5; American Psychiatric Association, 2013). Different ways of conceptualizing anxiety are reflected in perinatal research, which has examined worries about pregnancy through to state symptoms through to diagnostic disorders. In this chapter, we first look at why it is important to identify perinatal anxiety and whether diagnostic criteria are relevant to women during this time as well as general issues and provisos when screening for perinatal anxiety. The final section briefly outlines some questionnaire measures of anxiety symptoms and pregnancy-specific anxiety.

Why Is It Important to Identify Perinatal Anxiety?

There is increasing evidence that anxiety disorders and subthreshold symptoms negatively affect not only women's well-being but also child development. In addition, anxiety disorders before and during pregnancy predict postnatal anxiety and depression (Matthey, Barnett, Howie, & Kavanagh, 2003; Mauri et al., 2010; Milgrom et al., 2008; Sutter-Dallay, Giaconne-Marcesche, Glatigny-Dallay, & Verdoux, 2004). For example, anxiety in late pregnancy is associated with a more than threefold risk of depression 6–8 weeks' postpartum (Austin, Tully, & Parker, 2007; Milgrom et al., 2008). The relationship of antenatal anxiety with postnatal psychological disorders highlights the potential for antenatal screening to

Identifying Perinatal Depression and Anxiety: Evidence-Based Practice in Screening, Psychosocial Assessment, and Management, First Edition. Edited by Jeannette Milgrom and Alan W. Gemmill.

identify women who will continue to experience postnatal emotional difficulties. Even women who have symptoms of anxiety in pregnancy but do not fulfill diagnostic criteria are likely to report greater postnatal depressive symptoms (Skouteris, Wertheim, Rallis, Milgrom, & Paxton, 2009). Screening for high levels of anxiety in pregnant or postpartum women is therefore important in its own right and enables targeted interventions to help reduce women's distress.

Furthermore, anxiety in pregnancy is associated with poorer outcomes for infants and children (see Chapter 1). Poor birth and infant outcomes, such as complications in labor, low birth weight, low Apgar scores, and detrimental changes in the fetal heart rate and motor activity, are associated with anxiety in pregnancy (Berle et al., 2005; DiPietro, 2010; Field et al., 2010; Johnson & Slade, 2003; Teixeira, Fisk, & Glover, 1999). After birth, studies suggest that prenatal anxiety predicts child behavior problems from infancy through to teenage years, including attention problems, conduct disorder, and emotional problems aged 4–6 (O'Connor, Heron, Golding, Beveridge, & Glover, 2002; O'Connor, Heron, Golding, Glover, & The ALSPAC Study Team, 2003); ADHD and externalizing behavior problems aged 8–9 (Van den Bergh & Marcoen, 2004); and high impulsivity and low scores on cognitive tests aged 14–15 (Van den Bergh et al., 2005). Similarly, maternal anxiety after birth is associated with emotional and conduct problems and increased somatic symptoms in children (Glasheen, Richardson, & Fabio, 2010). Helping women who have high levels of anxiety during their pregnancy is therefore important for both women and their developing infant.

Much of the research on the impact of anxiety relies on self-report measures of anxiety *symptoms* as opposed to structured clinical interviews assessing anxiety *disorders*. This suggests that high anxiety symptoms are clinically significant in terms of the impact on women and their children (Glasheen et al., 2010; Rucci et al., 2003). It is likely that the effects of anxiety disorders may be even more severe. However, information on the prevalence and course of anxiety over the perinatal period is mixed.

Prevalence

Use of different time points and measures of perinatal anxiety means it is hard to draw an overall picture of the prevalence of perinatal anxiety. Large epidemiological studies of postnatal anxiety report varying prevalence rates and patterns of anxiety between pregnancy and the postpartum period. For example, a large epidemiological study of over 8000 women in the United Kingdom reported that women's symptoms of anxiety were stable throughout pregnancy with a small drop after birth (Heron et al., 2004). In contrast, a large cohort longitudinal study of maternal mental health in Australia found an increase in anxiety after birth, with 7.3% of women experiencing intense anxiety or panic attacks occasionally or often during pregnancy, increasing to 15.7% in the first three months' postpartum (Woolhouse, Brown, Krastev, Perlen, & Gunn, 2009).

In terms of anxiety disorders, research using structured clinical interviews suggests that GAD is most common and experienced by between 1.9% and 8.2% of women 6–8 weeks' postpartum (Ballard, Davis, Handy, & Mohan, 1993; Matthey et al., 2003; Wenzel, Haugen, Jackson, & Brendle, 2005). A study of women referred for perinatal psychiatric treatment found that the most common primary diagnosis was GAD followed by major depressive episode, with a high level of comorbidity (Grigoriadis et al., 2011). The prevalence of both GAD and obsessive–compulsive disorder is higher in perinatal samples than the general population (Ross & McLean, 2006). The prevalence of panic disorder (1.4%; Wenzel et al., 2005) and posttraumatic stress disorder (1.7–9%; Beck, Gable, Sakala, & Declercq, 2011) is comparable to the general population (Ross & McLean, 2006).

In addition, a substantial proportion of women experience high levels of anxiety but do not fulfill all diagnostic criteria. For example, in a study where 8.2% of postpartum women had GAD, a further 19.7% of women were classified as having subsyndromal GAD (Wenzel et al., 2005). This is consistent with evidence from the general population in primary care that an equal if not higher number of people experience subsyndromal anxiety (Olfson et al., 1996; Rucci et al., 2003) with similar levels of distress, disability, and poor subjective health as those who have the diagnosed disorder (Rucci et al., 2003).

Relevance of Standard Diagnostic Criteria to Perinatal Women

Given the prevalence of subthreshold anxiety symptoms in the perinatal population, it may be useful to develop and use other approaches in combination with standard diagnostic criteria. While the current "gold standard" of measuring mental health problems in the perinatal period is to use clinical diagnostic interviews based on DSM or ICD criteria for the relevant disorder, diagnostic criteria may not account for all perinatal-specific problems. Using diagnostic criteria for women in the perinatal period has been questioned by some (Liebowitz, 1993; Martini, Knappe, Beesdo-Baum, Lieb, & Wittchen, 2010; Matthey & Ross-Hamid, 2011; van Praag, Rodney, & Parker, 1998). For example, Phillips, Sharpe, Matthey, and Charles (2009) found that just as many women in their sample were diagnosed with "anxiety disorder not otherwise specified" as those with GAD.

There may be perinatal-specific problems which are not covered by standard psychiatric classifications. For example, Phillips et al. (2009) described maternally focused worry disorder with most women in this category experiencing uncontrollable worry about motherhood or their infant. Other perinatal-specific anxiety problems include severe fear of childbirth (tocophobia; Hofberg & Brockington, 2000) or bonding disorders (Klier, 2006). Scales focusing on specific perinatal anxiety may predict important outcomes and be relevant to targeting of primary and secondary interventions. For example, pregnancy-specific anxiety scales have been shown to be a better predictor of poor birth and developmental outcomes than general stress scales (Buss, Davis, Muftuler, Head, & Sandman, 2010; DiPietro, Hilton, Hawkins, Costigan, & Pressman, 2002; Huizink, Robles de Medina, Mulder, Visser, & Buitelaar, 2003; Roesch, Schetter, Woo, & Hobel, 2004; Wadhwa, Sandman, Porto, Dunkel-Schetter, & Garite, 1993).

A final concern is that perinatal symptoms and issues common among new mothers, such as sleep deprivation, can inflate diagnostic symptoms and be misinterpreted as pathological. For example, symptoms of GAD include feeling tired and having difficulty sleeping which are common for women looking after a new baby. Similarly, some somatic symptoms common in pregnancy can overlap with anxiety symptoms such as palpitations, numbness, and sweaty hands. The rates of anxiety disorders, particularly GAD, may therefore be overestimated if using diagnostic criteria (Matthey & Ross-Hamid, 2011). Conversely, such symptoms may be discounted as part of the common experience of being pregnant, resulting in underdiagnosis. Skilled clinicians therefore need to try to disentangle symptoms of mental health problems from nonpathological aspects of pregnancy and the postpartum.

The usefulness, or not, of standard diagnostic criteria to perinatal anxiety raises the possibility of other approaches to using diagnostic criteria as the gold standard against which to determine cutoff scores or criteria for probable anxiety. One alternative is to use norma-tive data for self-report anxiety measures to identify the top percentile of women with extreme anxiety. Which percentile is used needs further examination and could be based on different criteria such as expected prevalence of clinically significant anxiety or a woman's need for treatment. For example, if we expect 15% of women to have clinically significant anxiety, we would use the 85% percentile to determine the appropriate cutoffs. In order to use this approach, normative data need to be available on each measure for pregnancy.

Best-practice approach therefore suggests that provision of treatment should be based not only on diagnostic criteria but a full psychosocial assessment (see Chapter 8).

Issues to Consider When Measuring Perinatal Anxiety

When measuring anxiety during pregnancy and after birth, we need to consider measurement validity, what is meant by a "gold standard," the purpose and timing of measurement, whether we are measuring transient or enduring anxiety, and the conceptual overlap between anxiety and general measures of distress. These questions are considered in turn in the following text.

Purpose of measurement

The first issue to consider when contemplating measuring perinatal anxiety is the purpose of the measurement and the context in which it is applied. In a clinical context, the purpose of measurement is usually to identify women who require help or treatment. The focus at this stage is on detecting whether a woman is having difficulties with anxiety or psychological problems for which she would like help. Further detailed assessment can then ascertain the more precise nature of her difficulties and work out which referral or treatment is most appropriate.

In a research context, anxiety is commonly measured to examine the relationship bet-ween anxiety and other outcomes, or to report rates of women scoring "high," or who are "probably anxious." Use of different measures and cutoff scores means that rates of anxiety reported in different studies are often not comparable.

Transient versus enduring anxiety

Whether screening is used in clinical or research contexts, current evidence suggests that anxiety should be measured at least twice over a period of a few weeks to distinguish bet-ween transient and enduring distress (Ballestrem, Strauss, & Kächele, 2005; Matthey & Ross-Hamid, 2012; Wickberg & Hwang, 1996). Identifying women on the basis of a state measure of anxiety taken at one time point could result in many women being identified as anxious when this is not the case (i.e., false positives) as it is common to have a few anxious days which are not representative of general mood. Empirical studies have shown that such transient mood difficulties are common in the perinatal period. For example, studies of postnatal depression indicate that more than half of women who score as having "probable depression" on the Edinburgh Postnatal Depression Scale (EPDS) do not have ongoing mood difficulties (Ballestrem et al., 2005; Wickberg & Hwang, 1996). There is evidence that this is also true for anxiety in pregnancy, with Matthey and Ross-Hamid (2012) showing that around 50% of women scoring "high" on anxiety (or depression) measures are no longer highly anxious (or depressed) 2 weeks later.

Thus, whether screening for anxiety or depression, the distinction should always be made between transient and enduring symptoms. In the clinical context, questions such as "Why do you think you're feeling this way?" and "How do you think you may be feeling in 2 weeks or so?" can be asked in the context of a broader psychosocial assessment (see Chapter 8). Ignoring these questions and referring all "high scorers" to specialist health services, or reporting rates of women with "high anxiety" based upon single administration of an anxiety scale, may pathologize transient symptoms. A consequence of this is that health-care resources may not be used efficiently.

Timing of screening

An important consideration is when to screen for anxiety. Screening in pregnancy has the potential to identify women who are at risk of worse birth outcomes and postpartum psychological problems. This in turn would enable early intervention in pregnancy. However, the issue of transient anxiety is particularly pertinent. There is some consensus that during pregnancy, anxiety is higher in the first and third trimesters (e.g., Da Costa, Larouche, Dritsa, & Brender, 2000; Fertl, Bergner, Beyer, Klapp, & Rauchfuss, 2009; Figueiredo & Conde, 2011). In the second trimester, anxiety may be lower because normal stressors are likely to have dissipated, such as morning sickness, initial concern over the baby's development, and adjusting to the realization of being pregnant. In the third trimester, anxiety might increase as a result of increasing physical limitations and the prospect of labor and birth. However, there is substantial variation across women (Heron et al., 2004). For example, a woman who has had a previous late miscarriage or stillbirth is likely to continue to be highly anxious throughout pregnancy.

In the United Kingdom, screening for postnatal anxiety and depression has traditionally been done at six to eight weeks' postpartum which coincides with visits from health-care professionals and health reviews for the new baby (Department of Health, 2009). On the one hand, this is a time when women may have recovered physically from the birth and have become used to coping with the new baby, so ratings may be a better indication of enduring anxiety. On the other hand, this may be a time when support from family, partners, and health-care professionals is reduced and women may become anxious about being the sole carer of her child for much of the time. As with pregnancy, there is also considerable variability across women with respect to when and why they may feel highly anxious after birth, suggesting a need for further research.

It is therefore likely that, given current evidence, there is no "absolutely best" time to screen for anxiety in pregnancy or after birth. Rather, we need to be mindful of normal, potentially transient changes in anxiety. The following factors can be used as a guide for when to screen for anxiety: (i) from a pragmatic perspective, it is easier to screen at a time when most women are in contact with health services; (ii) screening early in pregnancy is preferable if the aim is to intervene to reduce levels of anxiety and impact on the fetus; and (iii) repeat testing is advisable for women scoring in the "highly anxious or distressed" range. This latter point can be facilitated by brief screening tools that can be used at antenatal and postnatal visits. This is examined in the next section which considers both diagnostic interviews and psychometric questionnaires, as well as the distinction between instruments designed specifically for screening and those designed to give a clinical reading of symptom severity.

Diagnostic Interviews to Assess Anxiety

As described previously, the current "gold standard" of measuring mental health problems in the perinatal period is to use clinical diagnostic interviews based on DSM or ICD criteria for the relevant disorder. Diagnosis takes place via use of a diagnostic interview with a practitioner trained in using the interview. Diagnostic interviews can be semistructured or highly structured. This section briefly outlines some of the diagnostic interviews commonly used in perinatal research and practice.

Structured Clinical Interview for DSM-IV Axis I Disorders diagnosis

The Structured Clinical Interview for DSM-IV Axis I Disorders (SCID-I) (First, Gibbon, Spitzer, & Williams, 2002) is a semistructured interview for current and lifetime history of DSM-IV disorders. Screening questions relating to current and lifetime experience of the individual anxiety disorders are asked, and women responding positively can then be interviewed using the relevant section(s) of the anxiety disorders module. In some studies, GAD duration criteria have been altered to identify generalized anxiety since childbirth (rather than the 6-month duration criterion usually used; Matthey et al., 2003; Wenzel et al., 2005).

Mini-International Neuropsychiatric Interview

The Mini-International Neuropsychiatric Interview (MINI) (Sheehan et al., 1998) was designed to be compatible with international diagnostic criteria to diagnose common mental health disorders and is considerably shorter (~15 min administration time) than other diagnostic interviews. It has shown reliability and established validity when compared to the SCID and expert professional opinion (Sheehan et al., 1998). It can be administered by lay interviewers who have undergone training as well as trained mental health professionals. The MINI can detect lifetime and current mania and panic disorder and current agoraphobia, social phobia, specific phobia, obsessive–compulsive disorder, GAD, and posttraumatic stress disorder. "Current" is defined as "in the past month" for all diagnoses except GAD, which has a 6-month time frame.

The Composite International Diagnostic Interview

Robins, Helzer, Croughan, and Ratcliff (1988) devised the Composite International Diagnostic Interview (CIDI) primarily for use in epidemiological studies across different cultures and settings. It is widely used in clinics and for research. Symptom questions, clinical probe questions, and time-related questions of first and last occurrence of a syndrome or diagnosis are highly standardized, resulting in a high level of consistency of symptom assessment and reliability of diagnostic decisions (Wittchen, 1993). The CIDI has highly detailed instructions allowing nonclinicians to use it reliably after a period of comprehensive training in a World Health Organization-designated center (Wittchen, 1993). Symptom questions assess mental disorders according to definitions and criteria of both the DSM and the ICD. Modules assessing anxiety disorders (panic, agoraphobia, social phobia, simple phobia, and GAD) and posttraumatic stress disorder are available. The CIDI has proven reliable in terms of consistency between two interviewers and is time efficient (Wittchen, 1993).

Questionnaire Measures of Anxiety

There are many questionnaire measures of anxiety—both for general anxiety symptoms and for pregnancy or postpartum-related anxiety. In this section, we outline a few of the most commonly used measures with information on reliability and validity. More detailed reviews can be found elsewhere (Meades & Ayers, 2011). New questionnaire measures of mental health are also being developed and evaluated in other populations, for example, the Kessler-10 (Kessler et al., 2002) and CORE-10 (Barkham et al., 2013). These are promising but not included here because they have not yet been widely used or evaluated with perinatal women.

State-Trait Anxiety Inventory

The State-Trait Anxiety Inventory (STAI) (Spielberger, Gorsuch, & Lushene, 1970) shows acceptable reliability and has been widely validated. It is one of the most commonly used measures of anxiety symptoms (Glasheen et al., 2010). It comprises two scales each with 20 items: a state anxiety scale and a trait anxiety scale. The state scale's instructions are for the respondent to indicate how he/she feels "*right* now, that is, *at this moment*" (original italics). Unfortunately, the state measure has been used frequently in perinatal studies where the exact "moment" being measured has not been standardized or controlled, thus making findings questionable. For example, Aktan (2012) reports having participants complete the STAI-S at home, and Paul, Downs, Schaefer, Beiler, and Weisman (2013) administered the measure to participants over the phone. In both cases, it is not possible to know what was happening for the women at the moment when they completed the scale—some may have been stressed if, for example, they had just had an argument, while others may have been more relaxed due to circumstances at that time.

In addition, items such as "I feel comfortable" and "I am relaxed" may be affected by the normal sequelae of the physical changes during pregnancy, such as becoming larger (and thus feeling uncomfortable, and not relaxed). Given the requirement for women to complete the items for how she is feeling "*right* now," it is likely that for some women, this will detect transient anxiety, much of which could be normal (e.g., concern over the health of the baby), and not just enduring anxiety. The state version should therefore only be used when assessing anxiety in a specific situation (e.g., just before an ultrasound scan) that can be standardized across all the participants. Further, consideration should be given to items that could be affected by normal physical changes of pregnancy (or the postpartum).

The trait subscale measures a more general or enduring individual tendency to react with heightened anxiety. Symptoms are endorsed on a four-point scale (1–4); thus, the maximum score on one scale is 80. Examples of items are "I am a steady person" and "I lack self-confidence." Both scales correlate highly with measures of depression (Stuart, Couser,

Schilder, O'Hara, & Gorman, 1998). A shorter six-item scale has been developed and validated for use in pregnant women with correlations of >0.90 between the original and shorter version scores (Marteau & Bekker, 1992).

In perinatal samples, the cutoff scores used for the 20-item trait scale vary. For example, Barnett and Parker (1985) used 32 or more for "moderate" anxiety and 45 or more for "high" anxiety in women 3 weeks' postpartum. However, Grant, McMahon, and Austin (2008) found that scoring 41 or more gave the best sensitivity, specificity, and positive and negative predictive values to identify cases of anxiety in late pregnancy and was associated with a sixfold increase in postnatal anxiety disorders and depression. The trait scale also seems to be affected by anxious state in perinatal samples, as test–retest correlations range between 0.37 and 0.85 and lower scores are found after birth (Hundley, Gurney, Graham, & Rennie, 1998).

Hospital Anxiety and Depression Scale-Anxiety subscale

The Hospital Anxiety and Depression Scale (HADS) (Zigmond & Snaith, 1983) consists of two subscales of depression and anxiety, which each have seven items. Anxiety items are general, for example, "I get sudden feelings of panic" and "Worrying thoughts go through my mind." However, a few items may be confounded by symptoms of pregnancy, for example, "I can sit at ease and feel relaxed" and "I feel restless as if I have to be on the move." Symptoms are endorsed on a four-point scale (0–3) over the last 7 days; thus, the maximum score is 21. Scores of 0–7 are considered "normal," 8–10 are suggestive of anxiety, and 11 or more indicates probable disorder (Snaith, 2003). Validation of cutoffs suggests a lack of consistency. In a nonperinatal sample, Bjelland et al. (2002) found that a score of 8 or above gives optimal sensitivity and specificity. This has subsequently been used in three studies validating the HADS-A (the anxiety scale) in pregnancy. However, this cutoff resulted in unusually high prevalence rates in UK (36–56%) and Uzbekistani (38–42%) samples (Jomeen & Martin, 2005; Karimova & Martin, 2003). A recent study found that a cutoff score of 9 or more identified the top 15% of English-speaking women on this measure in their sample (Matthey, Valenti, Souter, & Ross-Hamid, 2013b).

The HADS-A does not correlate highly with other measures of anxiety, for example, the Edinburgh Postnatal Depression Scale-Anxiety (EPDS-3A) (described in the following text) indicating these measures pick up different facets of anxiety (Matthey et al., 2013b). The factor structure of the HADS is also unclear with between 2 and 5 factors being found including both depression and anxiety items (Bjelland, Dahl, Haug, & Neckelmann, 2002; Jomeen & Martin, 2005; Karimova & Martin, 2003). However, internal reliability is usually good (Karimova & Martin, 2003). Studies validating the Hospital Anxiety and Depression Scale-Anxiety (HADS-A) in postpartum samples are scarce so that further work is needed.

EPDS-3A

Although not designed to detect anxiety, a review of research suggests that three items on the EPDS (Cox, Holden, & Sagovsky, 1987) can be used to detect anxiety in perinatal women (Matthey, Fisher, & Rowe, 2013a). The items are "I have blamed myself unnecessarily when things went wrong," "I have been anxious or worried for no good reason," and "I have felt scared or panicky for no very good reason." These load onto an anxiety subscale in factor analyses in ante- and postnatal populations, and there is also some evidence to suggest that the subscale can distinguish anxious and depressive disorders (Bowen, Bowen, Maslany, & Muhajarina, 2008; Matthey et al., 2013a; Ross, Evans, Sellers, & Romach, 2003). However, other studies suggest that separate subscale scores may not be accurate (Reichenheim, Moraes, Oliveira, & Lobato, 2011) and that using the usual total scale cutoff (i.e., 13 or more) might not identify all women with anxiety disorders (Matthey, 2008). Further research examining this is therefore needed. Scores range from 0 to 9 for the anxiety subscale and 0 to 30 for the total EPDS.

Pregnancy-Specific Measures of Anxiety

Specific measures of anxiety during pregnancy are available, although there is sometimes conceptual overlap between these and measures of pregnancy-related worries, stress, and distress, which often include anxiety-type affective items. For example, a review of pregnancy stress measures identified 15 questionnaires which broadly fell into either stressor measures, emotional response measures (e.g., anxiety), or multidimensional measures (Alderdice, Lynn, & Lobel, 2012). Three pregnancy-specific anxiety measures are outlined briefly in the following text.

Pregnancy-Related Anxiety Questionnaire

The Pregnancy-Related Anxiety Questionnaire (PRAQ) (Van den Bergh, 1989, 1990) is the longest scale available with 55 items covering five subscales of fear of delivery (9 items), fear of bearing a handicapped child (6 items), concerns about partner relations (11 items), concerns about mood (11 items), and fear of change (8 items). Responses are rated on a Likert scale from 1 to 7 giving a possible range of 55 to 385. Internal reliability is good (van Bussel, Spitz, & Demyttenaere, 2009), but no other psychometric information is available. Shorter 34-item and 10-item versions have been developed using factor analysis (Gutteling et al., 2006; Huizink, Mulder, Robles de Medina, Visser, & Buitelaar, 2004; Huizink, Robles de Medina, Mulder, Visser, & Buitelaar, 2002) with three subscales identified: fear of birth (e.g., "I am worried about the pain of contractions and the pain during delivery"), fear of bearing a handicapped child (e.g., "I am worried that the baby will be abnormal"), and pregnancy-related concerns about one's appearance (e.g., "I am worried about the fact that I shall not regain my figure after delivery"). The shorter versions of the PRAQ are associated with perceived stress, hassles, and alcohol use in pregnancy (Arch, 2013; Gutteling et al., 2006; Huizink et al., 2004, 2002).

Pregnancy Anxiety Scale

The Pregnancy Anxiety Scale (PAS) (Levin, 1991) is a brief and retrospective questionnaire of 10 items that measure anxiety about being pregnant (3 items, e.g., "Did you fear that you would fall and hurt your baby?"), giving birth (4 items, e.g., "Were you afraid the pain of childbirth would be bad?"), or being in hospital (3 items, e.g., "Were you afraid you would be alone the hospital?"). Responses are true/false giving a possible range of 0–10. The scale was extracted from 25 items using confirmatory factor analysis (Levin, 1991). Although the scale has been used in a few subsequent studies (e.g., Poikkeus et al., 2006), very little additional information on reliability and validity is available. There is also no information on optimal cutoffs or the point at which anxiety becomes clinically meaningful.

Pregnancy-Specific Anxiety Scale

The Pregnancy-Specific Anxiety Scale (PSAS) (Roesch et al., 2004) is a very short 4-item questionnaire which was extracted from a larger pool of items using factor analysis. Items are similar to the STAI in that they ask how often women have felt anxious, concerned, afraid, and panicky in the last week, but in the context of pregnancy. Responses are scored from 1 to 5, giving a possible range of 4 to 20. The PSAS has been used in various studies with inconsistent results. For example, it has been associated with shorter gestation (Roesch et al., 2004) and preterm birth (Kramer et al., 2009), but this was not replicated in a sample of African American women (Dominguez, Schetter, Mancuso, Rini, & Hobel, 2005). Internal reliability is also low in some instances (Roesch et al., 2004).

Whether to Measure Anxiety or General Distress

One further question that arises when measuring perinatal anxiety is whether it is more appropriate to use a specific measure of anxiety or a measure of general distress. This is likely to vary according to the purpose and context in which screening takes place. For research, a specific measure of anxiety with good criterion validity is essential if we are to further understand the causes and consequences of perinatal anxiety. However, in the clinical context, it may be useful to use one or two general questions to get a quick screen for any perinatal distress, regardless of whether it is "anxiety," "stress," or "depression" as a guide for later follow-up. Such questions are currently available, but further research is required to ascertain their sensitivity and specificity so that the clinician can have confidence in their use. Two examples are the Whooley questions for depression (Whooley, Avins, Miranda, & Browner, 1997) used by UK health services to screen for depression in pregnancy and after birth, and the Matthey Generic Mood Question (MGMQ) in Box 6.1 which have been developed and piloted in Australia (Matthey et al., 2013b).

Conclusion and Recommendations

In summary, anxiety symptoms are common in pregnancy and after childbirth, and some disorders, such as GAD, are more prevalent during this time. However, diagnostic criteria may be confounded by symptoms that are normal in pregnancy and the postpartum period and may not recognize perinatal-specific problems, such as fear of birth or worries about the baby. There is also evidence that those who do not fulfill diagnostic criteria but have subsyndromal symptoms may report similar levels of distress, disability, and poor subjective health.

Issues that need to be considered before screening for anxiety include considering what we are screening for, when the best time is to screen, and to ensure screening is not confounded by normal fluctuations in anxiety during pregnancy and after childbirth. In terms of screening tools, a range of general anxiety and pregnancy-specific anxiety questionnaires are available, with varying reliability and validity. Questionnaires vary in the symptoms

---

Box 6.1   The Matthey Generic Mood Question (MGMQ)

Q.1a	In the last 2 weeks, have you felt very stressed, anxious, or unhappy or found it difficult to cope,* for some of the time?	Yes *(go to Q.1b)* Possibly *(go to Q.1b)* No
Q.1b	How bothered have you been by these feelings?	Not at all A little bit Moderately *(go to Q.1c)* A lot *(go to Q.1c)*
Q.1c	Is there anything in particular that is making you feel this way?	*Describe*

From Matthey et al. (2013b). Reproduced with permission from Elsevier.
*The author is investigating the inclusion of the word "manage" to this question.

---

they focus on, and therefore, concordance between them can be poor. There is also often conceptual overlap with measures of stress, distress, and worry. Where cutoffs are available, these are usually determined by comparison with diagnostic criteria.

On the basis of the evidence covered in this chapter, we can make a number of recommendations. The first is that anxiety screening needs to be repeated to avoid overpathologizing transient distress. Secondly, in clinical contexts, it may be useful to use a 2-stage process where brief screening questions are used to identify women with *any* emotional distress who may benefit from a more detailed assessment at a subsequent stage, although further research evaluating this approach is needed. Finally, there are a number of anxiety questionnaires available that have different strengths and weaknesses. Choice of measure will be highly dependent on the purpose and context in which it is to be used. The STAI has been most validated and may be useful in research as a specific measure of anxiety. The HADS-A has shown good reliability in pregnancy. New measures are also being investigated which appear promising (e.g., Kessler-10). However, more research is needed on the validity of different measures in perinatal women and to provide normative data for measures at different time points so appropriate cutoffs can be identified. Similarly, research needs to examine men's anxiety during this time and consider the respective measurement issues.

References

Aktan, N. M. (2012). Social support and anxiety in pregnant and postpartum women: A secondary analysis. *Clinical Nursing Research, 21*, 183–194.

Alderdice, F., Lynn, F., & Lobel, M. (2012). A review and psychometric evaluation of pregnancy-specific stress measures. *Journal of Psychosomatic Obstetrics & Gynecology, 33*(2), 62–77.

American Psychiatric Association. (2013). *Diagnostic and statistical manual of mental disorders* (5th ed.). Arlington, VA: American Psychiatric Publishing.

Arch, J. J. (2013). Pregnancy-specific anxiety: Which women are highest and what are the alcohol-related risks? *Comprehensive Psychiatry, 54*(3), 217–228.

Austin, M. P., Tully, L., & Parker, G. (2007). Examining the relationship between antenatal anxiety and postnatal depression. *Journal of Affective Disorders, 101*(1–3), 169–174.

Ballard, C. G., Davis, R. E., Handy, S., & Mohan, R. M. C. (1993). Postpartum anxiety in mothers and fathers. *European Journal of Psychiatry, 7*, 117–121.

Ballestrem, C.-L. V., Strauss, M., & Kächele, H. (2005). Contribution to the epidemiology of postnatal depression in Germany—Implications for the utilization of treatment. *Archives of Women's Mental Health, 8*, 29–35.

Barkham, M., Bewick, B., Mullin, T., Gilbody, S., Connell, J., Cahill, J., … Evans, C. (2013). The CORE-10: A short measure of psychological distress for routine use in the psychological therapies. *Counselling and Psychotherapy Research: Linking Research with Practice, 13*(1), 3–13.

Barnett, B., & Parker, G. (1985). Professional and non-professional intervention for highly anxious primiparous mothers. *British Journal of Psychiatry, 146*, 287–293.

Beck, C. T., Gable, R. K., Sakala, C., & Declercq, E. R. (2011). Posttraumatic stress disorder in new mothers: Results from a two-stage U.S. National Survey. *Birth, 38*(3), 216–227.

Berle, J. O., Mykletun, A., Daltveit, A. K., Rasmussen, S. A., Holsten, F., & Dahl, A. A. (2005). Neonatal outcomes in offspring of women with anxiety and depression during pregnancy. A linkage study from the Nord-Trondelag Health Study (HUNT) and Medical Birth Registry of Norway. *Archives of Women's Mental Health, 8*, 181–189.

Bjelland, I., Dahl, A. A., Haug, T. T., & Neckelmann, D. (2002). The validity of the Hospital Anxiety and Depression Scale; an updated review. *Journal of Psychosomatic Research, 52*, 69–77.

Bowen, A., Bowen, R., Maslany, G., Muhajarina, N. (2008). Anxiety in a socially-high-risk sample of pregnant women in Canada. *Canadian Journal of Psychiatry, 53*, 435–440.

Buss, C., Davis, E. P., Muftuler, L. T., Head, K., & Sandman, C. A. (2010). High pregnancy anxiety during mid-gestation is associated with decreased gray matter density in 6–9-year-old children. *Psychoneuroendocrinology, 35*(1), 141–153.

Cox, J. L., Holden, J. M. C., Sagovsky, R. (1987). Detection of postnatal depression: Development of the 10-item Edinburgh Postnatal Depression scale. *British Journal of Psychiatry, 150*, 782–786.

Da Costa, D., Larouche, J., Dritsa, M., & Brender, W. (2000). Psychosocial correlates of prepartum and postpartum depressed mood. *Journal of Affective Disorders, 59*, 31–40.

Department of Health. (2009). *The Healthy Child Programme—Pregnancy and the first five years of life*. Retrieved from https://www.gov.uk/government/publications/healthy-child-programme-pregnancy-and-the-first-5-years-of-life. Accessed December 16, 2014.

DiPietro, J. A. (2010). Psychological and psychophysiological considerations regarding the maternal-fetal relationship. *Infant and Child Development, 19*, 27–38.

DiPietro, J. A., Hilton, S. C., Hawkins, M., Costigan, K. A., & Pressman, E. K. (2002). Maternal stress and affect influence fetal neurobehavioral development. *Developmental Psychology, 38*(5), 659–668.

Dominguez, T. P., Schetter, C. D., Mancuso, R. A., Rini, C. M., & Hobel, C. J. (2005). Stress in African American pregnancies: Testing the roles of various stress concepts in prediction of birth outcomes. *Annals of Behavioral Medicine, 29*, 12–21.

Fertl, K. I., Bergner, A., Beyer, R., Klapp, B. F., & Rauchfuss, M. (2009). Levels and effects of different forms of anxiety during pregnancy after a prior miscarriage. *European Journal of Obstetrics & Gynecology and Reproductive Biology, 142*, 23–29.

Field, T. A., Diego, M., Hernandez-Reif, M., Figueiredo, B., Deeds, O., Ascencio, A., … Kuhn, C. (2010). Comorbid depression and anxiety effects on pregnancy and neonatal outcome. *Infant Behavior and Development, 33*, 23–29.

Figueiredo, B., & Conde, A. (2011). Anxiety and depression symptoms in women and men from early pregnancy to 3-months postpartum: Parity differences and effects. *Journal of Affective Disorders, 132*, 146–157.

First, M. B., Gibbon, M., Spitzer, R. L., Williams, J. W. (2002). *Users Guide to the Structured Clinical Interview for DSM-IV-TR Axis I Disorders—Research Version (SCID-I for DSM-IV-TR, November 2002 revision)*. New York, NY: New York State Psychiatric Institute.

Glasheen, C., Richardson, G. A., & Fabio, A. (2010). A systematic review of the effects of postnatal maternal anxiety on children. *Archives of Women's Mental Health, 13*, 61–74.

Grant, K. A., McMahon, C., & Austin, M. P. (2008). Maternal anxiety during the transition to parenthood: A prospective study. *Journal of Affective Disorders, 108*, 101–111.

Grigoriadis, S., De Camps Meschino, D., Barrons, E., Bradley, L. S., Eady, A., Fishell, A., … Ross, L. E. (2011). Mood and anxiety disorders in a sample of Canadian perinatal women referred for psychiatric care. *Archives of Women's Mental Health, 14*(4), 325–333.

Gutteling, B. M., de Weerth, C., Zandbelt, N., Mulder, E. J. H., Visser, G. H. A., & Buitelaar, J. K. (2006). Does maternal prenatal stress adversely affect the child's learning and memory at age six? *Journal of Abnormal Child Psychology, 34*, 789–798.

Heron, J., O'Connor, T. G., Evans, J., Golding, J., Glover, V., & The ALSPAC Study Team. (2004). The course of anxiety and depression through pregnancy and the postpartum in a community sample. *Journal of Affective Disorders, 80*, 65–73.

Hofberg, K. R., & Brockington, I. (2000). Tokophobia: An unreasoning dread of childbirth. A series of 26 cases. *British Journal of Psychiatry, 176*, 83–85.

Huizink, A. C., Mulder, E. J. H., Robles de Medina, P. G., Visser, G. H. A., & Buitelaar, J. K. (2004). Is pregnancy anxiety a distinctive syndrome? *Early Human Development, 79*, 81–91.

Huizink, A. C., Robles de Medina, P. G., Mulder, E. J. H., Visser, G. H. A., & Buitelaar, J. K. (2002). Psychological measures of prenatal stress as predictors of infant temperament. *Journal of the American Academy of Child and Adolescent Psychiatry, 41*, 1078–1085.

Huizink, A. C., Robles De Medina, P. G., Mulder, E. J. H. Visser, G. H. A., & Buitelaar, J. K. (2003). Stress during pregnancy is associated with developmental outcome in infancy. *Journal of Child Psychology and Psychiatry, and Allied Disciplines, 44*(6), 810–818.

Hundley, V. A., Gurney, E., Graham, W. J., & Rennie, A. M. (1998). Can anxiety in pregnant women be measured using the State-Trait Anxiety Inventory? *Midwifery, 14*, 118–121.

Johnson, R. C., & Slade, P. D. (2003). Obstetric complications and anxiety during pregnancy: Is there a relationship? *Journal of Psychosomatic Obstetrics and Gynecology, 24*, 1–14.

Jomeen, J., & Martin, C. R. (2005). Confirmation of an occluded anxiety component within the Edinburgh Postnatal Depression Scale (EPDS) during pregnancy. *Journal of Reproductive and Infant Psychology, 23*, 143–154.

Karimova, G. K., & Martin, C. R. (2003). A psychometric evaluation of the Hospital Anxiety and Depression Scale during pregnancy. *Psychology, Health and Medicine, 8*, 89–103.

Kessler, R. C., Andrews, G., Colpe, L. J., Hiripi, E., Mroczek, D. K., Normand, S.-L., … Zaslavsky, A. M. (2002). Short screening scales to monitor population prevalences and trends in non-specific psychological distress. *Psychological Medicine, 32*, 959–976.

Klier, C. M. (2006). Mother-infant bonding disorders in patients with postnatal depression: The postpartum bonding questionnaire in clinical practice. *Archives of Women's Mental Health, 9*(5), 289–291.

Kramer, M. S., Lydon, J., Seguin, L., Goulet, L., Kahn, S. R., McNamara, H., … Platt, R. W. (2009). Stress pathways to spontaneous preterm birth: The role of stressors, psychological distress, and stress hormones. *American Journal of Epidemiology, 169*, 1319–1326.

Levin, J. S. (1991). The factor structure of the Pregnancy Anxiety Scale. *Journal of Health and Social Behavior, 32*, 368–381.

Liebowitz, M. R. (1993). Mixed anxiety and depression: Should it be included in DSM-IV? *Journal of Clinical Psychiatry, 54*(5 Suppl.), 4–7.

Marteau, T. M., & Bekker, H. L. (1992). The development of a six-item short form of the state scale of the Spielberger State-Trait Anxiety Inventory (STAI). *British Journal of Clinical Psychology, 31*, 301–306.

Martini, J., Knappe, S., Beesdo-Baum, K., Lieb, R., & Wittchen, H. U. (2010). Anxiety disorders before birth and self-perceived distress during pregnancy: Associations with maternal depression and obstetric, neonatal and early childhood outcomes. *Early Human Development, 86*(5), 305–310.

Matthey, S. (2008). Using the Edinburgh postnatal depression scale to screen for anxiety disorders. *Depression and Anxiety, 25*(11), 926–931.

Matthey, S., Barnett, B., Howie, P. M., Kavanagh, D. J. (2003). Diagnosing postpartum depression in mothers and fathers: Whatever happened to anxiety? *Journal of Affective Disorders, 74*, 139–147.

Matthey, S., Fisher, J. R. W., & Rowe, H. (2013a). Using the Edinburgh postnatal depression scale to screen for anxiety disorders: Conceptual and methodological considerations. *Journal of Affective Disorders, 146,* 224–230.

Matthey, S., & Ross-Hamid, C. (2011). The validity of DSM symptoms for depression and anxiety disorders during pregnancy. *Journal of Affective Disorders, 133*(3), 546–552.

Matthey, S., & Ross-Hamid, C. (2012). Repeat testing on the Edinburgh depression scale and the HADS-A in pregnancy: Differentiating between transient and enduring distress. *Journal of Affective Disorders, 141,* 213–221.

Matthey, S., Valenti, B., Souter, K., & Ross-Hamid, C. (2013b). Comparison of four self-report measures and a generic mood question to screen for anxiety during pregnancy in English-speaking women. *Journal of Affective Disorders, 148,* 347–351.

Mauri, M., Oppo, A., Montagnani, M. S., Borri, C., Banti, S., Camilleri, V., … Cassano, G. B. (2010). Beyond "postpartum depressions": Specific anxiety diagnoses during pregnancy predict different outcomes: Results from PND-ReScU. *Journal of Affective Disorders, 127*(1–3), 177–184.

Meades, R., & Ayers, S. (2011). Anxiety measures validated in perinatal populations: A systematic review. *Journal of Affective Disorders, 133*(1–2), 1–15.

Milgrom, J., Gemmill, A. W., Bilszta, J. L., Hayes, B., Barnett, B., Brooks, J., … Buist, A. (2008). Antenatal risk factors for postnatal depression: A large prospective study. *Journal of Affective Disorders, 108*(1–2), 147–157.

O'Connor, T. G., Heron, J., Golding, J., Beveridge, M., & Glover, V. (2002). Maternal antenatal anxiety and children's behavioral/emotional problems at 4 years. *British Journal of Psychiatry, 180,* 502–508.

O'Connor, T. G., Heron, J., Golding, J., Glover, V., & The ALSPAC Study Team. (2003). Maternal anxiety and behavioural/emotional problems in children: A test of a programming hypothesis. *Journal of Child Psychology and Psychiatry, 44,* 1025–1036.

Olfson, M., Broadhead, W. E., Weissman, M. M., Leon, A. C., Farber, L., Hoven, C. W., & Kathol, R. G. (1996). Subthreshold psychiatric symptoms in a primary care group practice. *Archives of General Psychiatry, 53,* 880–886.

Paul, I. M., Downs, D. S., Schaefer, E. W., Beiler, J. S., & Weisman, C. S. (2013). Postpartum anxiety and maternal-infant health outcomes. *Pediatrics, 131,* e1218–e1224.

Phillips, J., Sharpe, L., Matthey, S., & Charles, M. (2009). Maternally focussed worry. *Archives of Women's Mental Health, 12,* 409–418.

Poikkeus, P., Saisto, T., Unkila-Kallio, L., Punamaki, R. L., Repokari, L., Vilska, S., … Tulppala, M. (2006). Fear of childbirth and pregnancy-related anxiety in women conceiving with assisted reproduction. *Obstetrics and Gynecology, 108*(1), 70–76.

Reichenheim, M. E., Moraes, C. L., Oliveira, A. S. D., Lobato, G. (2011). Revisiting the dimensional structure of the Edinburgh Postnatal Depression Scale (EPDS): Empirical evidence for a general factor. *BMC Medical Research Methodology, 11,* 1–12, Article number 93.

Robins, L. N., Helzer, J. E., Croughan, J., & Ratcliff, K. S. (1988). The Composite International Diagnostic Interview: An epidemiological instrument suitable for use in conjunction with different diagnostic systems and in different cultures. *Archives of General Psychiatry, 45,* 1069–1077.

Roesch, S. C., Schetter, C. D., Woo, G., & Hobel, C. J. (2004). Modeling the types and timing of stress in pregnancy. *Anxiety, Stress, and Coping, 17*(1), 87–102.

Ross, L. E., Evans, S. E. G., Sellers, E. M., & Romach, M. K. (2003). Measurement issues in postpartum depression 1: Anxiety as a feature of postpartum depression. *Archives of Women's Mental Health, 6,* 51–57.

Ross, L. E., & McLean, L. M. (2006). Anxiety disorders during pregnancy and the postpartum period: A systematic review. *Journal of Clinical Psychiatry, 67,* 1285–1298.

Rucci, P., Gherardi, S., Tansella, M., Piccinelli, M., Berardi, D., Bisoffi, G., … Pini, S. (2003). Subthreshold psychiatric disorders in primary care: Prevalence and associated characteristics. *Journal of Affective Disorders, 76*(1–3), 171–181.

Sheehan, D. V., Lecrubier, Y., Sheehan, K. H., Amorim, P., Janavs, J., Weiller, E., … Dunbar, G. C. (1998). The Mini-International Neuropsychiatric Interview (MINI): The development and validation of a structured psychiatric interview for DSM-IV and ICD-10. *Journal of Clinical Psychiatry, 59*(Suppl 20), 22–33.

Skouteris, H., Wertheim, E. H., Rallis, S., Milgrom, J., & Paxton, S. J. (2009). Depression and anxiety through pregnancy and the early postpartum: An examination of prospective relationships. *Journal of Affective Disorders, 113*(3), 303–308.

Snaith, R. P. (2003). The hospital anxiety and depression scale. *Health and Quality of Life Outcomes, 1*(29). doi:10.1186/1477-7525-1-29.

Spielberger, C. D., Gorsuch, R. L., & Lushene, R. E. (1970). *Manual for the State-Trait Anxiety Inventory (STAI)*. Palo Alto, CA: Consulting Psychologists Press.

Stuart, S., Couser, G., Schilder, K., O'Hara, M., & Gorman, L. (1998). Postpartum anxiety and depression: Onset and comorbidity in a community sample. *Journal of Nervous and Mental Disease, 186*, 420–424.

Sutter-Dallay, A. L., Giaconne-Marcesche, V., Glatigny-Dallay, E., & Verdoux, H. (2004). Women with anxiety disorders during pregnancy are at increased risk of intense postnatal depressive symptoms: A prospective survey of the MATQUID cohort. *European Psychiatry, 19*, 459–463.

Teixeira, J. M. A., Fisk, N. M., & Glover, V. (1999). Association between maternal anxiety in pregnancy and increased uterine artery resistance index: Cohort based study. *British Medical Journal, 318*, 153–157.

van Bussel, J. C. H., Spitz, B., & Demyttenaere, K. (2009). Anxiety in pregnant and postpartum women. An exploratory study of the role of maternal orientations. *Journal of Affective Disorders, 114*, 232–242.

van den Bergh, B. R. H. (1989). *De emotionele toestand van de (zwangere) vrouw, obstretische complicaties en het gedrag en de ontwikkeling van de foetus en van het kind tot de leeftijd van zeven maanden* [The emotional state of the (pregnant) woman, obstetrical complications and the behavior and development of fetus and child until seven months after birth] (PhD dissertation), Universiteit Leuven, Belgium.

van den Bergh, B. R. H. (1990). The influence of maternal emotions during pregnancy on fetal and neonatal behavior. *Journal of Prenatal & Perinatal Psychological and Health, 5*, 119–130.

van den Bergh, B. R. H., & Marcoen, A. (2004). High antenatal maternal anxiety is related to ADHD symptoms, externalizing problems, and anxiety in 8- and 9-year-olds. *Child Development, 75*(4), 1085–1097.

van den Bergh, B. R. H., Mennes, M., Oosterlaan, J., Stevens, V., Stiers, P., Marcoen, A., & Lagae, L. (2005). High antenatal maternal anxiety is related to impulsivity during performance on cognitive tasks in 14- and 15- year olds. *Neuroscience and Biobehavioral Reviews, 29*, 259–269.

Van Praag, H. M., Rodney, J., & Parker, G. B. (1998). The diagnosis of depression in disorder. *Australian and New Zealand Journal of Psychiatry, 32*(6), 767–777.

Wadhwa, P. D., Sandman, C. A., Porto, M., Dunkel-Schetter, C., & Garite, T. J. (1993). The association between prenatal stress and infant birth weight and gestational age at birth: A prospective investigation. *American Journal of Obstetrics and Gynecology, 169*(4), 858–865.

Wenzel, A., Haugen, E. N., Jackson, L. C., & Brendle, J. R. (2005). Anxiety symptoms and disorders at eight weeks postpartum. *Journal of Anxiety Disorders, 19*, 295–311.

Whooley, M. A., Avins, A. L., Miranda, J., Browner, W. S. (1997). Case-finding instruments for depression: Two questions are as good as many. *Journal of General Internal Medicine, 12*, 439–445.

Wickberg, B., & Hwang, C. P. (1996). Counselling of postnatal depression: A controlled study on a population based Swedish sample. *Journal of Affective Disorders, 39*, 209–216.

Wittchen, H.-U. (1993). Reliability and validity studies of the WHO-Composite International Diagnostic Interview (CIDI): A critical review. *Journal of Psychiatric Research, 28*, 57–84.

Woolhouse, H., Brown, S., Krastev, A., Perlen, S., & Gunn, J. (2009). Seeking help for anxiety and depression after childbirth: Results of the Maternal Health Study. *Archives of Women's Mental Health, 12*(2), 75–78.

Zigmond, A. S., & Snaith, R. P. (1983). The hospital anxiety and depression scale. *Acta Psychiatrica Scandinavica, 67*, 361–370.

7

Diagnostic Assessment of Depression, Anxiety, and Related Disorders

Arianna Di Florio, John Seeley, and Ian Jones

Severe episodes of affective disorders occurring in relation to childbirth have been recognized for centuries. The first description of mood symptoms in the postpartum period can be traced back to the Corpus Hippocraticum around the first half of the fourth century BC. Despite improved obstetric care leading to organic causes of postpartum psychosis becoming much less prevalent in many parts of the world, the importance of perinatal psychiatry has been increasingly recognized in the last few decades. Specialized services and pathways of care have been established for women with psychiatric disorders occurring during pregnancy and after childbirth. Research in this field has flourished with, for example, over 4000 publications on postnatal depression in the last decade. Despite this considerable interest, the diagnosis and classification of perinatal psychiatric disorders are still subject to much debate.

This chapter discusses issues arising in the nosology and diagnosis of perinatal mood and anxiety disorders and is split into four sections. First, we will consider how they are dealt with in the most commonly used classification systems, the International Classification of Diseases, Tenth Edition (ICD-10), and the more recently published Diagnostic and Statistical Manual of Mental Disorders, Fifth Edition (DSM-5). Second, we will consider problems arising from current diagnostic approaches and, in particular, the central issue of whether there is a specific relationship between mood disorders and childbirth. Third, we will consider issues around the differential diagnosis of perinatal mood and anxiety disorders, and fourth and finally, we will look at the clinical evaluation of perinatal episodes and the use of diagnostic tools.

Perinatal Mood and Anxiety Disorders in the Current Diagnostic Systems

DSM, authored by the American Psychiatric Association, and ICD, by the World Health Organization (WHO), are the most widely used classification systems. They provide both researchers and clinicians with explicit criteria for disorders, improving communication

Identifying Perinatal Depression and Anxiety: Evidence-Based Practice in Screening, Psychosocial Assessment, and Management, First Edition. Edited by Jeannette Milgrom and Alan W. Gemmill.
© 2015 John Wiley & Sons, Ltd. Published 2015 by John Wiley & Sons, Ltd.

and enabling better diagnostic agreement (American Psychiatric Association, 2013; World Health Organization, 1992). In addition, as outlined in the introduction of the DSM-5, reliable diagnoses are "essential for guiding treatment recommendations, identifying prevalence rates for mental health service planning" and for research. The DSM-5 notes that the development of fully validated diagnoses continues to evolve. There is recognition that a too-rigid categorical system does not always capture clinical experience and the ongoing development of diagnostic classification systems attempts to strike a balance and be supplemented where appropriate by dimensional measures. Such an approach aims to provide diagnostic criteria which comprehensively describe a particular construct such as "major depression" or "generalized anxiety."

To encourage research into new definitions of disorders that take into account biology, imaging, and cognitive science, the NIMH has recently launched the Research Domain Criteria (RDoC) project, a "framework for collecting the data needed for a new nosology" (Insel, 2013). It has been argued that the current categorical diagnostic systems lack biological validity, as diagnoses are based on clusters of symptoms rather than pathophysiology. As the same symptoms can have different causes, a diagnostic system based on symptoms may not provide the patients with the best treatment. Although the RDoC are not designed for immediate clinical use and therefore do not replace DSM or ICD in clinical practice, the NIMH aims with this project to "reorient its research away from DSM categories." It is therefore likely that classification and nosology will remain an evolving area for some time to come.

Nowhere are the difficulties and inadequacies of current diagnostic approaches more clearly demonstrated than in their approach to the disorders of pregnancy and the postpartum period. Although the approach to perinatal episodes is different in ICD-10 and DSM-5, both assume that perinatal episodes of mood and anxiety disorders are not separate nosological entities. The underlying philosophy rather is that episodes of psychiatric illness occurring in the perinatal period should be classified in the same categories as are used for episodes that do not occur in relation to childbirth.

ICD-10

The ICD-10 category "mental and behavioural disorders associated with the puerperium, not elsewhere classified (F53)" includes mild (F53.0) or severe (F53.1) disorders commencing after delivery within 6 weeks' postpartum (World Health Organization, 1992). It is recommended to use this category only when "unavoidable," for disorders that cannot be classified elsewhere. ICD emphasizes that the clinical presentation of severe postnatal illness does not differ from that of disorders occurring at other times.

This residual category is aimed to aid clinicians and service providers in those countries in which it is very difficult to collect sufficient information to make a precise diagnosis of disorders occurring after delivery. It is clear, therefore, that the authors of ICD-10 would ideally not want this category of puerperal disorders to be used at all.

DSM-5

In DSM-5, mood episodes (depressive, manic, hypomanic) with onset in pregnancy or within 4 weeks' postpartum can be recorded via the specifier "with peripartum onset" (American Psychiatric Association, 2013). If a depressive episode presents at least three

Table 7.1   DSM-5 criteria for a major depressive episode. Changes from DSM-IV are highlighted in bold and described in the right column. Compared to the previous version, DSM-5 contains a broader definition of major depression, including hopelessness as a core symptom and depression only 2 weeks after bereavement

DSM-5 criteria (American Psychiatric Association, 2013)	Changes from DSM-IV (American Psychiatric Association, 2000)
A. 5 or more in the same 2-week period. Each of these symptoms represents a change from previous functioning and needs to be present nearly every day. At least one of these symptoms is (i) depressed mood, (ii) loss of interest or pleasure	Definition of depressed mood was narrower, including only sadness or emptiness
1. Depressed mood (subjective or observed) most of the day, defined as sad, empty or **hopeless**	
2. Loss of interest or pleasure, most of the day	
3. Change in appetite nearly every day or at least 5% change in weight over 1 month	
4. Insomnia or hypersomnia	
5. Psychomotor retardation or agitation (observed)	
6. Loss of energy or fatigue	
7. Worthlessness or guilt	
8. Impaired concentration or indecisiveness	
9. Recurrent thoughts of death or suicidal ideation or attempt	
B. Symptoms cause clinically significant distress or impairment in social, occupational, or other important areas of life	Distress and impairment were included in criterion A
C. Episode not attributable to a substance or medical condition. Depression can be present in addition to a normal response to **bereavement, according to clinical judgment**	Exclusion of symptoms better accounted for by bereavement

manic/hypomanic symptoms or a manic/hypomanic episode presents at least three depressive symptoms, the "mixed features specifier" should also be recorded.

Table 7.1 summarizes DSM-5 criteria for a major depressive episode and compares them to those of the previous version DSM-IV.

DSM-5 therefore does not distinguish between mood episodes occurring in pregnancy and those with a postpartum onset. Compared to the previous version, DSM-IV (American Psychiatric Association, 2000), that included only a postpartum onset specifier, the DSM-5 acknowledges the clinical importance of mood disorders, especially depression, occurring during pregnancy. However, if there is something specific about childbirth as a trigger of episodes, by including pregnancy in addition to postpartum onsets risks losing this specificity.

It has also been argued that a 4-week window for a postnatal onset is too narrow and, at least for depression, not supported by research evidence and clinical practice. Although DSM-5 mentions the presence of severe anxiety symptoms in perinatal depression and the association between anxiety in pregnancy and postpartum depression, the classification of anxiety disorders in DSM-5 does not include a peripartum onset specifier.

While the previous DSM-IV category Depressive Disorder NOS included "minor depression," DSM-5 now introduces the category of "other specified disorders." This is intended to encourage the clinicians to record the reason why a depressive illness causing distress or impairment does not meet the criteria for the full-blown disorder. This category includes depressive episodes lasting more than 4 days but less than 15 and "depressive episodes with insufficient symptoms" (depressed mood with at least one of the other eight symptoms of major depressive episode).

In summary, the diagnosis and classification of postnatal affective disorders are still controversial. In the next section, we will discuss the current challenges.

Diagnostic Challenges

Is there evidence of a specific relationship between episodes of illness with pregnancy and childbirth?

While for affective psychosis or mania, there is robust evidence of a relationship with childbirth (Di Florio et al., 2013; Munk-Olsen, Laursen, Meltzer-Brody, Mortensen, & Jones, 2012; Munk-Olsen, Laursen, Pedersen, Mors, & Mortensen, 2006; Munk-Olsen et al., 2009) that we will not consider in detail here, the link between pregnancy, childbirth, and other mental disorders is not so clear cut. Research on the pathogenesis of anxiety disorders in the perinatal period is particularly scarce.

Evidence from epidemiological studies
It has been hypothesized that there is a "selection into parenthood" by which women with lower risk of psychiatric disorders are more likely to have children (Munk-Olsen et al., 2006). After controlling for this effect, registry studies conducted on the entire Danish population found a threefold increased risk of admission for unipolar depression in the first two postpartum months compared to 11–12 months after childbirth (Munk-Olsen et al., 2006). While the Danish study investigated the most severe episodes requiring admission, another population-based study conducted in Norway assessed less severe episodes of depression with a cross-sectional questionnaire (Eberhard-Gran, Eskild, Tambs, Samuelsen, & Opjordsmoen, 2002). Using the Edinburgh Postnatal Depression Scale (EPDS) and the Hopkins Symptom Check List 25-item version, they found that rates of depression (defined as EPDS scores above 9) appeared to be lower in the postpartum group than in the nonpostpartum group. After controlling for a range of known risk factors for depression (including premenstrual tension, high score on the life event scale, and partner attachment), however, the risk of depression was twofold higher postpartum than at other times.

Evidence from phenomenological studies
Studies into the clinical presentation of postnatal depression have not consistently shown any difference between episodes of depression occurring after childbirth and those occurring at other times (Cooper, Campbell, Day, Kennerley, & Bond, 1988; Cooper et al., 2007; Eberhard-Gran, Tambs, Opjordsmoen, Skrondal, & Eskild, 2003; Evans, Heron, Francomb, Oke, & Golding, 2001; Pitt, 1968; Whiffen, 1991; Whiffen & Gotlib, 1993). It has been hypothesized that differences between postnatal and nonpostnatal depression symptomatology may be due to the context of new motherhood rather than to intrinsic differences in depression (Cooper et al., 2007).

Evidence from follow-up studies

There are only few studies comparing long-term outcomes of depression occurring within and outside the postpartum period, but they consistently suggest a specificity for puerperal episodes.

Women with a first incident episode of depression following childbirth have a heightened risk of further episodes of postnatal depression. They also have a lower risk of nonpuerperal depressive episodes compared to women with a first episode outside the childbirth period (Cooper & Murray, 1995). First incident depressive episodes occurring within the first month after delivery have also been linked to a bipolar diathesis. A Danish registry study followed up women with a first psychiatric admission for a nonbipolar diagnosis over the subsequent 15 years. It found that 14% of those with a first admission in the month after delivery subsequently received a diagnosis of bipolar disorder. In contrast, the 15-year conversion rates to bipolar disorder were similar, at around 4% for those with a first admission later in the puerperium or outside the first postpartum year (Munk-Olsen et al., 2012).

Evidence from etiological studies

At least in some women, a link between depression and childbirth may be specific. Bloch et al. (2000) pharmacologically simulated the high gonadal steroid levels of pregnancy and postpartum withdrawal in parous women with and without a history of postnatal depression. They found that over 60% of women with a history of postnatal depression developed depressive symptoms during the withdrawal phase and that these depressive symptoms improved with the restoration of gonad activity.

Evidence of a specific link between depression and childbirth has also been provided by a family study of sibling pairs with recurrent major depression which found that susceptibility to postpartum episodes is familial (Forty et al., 2006). Finally, a twin study found evidence of distinct genetic factors influencing vulnerability to postnatal and nonpostnatal depressive symptoms (Treloar, Martin, Bucholz, Madden, & Heath, 1999).

Childbirth is also likely to be a particularly potent precipitant of depression from a psychosocial perspective with vulnerability to a range of risk factors such as lack of social support, previous abuse, and domestic violence heightened.

Should the onset specifier cover pregnancy?

In ICD-10, there is no recognition of episodes occurring in pregnancy, while DSM has replaced the "postpartum onset specifier" of the previous edition (American Psychiatric Association, 2000) with a "peripartum onset specifier" for depressive disorders that includes both pregnancy and the postpartum period (American Psychiatric Association, 2013). According to DSM-5, specifiers aim to define more homogeneous groups of individuals with a disorder and, in turn, improve management (American Psychiatric Association, 2013).

Although there are consistent reports of depressive symptoms in pregnancy being as common as in the postpartum period (Fergusson, Horwood, & Thorpe, 1996), the risk of major depression in pregnancy is lower than after childbirth and at other times in a woman's reproductive years. In the Danish registry study, the relative risk of first admission for major depression in pregnancy was more than halved compared to other times in life (0.44, 95% CI 0.31–0.62), while it was more than threefold higher in the second month after delivery (3.53, 95% CI 2.47–5.05) (Munk-Olsen et al., 2006).

Although there is therefore no robust evidence of a specific link between depression and pregnancy, there are important clinical benefits, in flagging episodes occurring at this time. A pregnancy specifier would encourage the assessment and prevention of mental disorders in pregnancy, with important benefits for the mother and the baby. It has in fact been estimated that about 1 in 2 episodes of postnatal depression starts before childbirth (Wisner et al., 2013) and that depression in pregnancy is a risk factor for relapse after childbirth. Moreover, pregnancy represents a time of difficult choices about medications for a mother with mental illness. The possible teratogenic and long-term effects of some drugs need to be weighed against the high risk (68% in one study (Cohen et al., 2006)) of a recurrence if medications are stopped. Chapter 11 discusses both the pharmacological and psychological treatment options. There is also evidence that depression, stress, and anxiety during pregnancy are associated with an increased risk of a wide range of negative outcomes in the child, including emotional, cognitive, and behavioral problems (Glover, 2014). For these reasons, although the evidence of pregnancy as a specific trigger for mood episodes is lacking, there are good clinical reasons to support a pregnancy onset specifier. The question remains, however, of whether this should be part of a combined peripartum onset specifier or whether there should be separate pregnancy and postpartum specifiers.

What period after childbirth should the specifier cover?

Over 90% of severe episodes of postpartum psychosis have an onset within 2 weeks of delivery (Di Florio et al., 2013, Heron, McGuinness, Blackmore, Craddock, & Jones, 2008), and the association between bipolar disorder and childbirth is specific for the first month after delivery (Munk-Olsen et al., 2006, 2009, 2012). Episodes of major depression, in contrast, are more spread out in the postpartum period (Di Florio et al., 2013), and the increased risk of admission extends through the first 5 months' postpartum (Munk-Olsen et al., 2006). A family study also concluded that the specific familiarity for postnatal depression maximized when a 6–8-week onset definition was used and that the current DSM-5 4 weeks' onset specifier may be too narrow for depression (Forty et al., 2006).

From a clinical point of view, a 3–6-month onset definition has been advocated by many specialists (Jones & Cantwell, 2010; Sharma & Mazmanian, 2014; Wisner, Moses-Kolko, & Sit, 2010), and even onsets up to a year following childbirth may be labeled as postnatal depression in clinical practice (Musters, McDonald, & Jones, 2008). There are therefore good theoretical and clinical reasons to feel that the onset specifier should be extended beyond the current 4 weeks but how much extended is still subject to debate.

Should anxiety disorders include a peripartum onset specifier?

Anxiety and depressive symptoms in pregnancy are hard to disentangle, and comorbidity is common. The DSM-5 "peripartum onset" specifier cannot at present be used for anxiety disorders. There is a paucity of research investigating anxiety disorders in the perinatal period, despite the potential importance for the mother and the developing child. Anxiety and stress during pregnancy have been associated with long-term negative outcome in the offspring (Glover, 2014; King & Laplante, 2005).

A longitudinal clinical study using the Hospital Anxiety and Depression Scale questionnaire found that anxiety is more prevalent than depression during pregnancy and that it predicts postnatal depression (Lee et al., 2007). Using a two-stage screening design, Reck et al. (2008) assessed anxiety and depressive disorders 3 months after delivery using the SCID-4 interview. They found that anxiety disorders (panic disorder, agoraphobia, specific and social phobia, acute adjustment disorder with anxiety) were more prevalent than depressive disorders (minor or major depression, dysthymia). Despite these findings, the first incidence of episodes with onset in the postpartum was indeed higher for depressive disorders.

Obsessive–compulsive disorder

There is evidence of a relationship between postnatal depression and obsessive–compulsive symptoms, particularly unwanted intrusive thoughts of hurting the newborn (Ross & McLean, 2006).

A recent meta-analysis found that women during the perinatal period are at 1.5–2 times higher risk of obsessive–compulsive disorder than the general female population, with an aggregate risk ratio of 1.79 (Russell, Fawcett, & Mazmanian, 2013). Obsessive–compulsive symptoms are more prevalent after delivery than during pregnancy (Ross & McLean, 2006). Intrusive thoughts of harming the baby have, however, also been reported to be surprisingly common, over 80% (Russell et al., 2013), in parents with no mental disorders, and the majority of women with these thoughts will not act on them. One study, however, found that 5% of women with postnatal depression and aggressive obsessive thoughts had acted in an aggressive way toward their child (Wisner, Peindl, Gigliotti, & Hanusa, 1999, 199). For this reason, obsessive thoughts should always be explored in depth (Austin, Middleton, Reilly, & Highet, 2013) and must be differentiated from delusional thinking involving the baby.

Differential Diagnosis

Bipolar disorder

There is clear and compelling evidence of a link between bipolar disorder and childbirth. Women with no previous psychiatric history have a 23.33 (95% CI 11.52–47.24) increased risk of admission for bipolar disorder in the first month after childbirth (Munk-Olsen et al., 2006). The relative risk is even higher for women with a previous history of bipolar disorder (RR, 37.22; 95% CI, 13.58–102.04) (Munk-Olsen et al., 2009). A 15-year follow-up study on over 120,000 women with a first-time psychiatric contact for any type of mental disorder (excluding bipolar disorder) found that approximately 14% of those with a first contact within a month postpartum converted to a bipolar diagnosis and that an onset within 2 weeks of delivery predicted subsequent conversion to bipolar disorder (RR, 4.26; 95% CI 3.11–5.85) (Munk-Olsen et al., 2012). About 70% of parous women with bipolar disorder experience an episode of mood disorder after childbirth, including major depression (Di Florio et al., 2013). Although postnatal depression most often occurs in the context of a unipolar depressive illness, a recent study reported that more than 1 in 5 women with postnatal depression have a bipolar disorder of some description (Wisner et al., 2013).

The detection of manic features in postnatal depression is difficult, but important for clinical management, as the pharmacological treatment for unipolar and bipolar depression differs and antidepressants may be less effective and induce mania, mixed states, and rapid cycling in women with bipolar disorder (Sharma, Burt, & Ritchie, 2009).

There are few specific rating scales for hypomania/mania occurring in relation to pregnancy and childbirth. The Highs Scale (Glover, Liddle, Taylor, Adams, & Sandler, 1994) was developed to specifically measure hypomanic and subclinical high symptoms occurring in the postpartum period. It has been suggested that scales developed for use in bipolar disorder in general adult populations should be specifically validated for postpartum use (Smith et al., 2009). In a general obstetric ward, only 11% of women met the suggested threshold for hypomania on the Highs Scale in the immediate postpartum, while the prevalence of hypomania was fourfold higher at 44% using the Altman Mania Rating Scale (AMRS). It may therefore be that the Highs Scale is too conservative, while the AMRS overestimates hypomania at this time (Smith et al., 2009).

Physical disorders

When diagnosing mood and anxiety disorders, systemic physical illnesses should be ruled out, especially when significant distress and agitation are present. The lack of prompt diagnosis of any general medical condition can lead to a life-threatening delay of the appropriate treatment and, in the most tragic cases, to death (Cantwell et al., 2011). Conditions that need to be considered include thyroid dysfunction, anemia, substance-related disorders, and organic brain dysfunction due to primary cerebral or systemic disease (Gerace, Corsi, & Comanducci, 2013).

Perinatal symptoms unrelated to mood and anxiety disorders

Symptoms such as sleep disturbance, weight change, and loss of energy commonly occur in pregnancy and the puerperium without any associated mood disorder. As discussed in section "Obsessive–compulsive disorder," obsessive thoughts, especially of harming the baby, are common in puerperal women without mental disorder. In these cases, characteristic mood changes of depression are absent. Symptoms need to be assessed carefully and repetitively, as some may be transient and do not require medical treatment (Boyce, 2013).

Subthreshold symptoms

Research conducted on perinatal mood disorders using continuous measures for depressive and anxious symptomatology finds no points of rarity between subthreshold symptoms, mild depression, and more severe disorders. There does not seem to be a clear distinction between those women with subthreshold symptoms and those with disorders meeting criteria for a major disorder. The clinical validity and nosology of subthreshold syndromes therefore remain uncertain and subject to debate. Although categories may be needed to inform and improve standardized care, the current categorical approach has been widely criticized. Depressive symptoms lie on a continuum of severity (Rakofsky et al., 2013), and thresholds for the categorical diagnoses are arbitrarily defined and lack support from empirical evidence and clinical experience.

In order to encourage data collection in this area, ICD-10 introduced the diagnostic category of "recurrent brief depressive disorder" for episodes that meet the severity criteria but not the duration criterion for depressive episode (World Health Organization, 1992). Similarly, DSM-5 recognizes subthreshold syndromes such as recurrent brief depression with episodes lasting more than 4 days but less than 2 weeks and clusters of less than 5 symptoms that last more than 2 weeks (American Psychiatric Association, 2013). The arguments for including subthreshold syndromes in DSM-5 are both theoretical and practical. Using epidemiological data, Angst reported that over half of patients treated for depression did not formally meet the DSM-IV criteria for major depression (Angst et al., 2010), and it is argued that the broader approach taken by DSM-5 will provide individuals seeking treatment for subthreshold syndromes the appropriate care and support.

The main critique to DSM-5 inclusive approach is that it medicalizes negative emotions (Dowrick & Frances, 2013; Friedman, 2012). Overdiagnosis of anxiety and mood disorders is increasingly common in Western countries, with a dramatic rise in the prescription of antidepressants (Dowrick & Frances, 2013).

Evidence suggests that in individuals with minor depression, response to antidepressants and placebo are similar (relative risk of failure to respond 0.94, 95% CI 0.81–1.08) (Barbui, Cipriani, Patel, Ayuso-Mateos, & van Ommeren, 2011).

Considering the potential teratogenicity and long-term effects of antidepressant on the baby, nonpharmacological approaches are a more appropriate response to subthreshold and minor mood disorder symptoms. This level of symptomatology may need to be addressed, however, as it causes significant distress and may escalate into a more severe episode of illness.

Clinical Evaluation and Diagnostic Tools

Although the diagnosis of mood and anxiety disorder does not differ in major ways from that of disorders occurring at other times, the perinatal period poses particular problems for assessment. Postnatal disorders can interfere with the mother–baby relationship; impaired bonding with the baby, a lack of feeling of attachment toward the infant, and a sense of numbness are important features to consider (Musters et al., 2008). In addition to the aspects considered in the differential diagnosis section, crucial parts of the evaluation are the assessment of psychotic symptoms and the risk of suicide.

Psychotic symptoms occur in about 4% of women with postnatal depression (Cooper et al., 2007) and can substantially increase risk of harm to the women or her child, particularly if the content of the psychotic symptom is related to the baby. Suicide is a leading cause of maternal death (Cantwell et al., 2011). Assessment of the risk of suicide in the perinatal period is similar to that at any other time and involves inquiries into the extent of suicidal thoughts and intent (Work Group on Suicidal Behaviours, 2014). Consideration should also be given to a family and personal history of suicidal behavior, current misuse of alcohol or other drugs, social context and support, and the presence of specific symptoms such as agitation, shame, anger, guilt, impulsivity, hopelessness, despair, and psychosis. Whenever a woman is assessed for risk of suicide, inquiry should also be made about the risk to the infant. There is no evidence that raising these issues with women increases the risk of self-harm or suicide (Musters et al., 2008).

Diagnostic tools

Structured diagnostic interviews are strictly worded and do not allow clinical judgment. While they have made psychiatric diagnosis more reliable, enabling large-scale studies and comparisons between results from different researches, structured clinical tools are not used for the vast majority of assessments in clinical practice. Although no specific diagnostic interviews have been developed for perinatal disorders, a number of diagnostic interviews may be used, particularly in the context of research studies, and may include the following:

CIDI

The WHO Composite International Diagnostic Interview (CIDI) is a structured interview for the systematic assessment of mental disorders according to the ICD and DSM criteria (Robins et al., 1988). CIDI can be administered after specific training also by nonpsychiatrists. Its main aims are to measure the prevalence and severity of mental disorders and to assess their burden and management.

CIDI is organized in modules and covers both mood disorders (minor/subthreshold depression to major depression, hypomania, mania) and anxiety (agoraphobia, separation anxiety, panic disorder, generalized anxiety disorder, obsessive–compulsive disorder, social phobia, specific phobia, posttraumatic stress disorder). As every structured interview, CIDI does not allow clinical judgment or any liberty in wording or in eliciting the symptoms and does not account for their clinical significance. A thought-provoking study using the short form of the CIDI found that even minor changes in the symptoms definition lead to major differences in the identification of cases and therefore in prevalence estimates of major depression. Altering the diagnostic threshold for depressed mood from "all day" to "most of the day" doubled the prevalence estimate in the general population and more than tripled it in 15–24-year-olds (Karlsson, Marttunen, Karlsson, Kaprio, & Hillevi, 2010). For methodological issues related to CIDI, please refer to Kessler and Ustün (2004).

SCID

The Structured Clinical Interview for DSM-IV Axis I Disorders (SCID-I) is a semistructured interview for the diagnosis of psychiatric disorders, excluding personality disorders, according to the DSM-IV (First, Spitzer, Gibbon, & Williams, 2012). The next version, based on DSM-5 criteria, is planned to be available from early spring 2014. SCID can be used by any trained mental health professional, including nonclinical research assistants.

Similarly to CIDI, the SCID-I is organized into diagnostic modules that include all mood and anxiety disorders according to DSM-IV. While in CIDI the interviewer asks a rigid set of questions, SCID allows additional nonstructured follow-up to further explore a patient's answers.

Summary and Conclusions

Despite perinatal mood and anxiety disorders being recognized for hundreds, if not thousands, of years, there remains controversy over the nosology of these conditions. Current classification system does not recognize perinatal disorders as separate nosological entities, but mood episodes with onset in pregnancy or up to 4 weeks' postpartum can be highlighted by the perinatal onset specifier in DSM-5. Emerging evidence suggests that there is a specific relationship between childbirth and mood disorders and that postpartum episodes should be identified for the prognostic information this gives. There remain a number of issues with the perinatal onset specifier as it is currently employed. Arguments can be made for separate pregnancy and postpartum specifiers and that they should be extended to the diagnosis of anxiety disorders.

References

American Psychiatric Association. (2000). *Diagnostic criteria from DSM-IV-TR*. Washington, DC: The Association.

American Psychiatric Association. (2013). *Diagnostic and statistical manual of mental disorders* (5th ed.). Arlington, VA: American Psychiatric Association.

Angst, J., Gamma, A., Clarke, D., Ajdacic-Gross, V., Rössler, W., & Regier, D. (2010). Subjective distress predicts treatment seeking for depression, bipolar, anxiety, panic, neurasthenia and insomnia severity spectra. *Acta Psychiatrica Scandinavica, 122*(6), 488–498. doi:10.1111/j.1600-0447.2010.01580.x.

Austin, M.-P. V., Middleton, P., Reilly, N. M., & Highet, N. J. (2013). Detection and management of mood disorders in the maternity setting: The Australian Clinical Practice Guidelines. *Women and Birth: Journal of the Australian College of Midwives, 26*(1), 2–9. doi:10.1016/j.wombi.2011.12.001.

Barbui, C., Cipriani, A., Patel, V., Ayuso-Mateos, J. L., & van Ommeren, M. (2011). Efficacy of antidepressants and benzodiazepines in minor depression: Systematic review and meta-analysis. *The British Journal of Psychiatry: the Journal of Mental Science, 198*(Suppl 1), 11–16. doi:10.1192/bjp.bp.109.076448.

Bloch, M., Schmidt, P. J., Danaceau, M., Murphy, J., Nieman, L., & Rubinow, D. R. (2000). Effects of gonadal steroids in women with a history of postpartum depression. *The American Journal of Psychiatry, 157*(6), 924–930.

Boyce, P. (2013). Is too much caution enough? *The Australian and New Zealand Journal of Psychiatry, 47*(11), 1081–1082. doi:10.1177/0004867413502094.

Cantwell, R., Clutton-Brock, T., Cooper, G., Dawson, A., Drife, J., Garrod, D., … Springett, A. (2011, March). Saving Mothers' Lives: Reviewing maternal deaths to make motherhood safer: 2006–2008. The Eighth Report of the Confidential Enquiries into Maternal Deaths in the United Kingdom. *BJOG: An International Journal of Obstetrics and Gynaecology, 1*, 1–203. doi:10.1111/j.1471-0528.2010.02847.x.

Cohen, L. S., Altshuler, L. L., Harlow, B. L., Nonacs, R., Newport, D. J., Viguera, A. C., … Stowe, Z. N. (2006). Relapse of major depression during pregnancy in women who maintain or discontinue antidepressant treatment. *JAMA, the Journal of the American Medical Association, 295*(5), 499–507. doi:10.1001/jama.295.5.499.

Cooper, P. J., Campbell, E. A., Day, A., Kennerley, H., & Bond, A. (1988, June). Non-psychotic psychiatric disorder after childbirth. A prospective study of prevalence, incidence, course and nature. *The British Journal of Psychiatry: the Journal of Mental Science, 152*, 799–806.

Cooper, C., Jones, L., Dunn, E., Forty, L., Haque, S., Oyebode, F., … Jones, I. (2007). Clinical presentation of postnatal and non-postnatal depressive episodes. *Psychological Medicine, 37*(9), 1273–1280. doi:10.1017/S0033291707000116.

Cooper, P. J., & Murray, L. (1995). Course and recurrence of postnatal depression. Evidence for the specificity of the diagnostic concept. *The British Journal of Psychiatry: the Journal of Mental Science, 166*(2), 191–195.

Di Florio, A., Forty, L., Gordon-Smith, K., Heron, J., Jones, L., Craddock, N., & Jones, I. (2013). Perinatal episodes across the mood disorder spectrum. *JAMA Psychiatry (Chicago, IL), 70*(2), 168–175. doi:10.1001/jamapsychiatry.2013.279.

Dowrick, C., & Frances, A. (2013). Medicalising unhappiness: New classification of depression risks more patients being put on drug treatment from which they will not benefit. *BMJ (Clinical Research Ed), 347*, f7140.

Eberhard-Gran, M., Eskild, A., Tambs, K., Samuelsen, S. O., & Opjordsmoen, S. (2002). Depression in postpartum and non-postpartum women: Prevalence and risk factors. *Acta Psychiatrica Scandinavica, 106*(6), 426–433.

Eberhard-Gran, M., Tambs, K., Opjordsmoen, S., Skrondal, A., & Eskild, A. (2003). A comparison of anxiety and depressive symptomatology in postpartum and non-postpartum mothers. *Social Psychiatry and Psychiatric Epidemiology, 38*(10), 551–556. doi:10.1007/s00127-003-0679-3.

Evans, J., Heron, J., Francomb, H., Oke, S., & Golding, J. (2001). Cohort study of depressed mood during pregnancy and after childbirth. *BMJ (Clinical Research Ed), 323*(7307), 257–260.

Fergusson, D. M., Horwood, L. J., & Thorpe, K. (1996). Changes in depression during and following pregnancy. ALSPAC Study Team. Study of Pregnancy and Children. *Paediatric and Perinatal Epidemiology, 10*(3), 279–293.

First, M. B., Spitzer, R. L., Gibbon, M., & Williams, J. B. W. (2012). *Structured clinical interview for DSM-IV® Axis I Disorders (SCID-I), clinician version, administration booklet.* Washington, DC: American Psychiatric Publishing.

Forty, L., Jones, L., Macgregor, S., Caesar, S., Cooper, C., Hough, A., … Jones, I. (2006). Familiality of postpartum depression in unipolar disorder: Results of a family study. *The American Journal of Psychiatry, 163*(9), 1549–1553. doi:10.1176/appi.ajp.163.9.1549.

Friedman, R. A. (2012). Grief, depression, and the DSM-5. *The New England Journal of Medicine, 366*(20), 1855–1857. doi:10.1056/NEJMp1201794.

Gerace, C., Corsi, F. M., & Comanducci, G. (2013). Apathetic syndrome from carotid dissection: A dangerous condition. *BMJ Case Reports*, 1–3. doi:10.1136/bcr-2013-009686.

Glover, V. (2014). Maternal depression, anxiety and stress during pregnancy and child outcome; what needs to be done. *Best Practice & Research. Clinical Obstetrics & Gynaecology, 28*(1), 25–35. doi:10.1016/j.bpobgyn.2013.08.017.

Glover, V., Liddle, P., Taylor, A., Adams, D., & Sandler, M. (1994). Mild hypomania (the highs) can be a feature of the first postpartum week. Association with later depression. *The British Journal of Psychiatry: The Journal of Mental Science, 164*(4), 517–521.

Heron, J., McGuinness, M., Robertson Blackmore, E., Craddock, N., & Jones, I. (2008). Early post-partum symptoms in puerperal psychosis. *BJOG: An International Journal of Obstetrics and Gynaecology, 115*(3), 348–353. doi:10.1111/j.1471-0528.2007.01563.x.

Insel, T. (2013). Transforming diagnosis. Director's Blog. Retrieved from http://www.nimh.nih.gov/about/director/2013/transforming-diagnosis.shtml. Accessed December 16, 2014.

Jones, I., & Cantwell, R. (2010). The classification of perinatal mood disorders—Suggestions for DSMV and ICD11. *Archives of Women's Mental Health, 13*(1), 33–36. doi:10.1007/s00737-009-0122-1.

Karlsson, L., Marttunen, M., Karlsson, H., Kaprio, J., & Hillevi, A. (2010). Minor change in the diagnostic threshold leads into major alteration in the prevalence estimate of depression. *Journal of Affective Disorders, 122*(1–2), 96–101. doi:10.1016/j.jad.2009.06.025.

Kessler, R. C, & Üstün, T. B. (2004). The World Mental Health (WMH) Survey Initiative Version of the World Health Organization (WHO) Composite International Diagnostic Interview (CIDI). *International Journal of Methods in Psychiatric Research, 13*(2), 93–121.

King, S., & Laplante, D. P. (2005). The effects of prenatal maternal stress on children's cognitive development: Project Ice Storm. *Stress (Amsterdam, Netherlands), 8*(1), 35–45. doi:10.1080/10253890500108391.

Lee, A. M., Lam, S. K., Sze Mun Lau, S. M., Chong, C. S. Y., Chui, H. W., & Fong, D. Y. T. (2007). Prevalence, course, and risk factors for antenatal anxiety and depression. *Obstetrics and Gynecology, 110*(5), 1102–1112. doi:10.1097/01.AOG.0000287065.59491.70.

Munk-Olsen, T., Laursen, T. M., Meltzer-Brody, S., Mortensen, P. B., & Jones, I. (2012). Psychiatric disorders with postpartum onset: Possible early manifestations of bipolar affective disorders. *Archives of General Psychiatry, 69*(4), 428–434. doi:10.1001/archgenpsychiatry.2011.157.

Munk-Olsen, T., Laursen, T. M., Mendelson, T., Pedersen, C. B., Mors, O., & Mortensen, P. B. (2009). Risks and predictors of readmission for a mental disorder during the postpartum period. *Archives of General Psychiatry, 66*(2), 189–195. doi:10.1001/archgenpsychiatry.2008.528.

Munk-Olsen, T., Laursen, T. M., Pedersen, C. B., Mors, O., & Mortensen, P. B. (2006). New parents and mental disorders. *JAMA, the Journal of the American Medical Association, 296*(21), 2582–2589. doi:10.1001/jama.296.21.2582.

Musters, C., McDonald, E., & Jones, I. (2008). Management of postnatal depression. *BMJ (Clinical Research Ed), 337*, a736.

Pitt, B. (1968). "Atypical" depression following childbirth. *The British Journal of Psychiatry: The Journal of Mental Science, 114*(516), 1325–1335.

Work Group on Suicidal Behaviours. (2014). Practice guideline for the assessment and treatment of patients with suicidal behaviors. In American Psychiatric Association (Ed.), *APA practice guidelines for the treatment of psychiatric disorders: Comprehensive guidelines and guideline watches* (1st ed., Vol. 1). Arlington, VA: Author. Retrieved from http://psychiatryonline.org/pb/assets/raw/sitewide/practice_guidelines/guidelines/suicide.pdf. Accessed December 16, 2014.

Rakofsky, J. J., Schettler, P. J., Kinkead, B. L., Frank, E., Judd, L. L., Kupfer, D. J., … Rapaport, M. H. (2013). The prevalence and severity of depressive symptoms along the spectrum of unipolar depressive disorders: A post hoc analysis. *The Journal of Clinical Psychiatry, 74*(11), 1084–1091. doi:10.4088/JCP.12m08194.

Reck, C., Struben, K., Backenstrass, M., Stefenelli, U., Reinig, K., Fuchs, T., … Mundt, C. (2008). Prevalence, onset and comorbidity of postpartum anxiety and depressive disorders. *Acta Psychiatrica Scandinavica, 118*(6), 459–468. doi:10.1111/j.1600-0447.2008.01264.x.

Robins, L. N., Wing, J., Wittchen, H. U., Helzer, J. E., Babor, T. F., Burke, J., … Regier, D. A. (1988). The Composite International Diagnostic Interview. An epidemiologic instrument suitable for use in conjunction with different diagnostic systems and in different cultures. *Archives of General Psychiatry, 45*(12), 1069–1077.

Ross, L. E., & McLean, L. M. (2006). Anxiety disorders during pregnancy and the postpartum period: A systematic review. *The Journal of Clinical Psychiatry, 67*(8), 1285–1298.

Russell, E. J., Fawcett, J. M., & Mazmanian, D. (2013). Risk of obsessive-compulsive disorder in pregnant and postpartum women: A meta-analysis. *The Journal of Clinical Psychiatry, 74*(4), 377–385. doi:10.4088/JCP.12r07917.

Sharma, V., Burt, V. K., & Ritchie, H. L. (2009). Bipolar II postpartum depression: Detection, diagnosis, and treatment. *The American Journal of Psychiatry, 166*(11), 1217–1221. doi:10.1176/appi.ajp.2009.08121902.

Sharma, V., & Mazmanian, D. (2014). The DSM-5 peripartum specifier: Prospects and pitfalls. *Archives of Women's Mental Health, January, 17*(2), 171–173. doi:10.1007/s00737-013-0406-3.

Smith, S., Heron, J., Haque, S., Clarke, P., Oyebode, F., & Jones, I. (2009). Measuring hypomania in the postpartum: A comparison of the Highs Scale and the Altman Mania Rating Scale. *Archives of Women's Mental Health, 12*(5), 323–327. doi:10.1007/s00737-009-0076-3.

Treloar, S. A., Martin, N. G., Bucholz, K. K., Madden, P. A., & Heath, A. C. (1999). Genetic influences on post-natal depressive symptoms: Findings from an Australian twin sample. *Psychological Medicine, 29*(3), 645–654.

Whiffen, V. E. (1991). The comparison of postpartum with non-postpartum depression: A rose by any other name. *Journal of Psychiatry & Neuroscience: JPN, 16*(3), 160–165.

Whiffen, V. E., & Gotlib, I. H. (1993). Comparison of postpartum and nonpostpartum depression: Clinical presentation, psychiatric history, and psychosocial functioning. *Journal of Consulting and Clinical Psychology, 61*(3), 485–494.

Wisner, K. L., Moses-Kolko, E. L., & Sit, D. K. Y. (2010). Postpartum depression: A disorder in search of a definition. *Archives of Women's Mental Health, 13*(1), 37–40. doi:10.1007/s00737-009-0119-9.

Wisner, K. L., Peindl, K. S., Gigliotti, T., & Hanusa, B. H. (1999). Obsessions and compulsions in women with postpartum depression. *The Journal of Clinical Psychiatry, 60*(3), 176–180.

Wisner, K. L., Sit, D. K. Y., McShea, M. C., Rizzo, D. M., Zoretich, R. A., Hughes, C. L., … Hanusa, B. H. (2013). Onset timing, thoughts of self-harm, and diagnoses in postpartum women with screen-positive depression findings. *JAMA Psychiatry, 70*(5), 490–498. doi:10.1001/jamapsychiatry.2013.87.

World Health Organization. (1992). *ICD-10: The ICD-10 Classification of Mental and Behavioural Disorders: Clinical Descriptions and Diagnostic Guidelines*. Geneva, Switzerland: Author.

8

Psychosocial Assessment and Integrated Perinatal Care

Marie-Paule Austin, Jane Fisher, and Nicole Reilly

Background

The following section summarizes the concepts and practices that have been developed in the Anglophone, predominantly higher-income setting where much of the research has been done. The applicability and appropriateness of such practices in low-income countries is discussed in the subsequent section.

The perinatal period (pregnancy and the first postnatal year) is a time of increased psychological vulnerability for many women. Mental health conditions (recurrent or new onset) presenting in the postnatal period may be associated with negative outcomes for the mother, partner, infant, and family. Conversely, maternal mental health may be impacted by partner, infant, and family behaviors. It is well recognized that depressive symptoms are a common presentation for a number of underlying complex and serious psychosocial comorbidities such as interpersonal violence (IPV), substance misuse, and a history of adverse childhood experiences (e.g., childhood sexual abuse (CSA)). That is, depressive symptoms are often an indicator of distress which may be due to any number of scenarios across a spectrum from a diagnosable condition (e.g., major depression) through to more intractable psychosocial risk or adverse circumstance not necessarily associated with a diagnosable condition. It is also notable that unless the comorbidity is addressed, depression may not respond as well to the usual treatment modalities, and thus, the combination of factors in these "complex" cases is more likely to impact on consequences such as infant outcomes (Carter, Garrity-Rokous, Chazan-Cohen, Little, & Briggs-Gowan, 2001; Nanni, Usher, & Danese, 2012; Oei et al., 2009).

Population studies demonstrate an increased risk of *new* onset psychiatric episodes, especially major depression and puerperal psychoses, in the first few months postpartum (Munk-Olsen, Laursen, Pedersen, Mors, & Mortensen, 2006). In addition, risk of *relapse* of preexisting mood disorder (often following the cessation of medication in pregnancy) increases significantly across the perinatal period (Cohen et al., 2006; Viguera et al., 2000, 2007), especially bipolar disorder (Munk-Olsen et al., 2009). Maternal death associated with psychosocial morbidity (including substance misuse and IPV) has become one of the

Identifying Perinatal Depression and Anxiety: Evidence-Based Practice in Screening, Psychosocial Assessment, and Management, First Edition. Edited by Jeannette Milgrom and Alan W. Gemmill.
© 2015 John Wiley & Sons, Ltd. Published 2015 by John Wiley & Sons, Ltd.

leading causes of maternal deaths in higher-income countries (Austin, Kildea, & Sullivan, 2007; Oates, 2003). There is a 70-fold increased risk of suicide in the first postnatal year after admission for a severe psychiatric episode compared to at other times in a woman's life (Appleby, Mortensen, & Faragher, 1998).

It is increasingly acknowledged that perinatal mental health is multifaceted and encompasses far more than the simple diagnosis of "postnatal depression." The concept of *psychosocial assessment* promulgates a broad focus of inquiry about past and current risk factors underpinning a woman's presentation in the perinatal period while including screening for possible current depression (Austin, 2004). Key risk factors for poorer perinatal mental health outcomes are well documented (Beck, 1996; Boyce & Hickey, 2005; Collins, Dunkel-Schetter, Lobel, & Scrimshaw, 1993; Demyttenaere, Lenaerts, Nijs, & Van Assche, 1995; Fisher et al., 2013; Harlow et al., 2007; Lancaster et al., 2010; Milgrom et al., 2008; Munk-Olsen, Laursen, Pedersen, Mors, & Mortensen, 2007; Munk-Olsen et al., 2009; Nielsen Forman, Videbech, Hedegaard, Dalby Salvig, & Secher, 2000; Stuart, Couser, Schilder, O'Hara, & Gorman, 1998) and include:

- A past history of a mental health condition (including major depression, anxiety disorder, psychosis, personality disorder, etc.)
- Lack of supports
- Poor-quality intimate partner relationship including IPV
- Stressful life events, for example, poverty
- A history of childhood trauma or poor parenting
- Isolation (physical, mental, cultural)
- Substance misuse
- Long-standing personality vulnerabilities, for example, low self-esteem, high trait anxiety, or borderline traits

While the Australian Clinical Practice Guidelines for Perinatal Depression and Related Disorders (2011) note the use of universal psychosocial assessment as a good practice point (Austin, Highet, & The Guidelines Expert Advisory Committee, 2011), neither the Scottish (Scottish Intercollegiate Guidelines Network (SIGN), 2012) nor English and Welsh (National Institute for Health and Clinical Excellence (NICE), 2007) guidelines advocate a broad psychosocial assessment approach—although they do recommend inquiry about personal or family history of serious mental illness. The International Marcé Society Position Statement 2013 on "Psychosocial Assessment and Depression Screening in Perinatal Women" emphasizes the value of early identification of—and where appropriate—intervention to reduce maternal psychosocial risk or mental health morbidity (Austin and The Marcé Society Position Statement Advisory Committee, 2013). It emphasizes the importance of maternal emotional well-being in relation to the functioning of the family unit and the developing parent–infant relationship.

The presence of mental illness will very often affect a mother's role as caregiver for her infant, with the potential for impacting negatively on the development of infant attachment (Hipwell, Goossens, Melhuish, & Kumar, 2000; Martins & Gaffan, 2000; Poobalan et al., 2007). Irrespective of the presence of a mental health episode, maternal adjustment to parenthood and infant development will be affected by many of the other psychosocial risk factors noted earlier.

For example, the presence of high levels of anxiety and stress in pregnancy can adversely impact on fetal development with associated suboptimal cognitive, emotional, and behavioral outcomes in the offspring as identified in a number of large prospective cohort studies (Talge, Neal, & Glover, 2007). Postnatal depression may also impact on infant outcomes (Murray & Cooper, 1997).

The presence of IPV in pregnancy is associated with three times the rate of postnatal depression symptoms (Howard, Oram, Galley, Trevillion, & Feder, 2013) and poorer infant outcomes (Hungerford, Wait, Fritz, & Clements, 2012). The point prevalence of IPV in the general female population is reported as between 2% and 16.5%, with higher prevalences reported in low- and middle-income countries than in high-income settings (Devries et al., 2010). Lifetime experience of IPV (most often reported in terms of physical abuse) will occur in between 25% and 30% of the general population of women (Tjaden & Thoennes, 2000), rising to between 40% and 60% in women of low socioeconomic status (Tolman & Rosen, 2001). CSA is also well known to be associated with poor mental health outcomes in women generally (Mullen, Martin, Anderson, Romans, & Herbison, 1993), and in postpartum women, it is associated not only with increased risk for depression (Buist & Janson, 2001) but also increased parenting stress (Douglas, 2000) and poorer quality of maternal sensitivity and attachment (McMahon, Barnett, Kowalenko, & Tennant, 2006). Similarly, a controlling and affectionless experience of being parented is associated with mental health morbidity across the perinatal period (Grant, Bautovich, Reilly, McMahon, & Austin, 2012). These risk factors are deserving of more focus in the perinatal period, given their impact on maternal as well as infant outcomes.

Definitions Relevant to Integrated Psychosocial Assessment

We need to define the terminology and concepts that have arisen over the last decade around psychosocial assessment in the perinatal period, as undertaken in some high-income settings:

1 *Psychosocial risk factors:* cover the spectrum of psychosocial factors that have been empirically established as associated with a range of negative mental health outcomes, from a history of diagnosable psychiatric disorders (including high-prevalence disorders, i.e., major depression and anxiety disorders) and low-prevalence (but often more severe) disorders, such as psychosis, schizophrenia, personality, and bipolar disorder) to adverse circumstances (in particular intimate partner violence, substance misuse, and childhood abuse).

2 *Psychosocial assessment programs:* encompass the evaluation of current and long-standing psychological, social, and cultural risk factors impacting on the mental health and functioning of women across the perinatal period (Austin, 2004). Psychosocial assessment (as for depression screening) must be undertaken as part of an integrated care program, not as a stand-alone assessment (Barnett, 2011). It can be undertaken in a number of ways (e.g., by means of self-report assessment tool or structured interview), the key issue being that assessment is integrated with further mental health evaluation (if needed) and management (which may include psychiatric treatment, counseling, bolstering of social supports, or mother–infant therapy). Unlike mental health screening, psychosocial assessment does not set out to identify women with a possible diagnosis of a particular condition at the time of assessment. Rather it gives clinicians a *multidimensional* picture of the woman's circumstances which can then be used to make decisions about best care options. Given its

multidimensionality, it is important that it be undertaken as part of an integrated care program (see definition below).

3   *Integrated care*: the use of this concept is critical to the perinatal setting and has a number of interrelated applications:

   a   Integration *across health-care disciplines* and between primary and secondary/tertiary health-care systems

   b   Integration between *components of a psychosocial assessment program*: including the assessment itself (which incorporates depression screening) and clinician decision-making guidelines as to the need for mental health evaluation and the type of care plan and referral pathways

   c   Integration *across time periods* (antenatal and postnatal) and service settings (e.g., hospital and community)

   d   Integration of psychosocial assessment with "mainstream" (physical) maternity and postnatal care

The Debate: For and against Psychosocial Assessment

The potential clinical and economic value of inclusion of emotional and mental health as a routine component of maternal care has been recognized by the World Health Organization (2013).

In many countries, pregnancy and the postnatal period provide opportunistic periods for health education due to the frequency of contact with health-care providers. Expectant and new parents are often highly motivated to seek help in effecting change for the sake of their offspring and potential reduction in intergenerational family dysfunction. The perinatal period thus provides clinicians with a unique opportunity to address all aspects of their clients' health, and to consider *psychosocial assessment as part of universal, mainstream maternity and postnatal care*. Early identification and management of psychosocial morbidity are especially important in relation to the functioning of the family unit and the critical parent–infant relationship with potential to positively impact on the health of the next generation.

The key themes currently debated around psychosocial assessment in the perinatal period are: whether it should be universally undertaken, whether the potential benefits of universal assessment outweigh the harms (clinical and cost through overidentification), and the ethical implications of undertaking such activity in resource-constrained settings (Austin and The Marcé Society Position Statement Advisory Committee, 2013).

The case for psychosocial assessment is beset by many of the same challenges as for depression screening, in particular the potential for inaccuracy of self-report and the consequences of *false positives or false negatives*. Of note, *false positives* will be associated with increased cost to the system and potential stigmatization, while false negatives may mean women go undetected and untreated, adversely impacting on maternal and infant outcomes.

In favor of psychosocial assessment, inquiring about the woman's emotional state as part of broader maternity and postnatal care clearly indicates to the woman that her clinician is interested in her overall well-being. There is a strong argument for considering such inquiry as part of routine care—where physical and emotional care is integrated within the primary health-care context. While some question the routine use of a depression screening tool in isolation from other health system changes (for reasons outlined in earlier chapters), most clinicians would argue that psychosocial assessment has value in its own right as a means of:

1 *Opening up the conversation* about psychosocial issues including those that impact the family more broadly (e.g., intimate partner violence, supports, help seeking) and that can be addressed by non-mental health-trained care providers.
2 *Raising awareness and educating* pregnant women/mothers and their carers about the fact that psychiatric and psychosocial conditions may arise or relapse perinatally and deserve to be identified and treated, that difficulties in the parent–infant interaction may arise at this time, and that effective treatments and supports are available should these problems arise.

Further, in support of routine assessment of both depression and the broader psychosocial context, there is growing evidence that low-intensity interventions (e.g., Internet-based programs), social support, peer support, and self-help are effective in the management of social isolation, milder mood, or adjustment disorders (Dennis, 2006; Dennis & Hodnett, 2007; Dennis et al., 2009) and may circumvent the perceived increased workload for the health-care sector as a whole.

In summary, while there is no simple answer to the question of *whether there is a place for universal psychosocial assessment without the availability of comprehensive referral services,* not undertaking such assessment because of the complexity of issues or a lack of mental health resources overlooks the critical role of psychosocial well-being in maternal and infant outcomes. It is generally recognized by clinicians that such assessment holds intrinsic value in terms of educating women and families and "starting the conversation" about psychosocial issues. How exactly this takes place must be decided at a local health service level within the framework of appropriate policies and guidelines (see specific example in following section). Ultimately, long-term follow-up studies are needed to evaluate the benefits and costs for the well-being of mothers, infants, their families, and society.

Psychosocial Assessment Tools for Clinicians

To effectively undertake psychosocial assessment, primary health-care professionals will need a well-defined methodology that is suited to local circumstances. A number of approaches may be adopted from the use of structured questionnaires (self-report or clinician administered) to general unstructured inquiry as part of holistic care. The key issue is the need for these to be undertaken within an integrated care model (Austin, Priest, & Sullivan, 2008; Barnett, Glossop, Matthey, & Stewart, 2005). Unlike depression screening programs, psychosocial assessment tools are not targeting a single condition, and thus, it is challenging for these tools to have acceptable psychometric properties or be tested against diagnostic criteria such as the DSM system (American Psychiatric Association, 2013) for single diagnostic categories.

By definition, a *structured psychosocial assessment tool* will be multidimensional (Johnson et al., 2012; Jomeen, 2004). There are now a number of published examples of structured psychosocial assessment tools: these include the Antenatal Psychosocial Health Assessment (ALPHA) (Carroll et al., 2005), Antenatal Risk Questionnaire (ANRQ) (Austin, Colton, Priest, Reilly, & Hadzi-Pavlovic, 2013), Predictive Index of PND (Cooper, 1996), and the Antenatal Psychosocial Questionnaire (Matthey et al., 2004). The ANRQ and Predictive

Index of PND have been subjected to psychometric evaluation using a specific cutoff score when applied antenatally (late pregnancy) to predict which women would develop major depression (using diagnostic criteria) in the first postnatal weeks and months. Not surprisingly, given the interval of several weeks between assessment and diagnostic evaluation, these tools have limited positive predictive value (30% and 35%, respectively). While defining the psychometric properties of such tools in terms of their ability to predict the development of high-prevalence disorders may be useful in terms of identifying clinically meaningful cutoff score, the key value of these tools is their role as the first component of integrated, universal psychosocial intervention programs (Austin et al., 2013).

Principles for Establishing an Integrated Psychosocial Assessment Program in the Primary Health-Care Setting

The principles outlined below assume a certain level of resources. They are based on what has been feasible in an urban, medium sized, Australian maternity hospital. Once the level of resources is established, the following steps then need to be considered:

1   Develop a working party which includes all key managers and stakeholders in your local health setting; educating them about the value of psychosocial assessment and engaging their support (financial, strategic) will be critical to the viability of the program. Identify champions at management and clinician levels across the relevant disciplines, for example, midwifery, obstetrics, mental health, family physician practice, and community child health nursing.
2   Identify (or develop) appropriate local policy and/or guidelines to underpin the program with basic principles including frequency and timing of universal psychosocial assessment, for example, in pregnancy and again a few weeks postpartum, integrated with routine maternity and infant care, etc.
3   Identify (or develop) a validated, user-friendly, and acceptable psychosocial assessment tool or structured interview for primary care clinicians suited to the local setting.
4   Consider depression screening as part of the assessment, and decide which depression screening tool to use (see Chapter 5).
5   Ensure the program is suited to the available workforce and incorporates local referral options.
6   Include *decision-making rules* to aid clinicians in responding to the results of their assessment. This may include a decision-making algorithm (depending on the assessment method) and will usually entail a regular *multidisciplinary team meeting* where women identified as having a mental health condition (including current possible depression cases) and those at high psychosocial risk are discussed and an appropriate care plan is devised.
7   Develop or identify a *training program* suitable to your setting and clinician group; ensure all key staff have basic minimum training as part of their accreditation requirements.
8   Consider how to incorporate minimum training at undergraduate and postgraduate levels through the relevant professional training bodies.
9   Identify a mental health clinician available to provide ongoing support and clinical supervision to the primary clinicians undertaking the assessment.

10   Ensure integration between components of the program, including the psychosocial assessment, depression screening, clear clinician decision-making guidelines (including the need for mental health evaluation), a multidisciplinary approach, and type of care plan and referral pathways available within the specific local setting.

Integrated Psychosocial Assessment Program in the Maternity Setting: An Example

Many of the large metropolitan Australian maternity hospitals provide a working example of a universal integrated psychosocial assessment program. In this setting, midwives (but this could be other nurses or family physicians) undertake routine assessment using the EPDS and a structured psychosocial questionnaire (e.g., ARQ, ANRQ) with all women at their first antenatal clinic visit. Midwives discuss the self-harm question on the EPDS (question 10) as well as any past mental health episode, risk factors requiring further discussion (including IPV, substance use, current stressors, past abuse, supports, etc.), and any other matter the woman may wish to discuss. The midwife then makes a decision based on the EPDS score (total and self-harm question 10), the presence of specific risk items, and the number of risk factors as to the level of psychosocial risk (using a decision-making algorithm) and whether discussion at a weekly mental health intake meeting is required. An example of a woman with severe psychosocial risk and her management plan would be: single, homeless, substance using with a history of childhood abuse and recent IPV. Has a "borderline personality disorder" and two children have been removed in the past. This woman will need combined input from midwifery (e.g., continuity of care through group midwifery practice), mental health services (to review diagnosis and monitor for exacerbation/relapse of symptoms), drug and alcohol use services, and social work (IPV, housing, child protection services). Her care will be best integrated through complex case meetings involving all relevant clinicians/departments.

A woman with the presence of milder risk factors (e.g., presence of high trait anxiety and perfectionism and recent stress of moving house) may do well with supportive counseling from her midwife and/or antenatal CBT groups.

The intake meeting is attended by midwifery, mental health, social work, and nursing staff representing maternity and early childhood nurses. About 15% of new antenatal clinic attendees will need discussion at the meeting, with an additional 5–10% brought to the meeting later in the pregnancy (Priest, Austin, Barnett, & Buist, 2008). Referral pathways available in this setting include substance use services, social work, and individual counseling through private psychology services. Many women will benefit from antenatal groups (offered through the maternity hospital) including cognitive behavioral therapy, psychoeducation, and attachment-based interventions. Between 5% and 7% of those discussed will require psychiatric assessment and a smaller proportion of women will have a complex case plan devised with a case worker allocated (usually for women with multiple and complex issues).

The earlier example is outlined in detail as the Perinatal Risk Assessment Model (PRAM) (Priest et al., 2008). Practical steps involved in psychosocial assessment, including acting on identified psychosocial risk factors, are also outlined in the practice summary from the Australian Clinical Practice Guidelines (Austin, Highet, & The Guidelines Expert Advisory Committee, 2011) (see Table 8.1).

Where psychosocial assessment programs are undertaken, primary care clinicians will need adequate psychosocial assessment skills training and ongoing clinical supervision from the mental health sector. Ultimately, training and support for the primary health sector is likely to reduce the frequency of referrals to mental health services as these practitioners become more confident and skilled with managing women with milder psychosocial risk and depression or anxiety. An online training resource for the detection and management of perinatal mental health disorders by primary health-care providers has been developed in Australia (Beyondblue, 2013).

Integrated Perinatal Care for Women Living in Resource-Constrained Settings

Most of the world's women live in the 112 countries classified by the World Bank as low and lower-middle income (UNPF, 2013). There are very substantial disparities between the evidence available about the nature, prevalence, course, determinants, and consequences of severe and common perinatal mental disorders among women in these resource-constrained settings, than among women living in high-income countries. Almost all research in low- and lower-middle-income countries has been initiated only since the mid-1990s. This 30-year lag in generation of research evidence between high- and low-income settings is in part attributable to competing health priorities, including the urgent need to prevent pregnancy-related deaths due to hemorrhage, infection, and lack of skilled birth attendants. However, it is also because influential scientists had argued that in resource-constrained countries, women's mental health is protected because they have access to traditional cultural practices that provide an honored status, mandated rest for specified periods, relief from household work, and social and emotional support from female family members (Howard, 1993; Stern & Kruckman, 1983). This is now regarded as an oversimplification, and it is now understood that traditional practices are neither accessible to all women nor always welcome or helpful (Wong & Fisher, 2009).

There are thousands of studies about common and severe perinatal mental disorders among women in high-income countries on which policies and practices, including psychosocial assessment and integrated care, can be based. In contrast, a recent systematic review of the evidence from resource-constrained countries (Fisher et al., 2012) found only 13 studies related to antenatal and 34 to postnatal common mental disorders. There is no equivalent review yet available about severe perinatal mental disorders in these settings. This raises complex questions about the implementation of assessment of psychological symptoms, psychosocial risks for mental disorders, and integrated perinatal care in resource-constrained settings.

Patterns of severe and high-prevalence mental disorders in low-resource settings

There is evidence of some intercountry differences in diagnostic patterns, with more psychotic illnesses among women who have recently given birth in low-income settings compared to high-income settings. Some studies have reported more women being classified with schizophrenia and fewer with affective disorders in low-income countries, but these

Table 8.1   Psychosocial assessment: Practice summary

Psychosocial assessment

When—As early as practical in pregnancy and 6–12 weeks after the birth, integrated into existing antenatal and postnatal care. If it is not feasible to conduct the assessments the first time you see the woman (e.g., due to time constraints), explain the importance and purpose of the assessments and set aside time in a follow-up appointment. Should take place at least once, preferably twice, in both the antenatal and postnatal periods

Who—Midwife; maternal and child health nurse; GP; obstetrician; Aboriginal and Torres Strait Islander health worker; practice nurse; allied health professional

How—Self report or face-to-face

Before psychosocial assessment

Provide psychoeducation—Explain that pregnancy and early parenthood can be challenging and that some women experience symptoms of depression or anxiety at this time and may benefit from support. Give the woman appropriate written materials (e.g., *beyondblue* emotional health booklet)

Seek informed consent—Explain that checking for psychosocial factors and symptoms is a routine part of care during pregnancy and after a birth, much as medical checks are made at these times, and that they remain confidential (unless there is a significant risk that the woman may harm herself or others). Ask the woman for consent and, if given, explain the process of the assessment

After psychosocial assessment

Identify level of support needed—Base decisions on the need for further follow-up on clinical judgement and the woman's preferences, taking into account that not all women with an EPDS score of 13 or more will benefit from psychosocial monitoring and/or mental health assessment, and that low or high scores may reflect other factors

Consider safety—If concerned about the woman's mental health and safety, contact mental health services. A woman has a choice about her care but you may need to override that choice if you consider her safety or that of children in her care to be at risk. In some cases, notification to the relevant child protection agency may need to be considered

Assist women who decline further care—If a woman chooses not to seek further care, provide her with information about consumer-led and community-led supports. Wherever possible, maintain contact with the woman and encourage her trust and confidence. Suggest that if she is concerned about how she is feeling emotionally, she should approach her GP to discuss her concerns

Identify an appropriate health professional for the woman's ongoing care—Ideally, ongoing care will be provided by the woman's regular GP. Encourage women who do not have a regular GP to attend a family practice. In situations where this is not possible (e.g., woman's preferences, location or cultural considerations), assist the woman to identify an appropriate health professional

Arrange follow-up care—If you are the health professional who will provide ongoing care, plan follow-up appointments with the woman. If referral to another health professional is indicated, ensure that the woman understands the need for further care and ask for her consent. Explain any assistance that may be available to support the woman in accessing follow-up care

Continue to involve the woman's significant other(s)—If ongoing care is needed, ask the woman if there is anyone from her support network that she would like to be involved. Suggest that the woman invite her significant other to the next appointment or a separate appointment—help that person to understand what's happening and provide information

---

From ©Beyond Blue Ltd. Excerpt reproduced with permission from Table 3.1 of the Australian Clinical Practice Guidelines for Depression and Related Disorders in the Perinatal Period.

patterns may reflect intercountry differences in diagnostic criteria (Fisher, de Mello, & Izutsu, 2009; Howard, 1993; Kumar, 1994). There is also a higher incidence in poorly resourced countries of organic confusional postpartum states attributable to malnutrition and infection being labeled as psychoses (Howard, 1993; Kumar, 1994; Ndosi & Mtawali, 2002).

The prevalence of the common perinatal mental disorders of depression and anxiety may be up to 50% higher among women living in resource-constrained than high-income countries. A recent meta-analysis established a mean prevalence of nonpsychotic common mental disorders established either by diagnostic interviews or scores in the clinical range on locally validated screening instruments of 15.6% (95% CI: 15.4–15.9%) among pregnant women and 19.8% (95% CI: 19.5–20.0%) among those who have recently given birth (Fisher, de Mello, & Izutsu, 2009). In these settings, the same risk factors apply and rates of depression and anxiety are much higher among the poorest women living in rural areas or affected by critical, coercive, or generally unsupportive relationships with an intimate partner or other family members; family violence; poor reproductive health; or a past history of mental health problems. Mental health is protected among women with more years of education, with a permanent job, being of the ethnic majority, and who have a kind, trustworthy intimate partner.

Suicide and suicidal behaviors

There is a small body of evidence about perinatal suicide in resource-constrained settings, with up to 20% of deaths not related directly to pregnancy or childbirth being attributable to suicide (Granja, Zacarias, & Bergstrom, 2002; Lal et al., 1995). Suicide is disproportionately associated with adolescent pregnancy and has been conceptualized as the only alternative for young women who fear parental or social sanction or who lack access to legal pregnancy termination services in settings where reproductive choice is limited. Suicide has also been linked to women experiencing gender-based abuse (Fisher et al., 2009).

Associations between common mental disorders, health-care participation, and infant health

There is increasing evidence in these settings that women with perinatal mental health problems are less likely to participate in essential preventive health care like taking recommended micronutrient supplements (Fisher, Tran et al., 2011b). In these countries, maternal depression is associated with lower birth weight and higher rates of stunting, diarrheal diseases, infectious illnesses, hospital admissions, and reduced completion of recommended immunization schedules among infants (Patel & Prince, 2006; Patel, Rahman, Jacob, & Hughes, 2004; Rahman et al., 2013).

Screening for mental disorders in resource-constrained settings

There have been some systematic endeavors to establish the utility of brief screening questionnaires to detect symptoms of common perinatal mental disorders in resource-constrained settings. In general, it has been found that women can *recognize symptoms* when they are described even if they cannot identify them. However, there are major differences in how these scales can be used. In many countries, women have limited access to education and have low literacy. There is frequently low familiarity with test taking, including the completion of self-report questionnaires, and the experience can cause anxiety including about the possibility of identifying information being made available to government authorities (Fisher, Morrow, Ngoc, & Anh, 2004). In most settings, this requires that the instruments are administered as individual-structured interviews. Where formal validation against a gold standard diagnostic psychiatric interview has been undertaken, it has often been found that cutoff scores to detect clinically significant symptoms are much lower than those established in high-income settings. In northern Vietnam, for example, optimal sensitivity (69.7%) and specificity (72.9%) to detect common perinatal mental disorders among women using the Edinburgh Postnatal Depression Scale–Vietnam validation is a score greater than 3 (Tran et al., 2011). A number of reasons are advanced to account for relatively low cutoff scores compared to those established in high-income settings. First, questionnaires about psychological states can lack meaning for people with a limited emotional lexicon and who perhaps answer no if the question is about emotional states they cannot name. Expression of negative emotions can be socially proscribed and so there can be shame associated with acknowledging them. This might be more common in places where the well-being of the collective or group is of higher importance than the needs or experiences of individuals. Finally, many screening questionnaires ask about change from a usual emotional state, but for people whose lives are chronically difficult, this does not detect depression because people experiencing low mood say no to the question because it is not a change.

Together, these are indicators of a complex and serious situation. The prevalence of perinatal mental disorders among women is substantially higher in resource-constrained than high-income settings. However, recognition is generally low, and most such countries (85%) lack any local evidence to inform practice, policy, preservice education, or professional development. In many of these countries, there are insufficient health services or trained health workers to be able to provide safe pregnancy and birth care, and many women receive no or minimal health care and give birth at home. Their mental health services are often limited to custodial institutions, which provide, by world standards, poor-quality and even abusive care. There are risks that using psychopathological labels to describe the social suffering that is associated with poverty and gender-based violence increases the risk of marginalization and discrimination.

Screening requires acceptable, sensitive, feasible instruments. Integrated care requires a trained workforce, a service system into which the process can be integrated, and accessible secondary and tertiary health services to which people with identified needs can be referred and consideration of resource constraints (Fisher, de Mello, Izutsu, & Tran, 2011a).

Future Directions and Developing the Evidence Base

We now have acceptable, brief, structured psychosocial assessment tools that lend themselves to use in resource-rich (Schmied et al., 2013) and resource-constrained settings (Vythilingum et al., 2013). What we do not have is an evaluation of their effectiveness within an integrated assessment program, and in absolute terms, there is less published research evidence from resource-constrained settings. In addition and as a separate but closely related issue, there are no clear reproducible decision-making and referral processes for clinicians. Systematic reviews of depression screening embedded within an enhanced/integrated care setting indicate that overall this model can be effective in improving depression outcomes in the general population, and task forces on preventive health care in the United States and Canada have recommended such "interventions" (MacMillan et al., 2005; Pignone et al., 2002). One of the key studies, and the most strongly powered cluster randomized trials in which all participants (in a general population community study Wells et al., 2000) were screened for depression, found improved outcomes in those randomized to the enhanced depression care program ($N=913$) versus care as usual ($N=443$). At 6 months, approximately 60% of patients in the enhanced care program were engaged in appropriate therapy versus approximately 40% of patients who received care as usual, while around 40% of enhanced care patients and 50% of care as usual patients still met criteria for probable depressive disorder ($p=0.001$). These differences in treatment uptake and outcome were maintained at 12 months and 5 years (Wells et al., 2000).

The challenge with broader psychosocial assessment programs is how best to evaluate their impact on service uptake and clinical outcomes. In real-world settings, women will present with different psychosocial "risk" profiles triggering different interventions, and the journey from assessment to treatment may be influenced by a range of individual (e.g., maternal help-seeking behaviors), social (e.g., levels of practical and emotional support), and systemic factors (e.g., staff attitude to screening, training, availability of referral options, local policy).

A comprehensive evaluation of psychosocial assessment programs would (i) compare the service use and health outcomes of women exposed to an integrated psychosocial assessment intervention (program) compared to those not exposed, (ii) dissect the various components of the intervention in the exposed group (e.g., frequency, timing, and type of assessment; presence/type of referral; personal barriers/facilitators to care uptake), (iii) evaluate the moderating effect of women's preexisting psychosocial risk profiles on their health outcomes, and (iv) be inclusive of economic analyses, including an examination of the cost-effectiveness and cost–utility of the program.

Alternative ways of routinely administering psychosocial assessment also need to be considered. One promising method, where existing electronic database systems allow, is the use of e-screening or assessment tools which reduce the load on clinicians at the screening level so that greater time can be spent on referral or further assessment (see Chapter 15). Such an e-health method has been shown to address some of the key barriers identified by women and health-care providers, including acceptability in collection of sensitive issues e.g., IPV (MacMillan et al., 2006) and postpartum depression (Le, Perry, & Sheng, 2009). It is suited to busy clinical settings in that it offers consistency, avoids loss of data or incorrect scoring, and achieves similar rates of disclosure, in some cases being preferred by patients due to its anonymity (Turner et al., 1998).

Although at present it could not be recommended that protocols for screening and systems of integrated care are directly transferable from high- to low-income settings, a lack of action is not acceptable. A recent systematic review of the 11 community-based approaches to treating perinatal mental disorders in resource-constrained settings that were evaluated in randomized controlled trials yields promising findings (Rahman et al., 2013). Most used structured psychoeducational programs and were implemented by local health workers in routine services. The pooled effect size (Cohen's d) for maternal depression (according to diagnostic criteria) was -0.38 (95% CI: -0.56 to -0.21), and for those that assessed them, there were also benefits to the child.

Partnerships to reduce this disparity could focus on assistance to improve recognition, build local evidence about nature and prevalence, adapt and validate screening instruments, write and evaluate preservice curricula and professional development programs, and increase health service capacity. Psychosocial assessment tools are now being developed in resource-constrained settings. For example, in Cape Town, South Africa (Vythilingum et al., 2013), the risk factor assessment is an 11-item questionnaire which allows a measure of cumulative risk factors and is administered by local primary health-care workers at routine antenatal visits. Chowdhary et al. (2013), in a recent review, have also identified ways that psychological interventions for perinatal depression can be delivered by nonspecialist health workers in low- and middle-income countries. These developments suggest that, with appropriate support, routine psychosocial assessment is also feasible in less resource-rich regions of the world.

Acknowledgments

The authors thank St John of God Health Care Australia and the Jean Hailes Research Unit of the School of Public Health and Preventive Medicine at Monash University for infrastructure support. Discussions with members of the advisory group for the International Marcé Society Position Statement (2013) "Psychosocial Assessment and Depression Screening in Perinatal Women" helped shape some of the content of this chapter.

References

American Psychiatric Association. (2013). *Diagnostic and statistical manual of mental disorders* (5th ed.). Arlington, VA: American Psychiatric Publishing.

Appleby, L., Mortensen, P. B., & Faragher, E. B. (1998). Suicide and other causes of mortality after post-partum psychiatric admission. *British Journal of Psychiatry, 173*, 209–211.

Austin, M.-P. (2004). Antenatal screening and early intervention for "perinatal" distress, depression and anxiety: Where to from here? *Archives of Women's Mental Health, 7*, 1–6.

Austin, M. P., Colton, J., Priest, S., Reilly, N., & Hadzi-Pavlovic, D. (2013). The Antenatal Risk Questionnaire (ANRQ): Acceptability and use for psychosocial risk assessment in the maternity setting *Women & Birth 26*, 17–25. doi:10.1016/j.wombi.2011.06.002.

Austin, M. P., Highet, N. J., & The Guidelines Expert Advisory Committee. (2011). *Clinical practice guidelines for depression and related disorders—Anxiety, bipolar disorder and puerperal psychosis—In the perinatal period, a guideline for primary care health professionals providing care in the perinatal period*. Melbourne, Australia: beyondblue: the national depression initiative.

Austin, M. P., Kildea, S., & Sullivan, E. (2007). Maternal mortality and psychiatric morbidity in the perinatal period: Challenges and opportunities for prevention in the Australian setting. *The Medical Journal of Australia, 186*(7), 364–367.

Austin, M.-P., Priest, S. R., & Sullivan, E. (2008). Antenatal psychosocial assessment for reducing antenatal and postnatal mental health morbidity. *Cochrane Database of Systematic Reviews, (4)*, CD005124. doi:10.1002/14651858.CD005124.pub2.

Austin, M.-P., & The Marcé Society Position Statement Advisory Committee. (2013). Marcé International Society position statement 2013 psychosocial assessment and depression screening in perinatal women. *Best Practice & Research. Clinical Obstetrics & Gynaecology, 28*(1), 179–187. doi:10.1016/j.bpobgyn.2013.08.016.

Barnett, B. (2011). An integrated model of perinatal care. *European Psychiatric Review, 4*(2), 71–74.

Barnett, B., Glossop, P., Matthey, S., & Stewart, H. (2005). Screening in the context of integrated perinatal care. In C. Henshaw & S. Elliott (Eds.), Screening for perinatal depression. London, UK: Jessica Kingsley.

Beck, C. T. (1996). A meta-analysis of predictors of post-partum depression. *Nursing Research, 45*, 297–303.

Beyondblue. (2013). Beyond babyblues: Detecting and managing perinatal mental health disorders in primary care (online learning and resources). Retrieved from http://thinkgp.com.au/beyondblue. Accessed December 17, 2014.

Boyce, P., & Hickey, A. (2005). Psychosocial risk factors to major depression after childbirth. *Social Psychiatry and Psychiatric Epidemiology, 40*(8), 605–612. doi:10.1007/s00127-005-0931-0.

Buist, A., & Janson, H. (2001). Childhood sexual abuse, parenting and postpartum depression—A 3-year follow-up study. *Child Abuse & Neglect, 25*(7), 909–921. doi:10.1016/S0145-2134(01)00246-0.

Carroll, J. C., Reid, A. J., Biringer, A., Midmer, D., Glazier, R. H., Wilson, L., … Stewart, D. E. (2005). Effectiveness of the Antenatal Psychosocial Health Assessment (ALPHA) form in detecting psychosocial concerns: A randomized controlled trial. *Canadian Medical Association Journal, 173*(3), 253–259. doi:10.1503/cmaj.1040610.

Carter, A. S., Garrity-Rokous, F. E., Chazan-Cohen, R., Little, C., & Briggs-Gowan, M. J. (2001). Maternal depression and comorbidity: Predicting early parenting, attachment security, and toddler social-emotional problems and competencies. *Journal of the American Academy of Child & Adolescent Psychiatry, 40*(1), 18–26.

Chowdhary, N., Sikander, S., Atif, N., Ahmad, I., Fuhr, D. C., Rahman, A., & Patel, V. (2013). The content and delivery of psychological interventions for perinatal depression by non-specialist health workers in low and middle income countries: A systematic review. *Best Practice & Research. Clinical Obstetrics & Gynaecology, 28*(1), 113–133. doi:10.1016/j.bpobgyn.2013.08.013.

Cohen, L. S., Altshuler, L. L., Harlow, B. L., Nonacs, R., Newport, D. J., Viguera, A. C., … Stowe, Z. N. (2006). Relapse of major depression during pregnancy in women who maintain or discontinue antidepressant treatment. *JAMA: The Journal of the American Medical Association, 295*(5), 499–507. doi:10.1001/jama.295.5.499.

Collins, N. L., Dunkel-Schetter, C., Lobel, M., & Scrimshaw, S. C. M. (1993). Social support in pregnancy: Psychosocial correlates of birth outcomes and postpartum depression. *Journal of Personality and Social Psychology, 65*(6), 1243–1258. doi:10.1037/0022-3514.65.6.1243.

Cooper, P. J., Murray, L., Hooper, R., & West, A. (1996). The development and validation of a predictive index for postpartum depression. *Psychological Medicine, 36*, 627–634.

Demyttenaere, K., Lenaerts, H., Nijs, P., & Van Assche, F. A. (1995). Individual coping style and psychological attitudes during pregnancy predict depression levels during pregnancy and during postpartum. *Acta Psychiatrica Scandinavica, 91*(2), 95–102. doi:10.1111/j.1600-0447.1995.tb09747.x.

Dennis, C. L. (2006). Intensive postpartum support for postnatal depression has the most beneficial outcome—Meta-analysis. *Evidence-Based Obstetrics & Gynecology, 8*(3–4), 94–95. doi:10.1016/j.ebobgyn.2006.09.003.

Dennis, C. L., & Hodnett, E. (2007). Psychosocial and psychological interventions for treating postpartum depression. *Cochrane Database of Systematic Reviews,* (4), CD006116. doi:10.1002/14651858.CD006116.

Dennis, C. L., Hodnett, E., Kenton, L., Weston, J., Zupancic, J., Stewart, D. E., & Kiss, A. (2009). Effect of peer support on prevention of postnatal depression among high risk women: Multisite randomised controlled trial. *British Medical Journal, 338*(jan15_2), a3064. doi:10.1136/bmj.a3064.

Devries, K. M., Kishor, S., Johnson, H., Stöckl, H., Bacchus, L. J., Garcia-Moreno, C., & Watts, C. (2010). Intimate partner violence during pregnancy: Analysis of prevalence data from 19 countries. *Reproductive Health Matters, 18*(36), 158–170. doi:10.1016/S0968-8080(10)36533-5.

Douglas, A. R. (2000). Reported anxieties concerning intimate parenting in women sexually abused as children. *Child Abuse & Neglect, 24*(3), 425–434. doi:10.1016/S0145-2134(99)00154-4.

Fisher, J., de Mello, M. C., & Izutsu, T. (2009). Mental health aspects of pregnancy, childbirth and the postpartum period. In *Contemporary topics in women's mental health* (pp. 197–225). Hoboken, NJ: John Wiley & Sons, Ltd.

Fisher, J., de Mello, M., Izutsu, T., & Tran, T. (2011a). The Ha Noi Expert Statement: Recognition of maternal mental health in resource-constrained settings is essential for achieving the Millennium Development Goals. *International Journal of Mental Health Systems, 5*(1), 2. doi:10.1186/1752-4458-5-2.

Fisher, J., de Mello, M. C., Patel, V., Rahman, A., Tran, T., Holton, S., & Holmes, W. (2012). Prevalence and determinants of common perinatal mental disorders in women in low- and lower-middle-income countries: A systematic review. *Bulletin of the World Health Organization, 90*(2), 139G–149G. doi:10.2471/BLT.11.091850.

Fisher, J., Morrow, M. M., Ngoc, N. T., & Anh, L. T. (2004). Prevalence, nature, severity and correlates of postpartum depressive symptoms in Vietnam. *BJOG: An International Journal of Obstetrics and Gynaecology of India, 111*, 1353–1360.

Fisher, J., Tran, T., Biggs, B., Tran, T., Dwyer, T., Casey, G., … Hetzel, B. (2011b). Iodine status in late pregnancy and psychosocial determinants of iodized salt use in rural northern Viet Nam. *Bulletin of the World Health Organization, 89*(11), 813–820. doi: 10.2471/BLT.11.089763.

Fisher, J., Tran, T., Duc Tran, T., Dwyer, T., Nguyen, T., Casey, G. J., … Biggs, B.-A. (2013). Prevalence and risk factors for symptoms of common mental disorders in early and late pregnancy in Vietnamese women: A prospective population-based study. *Journal of Affective Disorders, 146*(2), 213–219. doi:10.1016/j.jad.2012.09.007.

Granja, A., Zacarias, E., & Bergstrom, S. (2002). Violent deaths: The hidden face of maternal mortality. *BJOG: An International Journal of Obstetrics and Gynaecology, 109*, 5–8. doi:10.1111/j.1471-0528.2002.01082.x.

Grant, K. A., Bautovich, A., Reilly, N., McMahon, C., & Austin, M. P. (2012). Parental care and control during childhood: Associations with maternal perinatal mood disturbance and parenting stress. *Archives of Women's Mental Health, 15*(4), 297–305. doi: 10.1007/s00737-012-0292-0.

Harlow, B. L., Vitonis, A. F., Sparen, P. P., Cnattingius, S., Joffe, H., & Hultman, C. M. (2007). Incidence of hospitalization for postpartum psychotic and bipolar episodes in women with and without prior prepregnancy or prenatal psychiatric hospitalizations. *Archives of General Psychiatry, 64*(1), 42–48. doi:10.1001/archpsyc.64.1.42.

Hipwell, A. E., Goossens, F. A., Melhuish, E. C., & Kumar, R. (2000). Severe maternal psychopathology and infant-mother attachment. *Development & Psychopathology, 12*, 157–175. doi:10.1017/S0954579400002030.

Howard, R. (1993). Transcultural issues in puerperal mental illness. *International Review of Psychiatry, 5*(2–3), 253–260. doi:10.3109/09540269309028315.

Howard, L., Oram, S., Galley, H., Trevillion, K., & Feder, G. (2013). Domestic violence and perinatal mental disorders: A systematic review and meta-analysis. *PLoS Medicine, 10*(5), 1–16. doi:10.1371/journal.pmed.1001452.

Hungerford, A., Wait, S. K., Fritz, A. M., & Clements, C. M. (2012). Exposure to intimate partner violence and children's psychological adjustment, cognitive functioning, and social competence: A review. *Aggression and Violent Behavior, 17*(4), 373–382.

Johnson, M., Schmeid, V., Lupton, S. J., Austin, M. P., Matthey, S. M., Kemp, L., … Yeo, A. E. (2012). Measuring perinatal mental health risk. *Archives of Women's Mental Health, 15*(5), 375–386. doi:10.1007/s00737-012-0297-8.

Jomeen, J. (2004). The importance of assessing psychological status during pregnancy, childbirth and the postnatal period as a multidimensional construct: A literature review. *Clinical Effectiveness in Nursing, 8*(3–4), 143–155. doi:10.1016/j.cein.2005.02.001.

Kumar, R. (1994). Postnatal mental illness: A transcultural perspective. *Social Psychiatry and Psychiatric Epidemiology, 29*(6), 250–264. doi:10.1007/bf00802048.

Lal, S., Satpathy, S., Khanna, P., Vashisht, B. M., Punia, M. S., & Kumar, S. (1995). Problem of mortality in women of reproductive age in rural area of Haryana. *Indian Journal of Maternal and Child Health, 6*(1), 17–21.

Lancaster, C. A., Gold, K. J., Flynn, H. A., Yoo, H., Marcus, S. M., & Davis, M. M. (2010). Risk factors for depressive symptoms during pregnancy: A systematic review. *American Journal of Obstetrics and Gynecology, 202*(1), 5–14. doi:10.1016/j.ajog.2009.09.007.

Le, H. N., Perry, D. F., & Sheng, X. (2009). Using the internet to screen for postpartum depression. *Maternal and Child Health Journal, 13*(2), 213–221. doi:10.1007/s10995-008-0322-8.

MacMillan, H., Patterson, C., Wathen, N., & The Canadian Task Force on Preventive Health Care. (2005). Screening for depression in primary care: Recommendation statement from the Canadian Task Force on Preventative Health Care. *Canadian Medical Association Journal, 172*(1), 33–35.

MacMillan, H. L., Wathen, C., Jamieson, E., Boyle, M., McNutt, L. A., Worster, A., … McMaster Violence Against Women Research. (2006). Approaches to screening for intimate partner violence in health care settings: A randomized trial. *JAMA: The Journal of the American Medical Association, 296*(5), 530–536. doi:10.1001/jama.296.5.530.

Martins, C., & Gaffan, E. A. (2000). Effects of early maternal depression on patterns of infant-mother attachment: A meta-analytic investigation. *Journal of Child Psychology & Psychiatry, 41*(6), 737–746.

Matthey, S., Phillips, J., White, T., Glossop, P., Hopper, U., Panasetis, P., … Barnett, B. (2004). Routine psychosocial assessment of women in the antenatal period: Frequency of risk factors and implications for clinical services. *Archives of Women's Mental Health. 7*(4), 223–229. doi:10.1007/s00737-004-0064-6.

McMahon, C. A., Barnett, B., Kowalenko, N. M., & Tennant, C. C. (2006). Maternal attachment state of mind moderates the impact of postnatal depression on infant attachment. *Journal of Child Psychology and Psychiatry, 47*(7), 660–669. doi:10.1111/j.1469-7610.2005.01547.x.

Milgrom, J., Gemmill, A. W., Bilszta, J. L., Hayes, B., Barnett, B., Brooks, J., … Buist, A. (2008). Antenatal risk factors for postnatal depression: A large prospective study. *Journal of Affective Disorders, 108*(1–2), 147–157. doi:10.1016/j.jad.2007.10.014.

Mullen, P. E., Martin, J. L., Anderson, J. C., Romans, S. E., & Herbison, G. P. (1993). Childhood sexual abuse and mental health in adult life. *The British Journal of Psychiatry, 163*(6), 721–732. doi:10.1192/bjp.163.6.721.

Munk-Olsen, T., Laursen, T. M., Mendelson, T., Pedersen, C. B., Mors, O., & Mortensen, P. B. (2009). Risks and predictors of readmission for a mental disorder during the postpartum period. *Archives of General Psychiatry, 66*(2), 189–195. doi:10.1001/archgenpsychiatry.2008.528.

Munk-Olsen, T., Laursen, T. M., Pedersen, C. B., Mors, O., & Mortensen, P. B. (2006). New parents and mental disorders: A population-based register study. *JAMA: The Journal of the American Medical Association, 296*(21), 2582–2589. doi:10.1001/jama.296.21.2582.

Munk-Olsen, T., Laursen, T. M., Pedersen, C. B., Mors, O., & Mortensen, P. B. (2007). Family and partner psychopathology and the risk of postpartum mental disorders. *Journal of Clinical Psychiatry, 68*(12), 1947–1953.

Murray, L., & Cooper, P. J. (1997). Postpartum depression and child development. *Psychological Medicine, 27*(2), 253–260. doi:10.1136/adc.77.2.99.

Nanni, V., Usher, R., & Danese, A. (2012). Childhood maltreatment predicts unfavorable course of illness and treatment outcome in depression: A meta-analysis. *The American Journal of Psychiatry, 169*(2), 141–151. doi:10.1176/appi.ajp.2011.11020335.

National Institute for Health and Clinical Excellence (NICE). (2007). Antenatal and postnatal mental health: The NICE guidelines on clinical management and service guidance CG45. National Collaborating Centre for Mental Health. The British Psychological Society & The Royal College of Psychiatrists.

Ndosi, N. K., & Mtawali, M. L. W. (2002). The nature of puerperal psychosis at Muhimbili National Hospital: Its physical co-morbidity, associated main obstetric and social factors. *African Journal of Reproductive Health, 6*(1), 41–49.

Nielsen Forman, D., Videbech, P., Hedegaard, M., Dalby Salvig, J., & Secher, N. J. (2000). Postpartum depression: Identification of women at risk. *BJOG: An International Journal of Obstetrics & Gynaecology, 107*(10), 1210–1217.

Oates, M. (2003). Suicide: The leading cause of maternal death. *British Journal of Psychiatry, 183*, 279–281. doi:10.1192/02-488.

Oei, J. L., Abdel-Latif, M. E., Craig, F., Kee, A., Austin, M.-P., Lui, K., & on behalf of the N. S. W. and A. C. T. N. A. S. Epidemiology Group. (2009). Short-term outcomes of mothers and newborn infants with comorbid psychiatric disorders and drug dependency. *Australian and New Zealand Journal of Psychiatry, 43*(4), 323–331. doi:10.1080/00048670902721087.

Patel, V., & Prince, M. (2006). Maternal psychological morbidity and low birth weight in India. *The British Journal of Psychiatry, 188*(3), 284–285. doi:10.1192/bjp.bp.105.012096.

Patel, V., Rahman, A., Jacob, K. S., & Hughes, M. (2004). Effect of maternal mental health on infant growth in low income countries: New evidence from South Asia. *British Medical Journal*, *328*(7443), 820–823. doi:10.1136/bmj.328.7443.820.

Pignone, M. P., Gaynes, B. N., Rushton, J. L., Burchell, C. M., Orleans, C. T., Mulrow, C. D., & Lohr, K. N. (2002). Screening for depression in adults: A summary of the evidence for the U.S. Preventive Services Task Force. *Annals of Internal Medicine*, *136*(10), 765–776. doi:10.7326/0003-4819-136-10-200205210-00013.

Poobalan, A. S., Aucott, L. S., Ross, L., Smith, W. C., Helms, P. J., & Williams, J. H. (2007). Effects of treating postnatal depression on mother infant interaction and child development: Systematic review. *The British Journal of Psychiatry*, *191*, 378–386.

Priest, S., Austin, M. P., Barnett, B., & Buist, A. (2008). A psychosocial risk assessment model (PRAM) for use with pregnant and postpartum women in primary care settings. *Archives of Women's Mental Health*, *11*(5–6), 307–317. doi:10.1007/s00737-008-0028-3.

Rahman, A., Fisher, J., Bower, P., Luchters, S., Tran, T., Yasamy, M. T., … Waheed, W. (2013). Interventions for common perinatal mental disorders in women in low- and middle-income countries: A systematic review and meta-analysis. *Bulletin of the World Health Organization*, *91*(8), 18.

Schmied, V., Johnson, M., Naidoo, N., Austin, M. P., Matthey, S., Kemp, L., … Yeo, A. (2013). Maternal mental health in Australia and New Zealand: A review of longitudinal studies. *Women and Birth*, *26*(3), 167–178. doi:10.1016/j.wombi.2013.02.006.

Scottish Intercollegiate Guidelines Network (SIGN). (2012). Management of perinatal mood disorders (SIGN Publication no. 127). Edinburgh, Scotland: Author. Retrieved from http://www.sign.ac.uk Accessed December 17, 2014.

Stern, G., & Kruckman, L. (1983). Multi-disciplinary perspectives on post-partum depression: An anthropological critique. *Social Science and Medicine*, *17*: 1027–1041.

Stuart, S., Couser, G., Schilder, K., O'Hara, M. W., & Gorman, L. (1998). Postpartum anxiety and depression: Onset and comorbidity in a community sample. *Journal of Nervous & Mental Disease*, *186*(7), 420–424.

Talge, N. M., Neal, C., & Glover, V. (2007). Antenatal maternal stress and long-term effects on child neurodevelopment: How and why? *Journal of Child Psychology and Psychiatry, and Allied Disciplines*, *48*(3–4), 245–261. doi:10.1111/j.1469-7610.2006.01714.x.

Tjaden, P., & Thoennes, N. (2000). Prevalence and consequences of male-to-female and female-to-male intimate partner violence as measured by the National Violence Against Women Survey. *Violence Against Women*, *6*(2), 142–161. doi:10.1177/10778010022181769.

Tolman, R. M., & Rosen, D. (2001). Domestic violence in the lives of women receiving welfare: Mental health, substance dependence, and economic well-being. *Violence Against Women*, *7*(2), 141–158. doi:10.1177/1077801201007002003.

Tran, T. D., Tran, T., La, B., Lee, D., Rosenthal, D., & Fisher, J. (2011). Screening for perinatal common mental disorders in women in the north of Vietnam: A comparison of three psychometric instruments. *Journal of Affective Disorders*, *133*(1–2), 281–293. doi:10.1016/j.jad.2011.03.038.

Turner, C. F., Ku, L., Rogers, S. M., Lindberg, L. D., Pleck, J. H., & Sonenstein, F. L. (1998). Adolescent sexual behavior, drug use, and violence: Increased reporting with computer survey technology. *Science*, *280*(5365), 867–873. doi:10.1126/science.280.5365.867.

United Nations Population Fund. (2013). *State of the world's population.* Retrieved from https://www.unfpa.org/swp

Viguera, A., Nonacs, R., Cohen, L. S., Tondo, L., Murray, A., & Baldessarini, R. (2000). Risk of recurrence of bipolar disorder in pregnant and nonpregnant women after discontinuing lithium maintenance. *American Journal of Psychiatry*, *157*, 179–184. doi:10.1176/appi.ajp.157.2.179.

Viguera, A. C., Whitfield, T., Baldessarini, R. J., Newport, D. J., Stowe, Z., Reminick, A., … Cohen, L. S. (2007). Risk of recurrence in women with bipolar disorder during pregnancy: Prospective study of mood stabilizer discontinuation. *The American Journal of Psychiatry*, *164*(12), 1817–1824. doi:10.1176/appi.ajp.2007.06101639.

Vythilingum, B., Field, S., Kafaar, Z., Baron, E., Stein, D. J., Sanders, L., & Honikman, S. (2013). Screening and pathways to maternal mental health care in a South African antenatal setting. *Archives of Women's Mental Health, 16*, 371–379. doi:10.1007/s00737-013-0343-1.

Wells, K. B., Sherbourne, C., Schoenbaum, M., Duan, N., Meredith, L., Unutzer, J., … Rubenstein, L. V. (2000). Impact of disseminating quality improvement programs for depression in managed primary care: A randomized controlled trial. *JAMA: The Journal of the American Medical Association, 283*(2), 212–220. doi:10.1001/jama.283.2.212.

Wong, J., & Fisher, J. (2009). The role of traditional confinement practices in determining postpartum depression in women in Chinese cultures: A systematic review of the English language evidence. *Journal of Affective Disorders, 116*(3), 161–169. doi:10.1016/j.jad.2008.11.002.

World Health Organization (WHO). (2013). Mental Health Action Plan 2013–2020: Report by the Secretariat. Sixty-sixth World Health Assembly. WHA66.8. (Agenda item 13.3)., Geneva, Switzerland: World Health Organization.

9

Postnatal Depression, Mother–Infant Interactions, and Child Development
Prospects for Screening and Treatment

Lynne Murray, Pasco Fearon, and Peter Cooper

Overview

Depression is common among women of childbearing age, with over 8% being affected at any one time (Weissman, Warner, Wickramaratne, & Prusoff, 1988). Depression occurring specifically in the postnatal period affects around 14% of women in developed world samples (O'Hara & Swain, 1996) and is substantially more common in some developing world populations (Cooper et al., 1999; Parsons, Young, Rochat, Kringelbach, & Stein, 2012; Wachs, Black, & Engle, 2009). Although postnatal depression (PND) may affect women across the social spectrum, rates are increased among those experiencing stressful life events, poor social support, and a history of depression (Beck, 2001; O'Hara & Swain, 1996; Robertson, Grace, Wallington, & Stewart, 2004). Typically, symptoms of PND resolve by around 6 months postpartum, but some women are affected throughout the first year and beyond. Overall, depression-related impairments can be wide-ranging and persistent and may have a profound effect on interpersonal functioning.

Concern about the possible adverse consequences of exposure to PND for the developing child has arisen principally as a result of evidence from nondepressed populations of both the sensitivity of young infants to their interpersonal environment and the importance of social interactions in fostering optimal child psychological development (see Murray, 2014). The fact that the infant's primary environment in the early weeks and months is, in many cases, largely constituted by their mother has added to concern about the possible effects of PND on the child. Accumulating evidence from both animal and human studies of the role of caretaking in the development of neurobiological systems has provided further research impetus.

In this chapter, a careful review of the effects of PND on the mother–infant relationship is conducted in order to inform the need for intervention and screening. We review research on the effects of PND on maternal interactions with the infant and young child and on biological outcomes. We then consider what is known about the development of children of postnatally depressed mothers in the domains of cognitive, emotional–behavioral, and

Identifying Perinatal Depression and Anxiety: Evidence-Based Practice in Screening, Psychosocial Assessment, and Management, First Edition. Edited by Jeannette Milgrom and Alan W. Gemmill.
© 2015 John Wiley & Sons, Ltd. Published 2015 by John Wiley & Sons, Ltd.

psychiatric functioning. We note throughout the role of other factors commonly occurring with PND and those that are also associated with adverse child outcome (i.e., socioeconomic adversity, marital conflict, and subsequent maternal depression). We also address the question of more proximal mechanisms mediating associations between PND and adverse child outcome, giving particular attention to the role of parent–child interactions. Finally, we review intervention studies and prospects for screening for mother–infant difficulties.

Effects of Postnatal Depression on Mother–Child Relationships

Early infancy

The seminal work in the 1980s by Field, Cohn, and Tronick and colleagues (Cohn, Matias, Tronick, Connell, & Lyons-Ruth, 1986; Field, 1984; Field et al. 1985, 1988) was largely conducted with high adversity populations. It showed marked differences between depressed and well women during face-to-face play with their infants. The depressed mothers deviated from the normal pattern of interaction, where parents respond to infant cues by imitating and elaborating infant expressions and gestures and adjusting the timing and form of response to help regulate the infant's attention and affect (Brazelton, Koslowski, & Main, 1974; Papousek & Papousek, 1987; Stern, Beebe. Jaffe, & Bennett, 1977; Trevarthen, 1979). Instead, depressed mothers were generally insensitive, with the form of insensitivity varying from intrusive and hostile communication at one extreme to flat, withdrawn, and disengaged behavior at the other. In turn, the infants of depressed mothers showed high rates of distress and avoided social interaction with their mothers.

While subsequent research with lower-risk samples has shown less marked disturbance in the interactions between depressed mothers and their infants, more subtle effects of depression *have* been found (Campbell, Cohn, & Meyers, 1995; Murray, Fiori-Cowley, Hooper, & Cooper, 1996; Weinberg, Olson, Beeghly, & Tronick, 2006). These mainly involve reductions in depressed mothers' behavioral responsiveness and sensitivity to infant signals (Murray, Stanley, Hooper, King, & Fiori-Cowley, 1996; Stanley, Murray, & Stein, 2004), less physical touching of the infant, and fewer signs of overt affection (Ferber, Feldman & Makhoul, 2008; Herrera, Reissland, & Shepherd, 2004). These interactive disturbances are most evident when the depression persists (Campbell et al., 1995) or when the interaction takes place under challenging circumstances (Weinberg et al., 2006). Depressed mothers' speech to their infants has also been found to differ from that of nondepressed mothers. Slower and less responsive speech has been reported (Bettes, 1988; Breznitz & Sherman, 1987; Murray, Kempton, Woolgar, & Hooper, 1993; Zlochower & Cohn, 1996), as have a reduction in the use of both prosodically "exaggerated" intonation contours (Fernald, 1989) and modulations in fundamental frequency (Kaplan, Bachorowski, Smoski, & Hudenko, 2002; Kaplan, Bachorowski, Smoski, & Zinser, 2001) and an increased frequency of falling intonations (Murray, Marwick, & Arteche, 2010). In these relatively low-risk samples, infants of depressed mothers do not show the gross disturbances apparent in high-risk groups, although disruptions in attention and behavioral regulation have been observed in response to maternal insensitivity (Murray, Fiori-Cowley et al., 1996), particularly among boys (Weinberg et al., 2006).

Late infancy and beyond

Two meta-analyses have shown an overall reduced likelihood of attachment security in infants and young children of depressed mothers (Atkinson et al., 2000; Martins & Gaffan, 2000), although effects were not substantial. Subsequent studies (Campbell et al., 2004; McMahon, Barnett, Kowalenko, & Tennant, 2006) indicated that depressed mothers' functioning may be highly variable, with the degree of disturbance being linked to background risk. This variability appears significant in determining the impact on the child's developing attachment. The Campbell study showed that the chronicity of maternal depression, rather than early depression per se, was important in predicting child attachment insecurity and that when depressed mothers were able to be sensitive with their infant, the child generally escaped the risk for insecure attachment. Similarly, McMahon found that children of depressed mothers who were themselves securely attached were buffered from the otherwise adverse effect of maternal depression on child attachment.

Other studies examining mother–child interactions in late infancy and early childhood have found residual impairments in child responsiveness to maternal communication. Thus, Stein et al. (1991), conducting home-based observations in a UK sample, found that, compared to controls, 19-month-old infants of postnatally depressed women showed less sharing of emotion with their mothers and more anger. While this pattern of behavior was particularly evident if the mother was still depressed, the effect was also present where the mother's depression had remitted, particularly where there was marital conflict. A similar profile of less responsive engagement with the mother was found in children of postnatally depressed mothers in a follow-up at 5 years of the Cambridge (UK) longitudinal sample (Murray, Sinclair et al., 1999). In this study, postnatal depression (PND) was associated with reduced engagement, even when controlling for current and chronic maternal depression, marital conflict, and the quality of the mother's current behavior toward the child, and this association was wholly mediated by the development of an insecure pattern of attachment in infancy.

Overall, research on the effects of maternal PND on the mother–infant relationship indicates that there may be long-term effects of early difficulties, especially in contexts of marked adversity, where depression is more likely to be chronic and where maternal responsiveness and sensitivity to the child is particularly impaired. Insecure infant attachment may be a particular risk and may mediate longer-term effects of PND on difficulties in mother–child relationships. This research suggests that intervening early may play an important role in helping to prevent longer-term difficulties.

Effects of PND on Biological Outcomes

Neural development

Emerging research suggests that the marked difficulties in social interactions of PND mothers with their infant may have direct effects on developing infant and child neurophysiological systems. EEG recordings taken from children of PND mothers have shown reduced left frontal activation from 1 to 3 months (Jones, Field, Fox, Lundy, & Davalos, 1997) through to six (Field, Fox, Pickens, & Nawrocki, 1995) and 15 months (Dawson, Frey, Panagiotides, Osterling, & Hessl, 1997; Dawson et al., 1999), with evidence of some stability through to early childhood (Jones, Field, Davalos, & Pickens, 1997).

Meta-analysis shows this association to be quite robust (Thibodeau, Jorgensen, & Kim, 2006). This pattern of activation, observed in infants of depressed mothers from both low- and high-risk samples, shows systematic associations with the severity of the maternal disorder, and it is not accounted for by prenatal depression (Dawson, Frey, Panagiotides, Osterling et al., 1997). There is evidence that the association between reduced left frontal activation and maternal depression is mediated by the infant's experience of interaction with the mother, particularly by her noncontingent (Dawson, Frey, Panagiotides, Self et al., 1997; Dawson et al., 1999) and withdrawn behavior (Diego, Field, & Hernandez-Reif, 2001). Longitudinal cross-panel data in childhood suggest that earlier maternal depression predicts changes in EEG asymmetry later on, consistent with a potential causal influence (Forbes et al., 2008). Notably, by 13–15 months, differences between index and control infants in frontal activity are not confined to periods when the infant interacts with the mother, but extend to both baseline conditions and positive interactions with a stranger (Dawson et al., 1999). Importantly, evidence indicates that EEG asymmetry may partially mediate the association between withdrawn parenting in depressed mothers and adverse child outcomes (Dawson et al., 2003).

HPA axis functioning

A second area of investigation concerns infant and child stress responses, with the functioning of the HPA axis system being a particular focus. The suggestion that maternal depression may influence the development of the HPA axis arises from animal studies indicating its early programming by maternal behavior. In rodents, reduced levels of maternal tactile stimulation can result in a more reactive HPA axis, at least in part due to reduced levels of central glucocorticoid receptors which provide negative feedback to the system (see review of Kaffman & Meaney, 2007). These changes in glucocorticoid receptor density appeared to be controlled by epigenetic mechanisms that are regulated by parental caregiving (Weaver et al., 2004). While nonhuman primate research is at an earlier stage, findings are consistent with the rodent model (Coplan et al., 1996, 2001, 2006; Rosenblum et al., 1994). Studies have also examined human cortisol secretion in relation to maternal PND, again with broadly consistent findings. Field et al. (1988) observed elevated cortisol levels in both PND mothers and their infants during face-to-face interactions; and they attributed these findings to the fact that interactions were nonsynchronous and therefore stressful. Studies have also demonstrated longitudinal associations between PND and offspring cortisol secretion, with elevations being observed in basal measures in children at 18 months (Bugental, Martorell, & Barraza, 2003), 3 years (Hessl et al., 1998), and 4.5 years of age (Essex, Klein, Cho, & Kalin, 2002). Finally, evidence for long-term effects of depressed mothers' early interactions was found in a follow-up of the Cambridge sample: here, elevated morning cortisol secretion observed in the postnatally depressed mothers' children at 13 years (Halligan, Herbert, Goodyer, & Murray, 2004) was predicted by maternal withdrawal during early interactions, rather than by later interaction difficulties (Murray, Marwick et al., 2010). Few studies have addressed HPA reactivity in response to *challenge* among children exposed to PND, although Waters et al. (2013) found *reduced* cortisol responsiveness to mild challenges in infants whose mothers had experienced depression (antenatally or postnatally) relative to controls.

While consistency in findings regarding biological outcomes of children of PND mothers is notable given the methodological variability, some caution is required in their interpretation. Thus, in relation to cortisol, although there have been attempts to examine the relevance of early versus later exposure to maternal depression (Essex et al., 2002; Halligan et al., 2004) and associated disturbances in maternal interactions (Murray, Marwick et al., 2010), there is evidence to suggest that *any* parental history of depression may have an impact on HPA reactivity in the child (Mannie, Harmer, & Cowen, 2007; Young, Vazquez, Jiang, & Pfeffer, 2006). The same possibility, in principle, exists for EEG effects. Antenatal exposures may also be influential (Field et al., 2004; O'Connor et al., 2005), and genetic effects are likely (Bartels, Van den Berg, Sluyter, Boomsma, & de Geus, 2003). Further clarity requires studies that differentially link exposure to maternal depression during particular periods of development to biological changes in the offspring, as well as further research into the mechanisms by which effects are brought about.

Effects of PND on Cognitive Development

Outcome studies

A number of prospective longitudinal studies of community samples have examined the effects of PND on preschool and school-aged children, and several have identified associations with poor child cognitive functioning. Sutter-Dallay et al. (2011) examined cognitive outcome in 2-year-olds in a French sample of almost 600 mothers whose depression was carefully monitored throughout. Depression at 6 weeks postpartum was associated with significantly poorer child cognitive outcome, even when controlling for other risk factors and intervening depression. Cogill, Caplan, Alexandra, Robson, and Kumar (1986) assessed child IQ at four years in a London community sample. Boys and girls whose mothers had been depressed in the first postnatal year had poorer scores than both children of well mothers and children of mothers who had been depressed later on. However, the adverse effects of PND were confined to children whose mothers had a low level of education (Hay & Kumar, 1995). A second study of a largely disadvantaged London sample (Sharp et al., 1995) found that, while girls' IQ was unaffected by PND, boys whose mothers had been depressed in the first year had significantly lower scores compared to both those never exposed to maternal depression and those exposed to maternal depression subsequent to the postnatal period. A follow-up of this sample at 11 found persistent effects on boys' IQ, taking account of subsequent maternal depressive episodes, although the number of children exposed only in the early months was small (Hay et al., 2001). Similar findings were obtained in a follow-up by Milgrom, Westley, and Gemmill (2004) of an Australian inpatient sample who were depressed at 6 months, with index group boys having lower IQ at 42 months than both index group girls and control children. Murray and colleagues examined this issue in their Cambridge longitudinal sample. As in the studies of Sharp and Milgrom, boys of PND mothers had lower scores than both exposed girls and control group infants on the Bayley Mental Development Index at 18 months (Murray, 1992; Murray, Fiori-Cowley et al., 1996). Further, at 16 years, these boys had significantly poorer school results (on UK GCSE public examinations); and these showed substantial continuity with their poorer cognitive performance in infancy (Murray, Arteche et al., 2010).

Other studies have failed to identify adverse long-term effects of maternal PND on child cognitive development or have shown smaller effects. In a large Bavarian sample, Kurstjens and Wolke (2001) assessed cognitive development at 20 months and 4 and 6 years and found no adverse effects of PND per se. However, boys with additional risk factors (low SES, neonatal risk), as well as those whose mothers experienced subsequent depression in addition to the postnatal episode, did have poorer scores at the final assessment (Kurstjens & Wolke, 2001). Cornish et al. (2005) assessed cognitive functioning in 15-month-old infants of Australian mothers and found no effect on infant outcome of maternal depression occurring only at 4 months postpartum. However, infants of mothers whose depression persisted did have reduced scores on the Bayley Scales.

The importance of the chronicity and severity of maternal depression for infant and child cognitive functioning is also shown by two large-scale studies. The US National Maternal and Child Health survey found only modest associations between maternal depression after the birth and child cognitive functioning at 3 years, whereas severe and chronic maternal depression was associated with substantially poorer child cognitive outcome, independent of family income (Petterson & Burke-Albers, 2001). In an Australian sample of almost 5000 mothers, assessments of maternal mood were made in pregnancy, shortly after the birth, and at 6 months and 5 years (Brennan et al., 2000). At 5 years, both severity and chronicity of depression were associated with poorer child vocabulary, although these effects were not substantial. Further, the US NICHD sample of more than 1000 families showed that, compared to nonexposed children, children whose mothers were chronically depressed over the first 3 years were adversely affected on a range of cognitive measures, while those exposed intermittently were less affected (NICHD, 1999).

The findings from these diverse studies suggest that maternal depression in the postnatal period poses a risk for long-term poor cognitive functioning in the child where the depression is chronic. They also suggest that this effect principally obtains in the context of wider socioeconomic difficulties and for male offspring. In low-risk samples, long-term effects of PND on child cognitive development are not so evident and are principally confined to subgroups experiencing additional risks. Recent studies are beginning to examine whether antenatal depression may also have effects on child cognitive outcomes (e.g., Evans et al., 2012).

Mechanisms mediating cognitive effects of PND

General responsiveness
Substantial evidence with normal populations has shown the overall level of child-centered parental responsiveness, or *contingency*, during social interactions to be important for child cognitive development (Eshel, Daelmans, Cabral De Mello, & Martines, 2006). This kind of responsiveness concerns the parent's ability to notice and respond to their infant's cues—such as their direction of attention or their efforts to engage with the environment. As noted earlier, depressed mothers' awareness of their infant's experience can be quite reduced, in all likelihood due to symptoms such as rumination. Accordingly, such impairments in maternal responsivity may contribute to poor cognitive functioning for their children. This possibility has been investigated in four studies. Stanley et al. (2004) found reduced maternal contingent responsiveness during interactions in the first 2–3 postnatal months predicted infant performance in an operant learning task. In the Cambridge longitudinal study, Murray and colleagues (1993, 1996) showed that reduced maternal responsiveness to the infant at 2 months mediated the adverse effects of PND on boys' performance on the Bayley Scales at 18 months. Furthermore, those children whose mothers had shown a particularly marked reduction in responsiveness postnatally were continued on a trajectory of poor cognitive functioning to 5 years (Murray, Hipwell, Hooper, Stein, & Cooper, 1996) and later childhood and adolescence (Murray, Arteche et al., 2010).

In the NICHD study, variability in the interactions of depressed mothers was also highlighted, with those experiencing adversity having markedly lower levels of responsiveness. Where the interactions of depressed mothers were particularly poor, risk for poor child cognitive outcome was substantial. In contrast, children whose mothers maintained good interactions despite their depression were buffered from the potentially negative effects of the maternal disorder. Finally, in their clinic-based Australian sample, Milgrom et al. (2004) found that low maternal responsiveness at 6 months mediated the adverse effect of maternal depression on boy's IQ at 42 months.

Attention regulation
Difficulties in depressed mothers' interactions that concern infant attention regulation may also contribute to poorer infant cognitive performance, since the infant's ability to sustain attention is a robust predictor of later childhood IQ (Slater, 1995). The mother's ability to support the infant's attention is one element of contingent responsiveness that typically involves vocal modulations that help both attract and maintain infant attention (Stern, Spieker, & MacKain, 1982). Kaplan, Bachorowski, and Zarlengo-Strouse (1999), for example, found that segments of child-directed speech recorded from postnatally depressed mothers, in contrast to that of nondepressed mothers, failed to promote associative learning in their infants in a conditioned attention paradigm. Notably, the fundamental frequency of the final portion of the speech segments of mothers with more depressive symptoms was less modulated than that of other mothers, and this reduced modulation may have failed to increase infant arousal sufficiently to enable efficient processing of, and attention to, the information required.

Dysregulation of emotion
Emotion regulation processes during parent–infant interactions may also be important. Dysregulated affect is likely both to impair attention and disrupt infant information retrieval (Fagen, Ohr, Fleckenstein, & Ribner, 1985). The increase in infant and child cortisol levels associated with depressed mothers' withdrawal and lack of support for infant emotion regulation (Field et al., 1988; Murray, Halligan, Goodyer, & Herbert, 2010) may also be relevant. This mechanism requires further investigation.

Conclusions
Studies on the cognitive development of postnatally depressed mothers' children suggest that particularly poor mother–child interactions are likely to occur when the maternal disorder is accompanied by wider adversity and they may also be more impaired with male infants, whose regulation of their state and behavior may be more dependent on maternal support than that of girls. Where this is the case, child cognitive functioning may be affected in the longer term. While general deficits in maternal responsiveness have been widely linked to poor child outcome, research also indicates more specific features of parent–child interactions that may have differential effects on particular psychological processes underpinning optimal cognitive development. Further research is needed to investigate these specific processes in the context of maternal depression and to explore the role of biological changes. These findings suggest that intervention may need to be targeted not only on the early mother–child interaction but also at later points to prevent long-term effects. *Maternal responsiveness* (or contingency) appears to be an important target for child cognitive development, and other characteristics such as supporting the infant's attention and regulation of affect may also be important.

Effects of PND on Behavioral, Socioemotional, and Psychiatric Problems

Outcome studies

Maternal reports in infancy and the preschool and early school years
Using maternal report measures, Murray (1992) found that mothers who had been depressed in the first few postnatal months reported increased behavior problems in their infants at 18 months on an age-adjusted version of the Behavior Screening Questionnaire (BSQ; Richman & Graham, 1971), despite most mothers having recovered by the time of assessment. Reported problems mainly concerned behavioral regulation difficulties (e.g., sleep disturbance, separation difficulties, temper tantrums). Similarly, Cicchetti, Rogosch, and Toth (1998) found raised child behavior problem scores at 20 months on the Child Behavior Checklist (CBCL; Achenbach, 1991) to be associated with maternal depression occurring at some point following childbirth. In this sample, the relationship between maternal depression and child behavior disturbance was accounted for by general contextual risk. Avan, Richter, Ramchandani, Norris, and Stein (2010), in a large socioeconomically deprived longitudinal cohort in Soweto, Johannesburg, South Africa, also found associations between postnatal depressive symptoms and child behavioral problems at age 2.

With regard to older, preschool-aged children, Ghodsian, Zajicek, and Wolkind (1984) found that depression at both 4 and 14 months predicted maternal reports of child behavior problems (BSQ) at 42 months in a London sample, although only the effects of 14-month depression were significant when current maternal mental state was taken into account. Caplan et al. (1989) also investigated maternal reports of child behavior at four years in another London sample. In addition to effects of current depression, postnatal episodes showed some association with child disturbance. However, as in the study of Cicchetti et al. (1998), this was principally accounted for by chronic difficulties co-occurring with PND (marital conflict and paternal psychiatric history).

The importance of chronic and later maternal depression for child behavior problems, rather than depression confined to the postnatal period, is suggested by four further studies of community samples. In the Australian study, maternal reports of child disturbance on the CBCL at 5 years were associated with both chronicity and severity of maternal depression, and these effects were additive (Brennan et al., 2000). There was little evidence for the impact of disorder in the immediate postpartum period, whereas later depressions were significantly associated with child behavior problems. Philipps and O'Hara (1991), following up a community sample in the United States, also found no effect of PND on child behavior problems (assessed on the CBCL) at 4½ years, but did find that subsequent maternal depression was associated with child disturbance. Finally, in a disadvantaged London sample, compared to children of never-depressed women, maternal reports of "violent" behavior in 11-year-olds were associated with postnatal episodes but only if the mother experienced subsequent depression (Hay, Pawlby, Angold, Harold, & Sharp, 2003). A more recent nationally representative study from Norway (Bekkhus, Rutter, Barker, & Borge, 2011) examined the effects of antenatal and postnatal depressive symptoms on age 3 crying and aggressive behavior. Robust associations were found for postnatal, but not prenatal, depressive symptoms (see also Bagner, Pettit, Lewinsohn, Seeley, & Jaccard, 2013). Notably, there was substantial continuity in postnatal depressive symptoms, and it seemed that this quite stable trajectory was the most significant predictor of later child problems.

In contrast, at least five studies have found positive associations with PND and maternally reported child behavior problems. In the high-risk US sample studied by Alpern and Lyons-Ruth (1993), both chronic (18 months and at 5 years) and recent maternal depression were associated with increased problems at age 5. Three further studies of low-risk samples of preschool children have reported similar findings. In a study of a Scottish community sample, Wrate, Rooney, Thomas, and Cox (1985) found PND episodes of relatively short duration (1 month) were associated with maternal reports of child behavior problems at 3 years, even when controlling for current and recent depression. Similarly, in the Cambridge longitudinal study (Murray, Sinclair et al., 1999), maternal reports of child behavior problems on the Rutter Scale at age 5 showed a significant association with PND, even when account was taken of the recent and chronic episodes, the presence of marital conflict, and the current quality of the mother's interaction with the child. In similar vein, Dawson et al. (2003) found that exposure to maternal depression during the child's first 2 years was the strongest predictor of maternal reports of behavior problems at 3½ years. Once early depression was taken into account, the degree of subsequent exposure was unrelated to child outcome. Finally, Bagner et al. (2013) also found that postnatal major depression predicted later child internalizing problems after controlling for later depressive episodes, while later depression did not.

These maternal report studies indicate that chronic depressive disorder, particularly in the context of general adversity, generally emerges as a strong predictor of poor child outcome. Nevertheless, there is evidence of behavior difficulties in children of mothers who were depressed in the first 1–2 postnatal years, independent of subsequent depression.

Independent assessments in the preschool and early school years
The findings from some maternal reports of persistent effects of early exposure to depression are in line with a number of studies that have used independent evidence concerning child behavior. These include teacher reports, direct observations, and child reports.

Using teacher reports, Alpern and Lyons-Ruth (1993) found that recent and chronic maternal depression was linked to raised rates of child behavior problems in school. Children who had been exposed to depression by 18 months, but not those exposed at 5 years, were reported to be more withdrawn and anxious than children whose mothers had been well. Similar findings have emerged from a prospective study of a low-risk US community sample, where teacher reports at 6 years showed significant effects of the timing of the child's exposure to depression (Essex, Klein, Miech, & Smider, 2001). Children who had initially been exposed during their first year had high rates of both internalizing and externalizing symptoms. In contrast, first exposure to maternal depression beyond infancy increased the risk only of externalizing problems (a finding confined to girls). These associations were not altered when the overall chronicity of maternal depression was taken into account. Boys who were exposed only to early maternal depression had raised rates of internalizing problems (assessed by combined teacher and mother reports) but developed externalizing difficulties if early maternal depression was followed by marital conflict (Essex, Klein, Cho, & Kraemer, 2003). Teacher reports of child adjustment in the Cambridge longitudinal study (Sinclair & Murray, 1998) revealed an association between PND and boys' behavior problems (antisocial and hyperactive symptoms), particularly in the context of low SES. Finally, in a small sample study of clinic-referred women, Wright, George, Burke, Gelfand, and Teti (2000) found that 5- to 8-year-old children of mothers who experienced depression between 3 and 30 months had more adverse outcomes on teacher reports of adjustment than children of well mothers, especially on measures of aggression and poor peer relationships, even when controlling for current symptoms.

Direct assessments of children of PND mothers were made in several contexts in the longitudinal study of Murray and colleagues. In school-based observations, both boys and girls of postnatally depressed mothers showed low levels of creative play, and they were relatively unresponsive to the positive approaches of other children (Murray, Sinclair et al., 1999), effects that were still obtained when both recent depression and marital conflict were taken into account. More extreme social difficulties in the form of marked aggression were also shown by the children of postnatally depressed mothers in this sample during peer play, although in this case the presence of marital conflict accounted for the association (Hipwell, Murray, Ducournau, & Stein, 2005).

Research has also identified child sociocognitive disturbances relevant to the development of depression. Thus, when children in the Cambridge longitudinal study were exposed to a mild stressor, those who had been exposed to early maternal depression were more likely than nonexposed children to show evidence of depressive thinking, even when controlling for the effects of recent maternal depression (Murray, Woolgar, Cooper, & Hipwell, 2001). A similar finding emerged from the study of Maughan, Cicchetti, Toth, and Rogosch (2007), where early maternal depression (before 21 months) was significantly associated with child reports of low self-competence at 5 years.

The findings derived from independent assessments, while often consistent with maternal reports in showing effects of current difficulties, are notable in that all show persistent effects of early maternal depression, even when controlling for later episodes, with the majority showing an impact on child internalizing problems in the preschool or early school years.

Psychiatric disturbance in adolescence
Children whose parents experience depression are at substantially raised risk themselves for depression and anxiety (Weissman et al., 2006). However, since first episodes of depression typically occur only from adolescence onward, long-term follow-up is required to examine associations between maternal PND and offspring disorder. To date, three studies have been reported involving children below the age of greatest risk for occurrence of depression. Hammen and Brennan (2003) examined the psychiatric status of 15-year-old children of mothers in a large Australian community sample, overselected for maternal depression. Both severity and chronicity of maternal depression were important, with adolescent disorder (and particularly depression) being more likely in the context of severe maternal episodes, even of short duration. Milder maternal depression posed risk only if it was prolonged. Timing of maternal depression was also considered. They found the occurrence of maternal depression at any time in the first 10 years to be associated with adolescent risk for depressive disorder, but there was no specific risk from exposure in infancy.

Offspring psychiatric disorder was also assessed in the Cambridge longitudinal sample. At 13 years, those who had been exposed to PND were at increased risk of both depression and anxiety disorder, although the number of episodes of depression by this age was small. In a later follow-up when offspring were aged 16, the risk for depression in the index group was confirmed, with almost half having experienced an episode of depression, more than four times the rate among controls (Murray et al., 2011). Adolescent depression was predicted by low levels of resilience in childhood, itself predicted by insecure infant attachment. Other factors of importance were further prolonged maternal depression and the occurrence of marital conflict. Although both of these factors were associated with the original PND, neither of them fully accounted for the impact of the postnatal episode on adolescent offspring mental state.

Finally, assessments were made of psychiatric disorder in the disadvantaged London sample of Sharp and colleagues. At 11 years, PND was associated with a raised risk of child disorder (SAD, social anxiety, depression, and behavior disorders combined). However, since subsequent maternal depression was not considered, conclusions regarding specific links to the postpartum episode cannot be drawn (Pawlby, Hay, Sharp, Waters, & O'Keane, 2009). A subsequent report of offspring depression at 16 years in this sample focused on the effects of timing of *new onsets*, rather than on exposure to maternal depression per se during particular time periods (Pawlby et al., 2009). As in the Cambridge sample, this study found chronicity of child exposure to maternal depression to be important.

Mechanisms mediating socioemotional outcomes

Some individual differences in infant emotional expressiveness and reactivity through the first year, such as crying levels, appear relatively independent of parenting (James-Roberts & Plewis, 1996). However, capacities concerned with the self-regulation of behavioral and emotional states, which are key to subsequent good adjustment (DeGangi, Breinbauer, Roosevelt, Porges, & Greenspan, 2000; Kochanska, Murray, & Harlan, 2000; Kochanska, Tjebkes, & Forman, 1998), develop only gradually (Posner & Rothbart, 2000) and appear more responsive to parental intervention (Sameroff & Emde, 1989). Whereas good cognitive outcome is primarily promoted by contingent responsiveness to infant attention and engagement with the environment, good behavioral and emotional regulation appears to be particularly affected by parental sensitivity to the infant's emotions. This includes the ability to be appropriately and affectively attuned to the child's behavior and to provide "emotional scaffolding" where the child's difficult emotions are supportively contained. This association holds in both depressed and normal samples. In the NICHD study, for example, behavior problems (poor cooperation) were predicted by maternal depression that was accompanied by insensitivity (NICHD, 1999). Three specific ways in which parental interaction difficulties associated with PND may reflect poor emotional scaffolding and impede the development of emotional and behavioral are proposed.

Contagion of distress
Field (1995) suggested a contagion effect, whereby infants show increased sad affect and distress, either through modeling their mothers' depressed behavior or else being directly affected by the mother's manifest sadness. This suggestion is consistent with the high levels of matching of negative emotional expressions in depressed mother–infant interactions (Field, Healy, Goldstein, & Guthertz, 1990). To date, direct evidence for the effects of distress contagion on longer-term regulatory problems is lacking, although findings from studies with older children and adolescents of depressed parents are consistent with this mechanism (Joormann, Talbot, & Gotlib, 2007; Monk et al., 2008).

Failures of interactive repair
In normal populations, mother and infant repeatedly shift during social interactions from miscoordinated to coordinated states, as the mother supports the infant's immature capacities to regulate their behavior and affect (Jaffe, Beebe, Feldstein, Crown, & Jasnow, 2001; Tronick, 1989; Tronick & Gianino, 1986). Postnatally depressed mothers may fail to provide

such experience (Tronick & Weinberg, 1999; Weinberg et al., 2006), as do depressed mothers of older children (Jameson, Gelfand, Kulcsar, & Teti, 1997). While there is evidence from normal populations for the longer-term beneficial effects of parental strategies to promote infant self-regulation, as assessed by secure attachment (Isabella & Belsky, 1991; Jaffe et al., 2001) and good sleep outcomes (Murray & Ramchandani, 2007), further research is required to investigate the role of parenting in infant self-regulation outcomes in the context of PND.

Maternal hostility and coercion

The hostile and intrusive, or coercive, behavior that characterizes some depressed mothers may directly provoke infant distress and behavioral dysregulation. A microanalysis of face-to-face interactions between depressed and well mothers and their infants in the Cambridge study showed that episodes of infant behavioral dysregulation were immediately preceded by the mother's negating the infant's experience, often through intrusive or hostile interventions (Murray, Fiori-Cowley et al., 1996). Long-term associations were also found, with early maternal hostility predicting negative child self-cognitions at 5 years (Murray et al., 2001). Such an association was similarly identified in the study of Maughan et al. (2007). In the Cambridge study, a path analysis of mother–infant/child interactions and child behavior assessed over 8 years showed that infant emotional and behavioral dysregulation at 2 months, assessed independently of the mother, was unrelated to depressed mothers' hostile and coercive interactions at this time; but by 4 months, an association was present. This difficult infant behavior began to show continuity over time and in turn appeared to provoke further maternal negativity and intrusiveness, with the ensuing vicious cycle culminating in raised rates of conduct problems and ADHD symptoms by age 5–8 years (Morrell & Murray, 2003). Such findings are consistent with more general research with older children, showing the occurrence of disruptive behavior disorders to be associated with parental hostility and coercive control (see review by Hill, 2002).

Conclusions

Research on the effects of maternal PND on child behavioral and socioemotional development indicates the importance of the general parenting characteristic of emotional scaffolding sensitivity. This may be an important target for intervention and includes the ability to be affectively attuned to the child's behavior and contain the child's difficult emotions. In addition, a number of specific dimensions of interactions between depressed mothers and their infants in the postnatal months are implicated. Further longitudinal work is needed that directly examines the role of early mother–infant interactions in longer-term child outcomes.

Mediators of poor psychiatric outcomes

While preliminary research indicates that PND is associated with increased rates of offspring psychiatric disorder, longer-term follow-up studies are required for more definitive estimation of risks. Furthermore, the limited nature of the evidence to date necessarily constrains conclusions regarding the mechanisms underlying any increased risk. What does seem apparent, however, at least for offspring depression, is that the chronicity and severity of maternal depression are important. This may, in part, reflect genetic liability, since both these dimensions are associated with genetic risk (Kendler, 1996). Nevertheless, recent adoption study data suggest that any genetic vulnerability is likely to be environmentally mediated (Silberg, Maes, & Eaves, 2010), a conclusion consistent with the well-established role of environmental adversity in the etiology of depression (Brown & Harris, 1978). In addition to these broad influences, a number of specific processes initiated in the postnatal period itself are also suggested.

Biological processes
As noted earlier, the unresponsive or withdrawn interactions with the infant seen in some postnatally depressed mothers predict particular infant EEG profiles (i.e., reduction in left vs. right prefrontal EEG activity) (Dawson, Frey, Panagiotides, Osterling et al., 1997; Dawson et al., 1999; Diego et al., 2001). In adults, this EEG profile is induced by observing negative emotion stimuli (Davidson, Ekman, Saron, Senulis, & Friesen, 1990; Tomarken, Davidson, & Henriques, 1990) and is also associated with adult depressive disorder itself (Henriques & Davidson, 1990; Schaffer, Davidson, & Saron, 1983). While the parallels between EEG responses in infants of depressed mothers and those of adults experiencing depression are notable, it is important that follow-up studies of infant populations be conducted to establish whether there are indeed direct links between early EEG functioning and subsequent disorder.

Research on HPA axis functioning has also begun to show associations with disturbances in parenting in the context of PND (Murray, Halligan et al., 2010). The previously noted pattern of increased basal cortisol secretion among children exposed to PND has also been associated with both risk for depression (Goodyer, Tamplin, Herbert, & Altham, 2000; Harris et al., 2000; Mannie et al., 2007) and the occurrence of adolescent and adult depressive disorder (Southwick, Vythilingam, & Charney, 2005). For example, the age 13 cortisol elevations in offspring of PND mothers in the Cambridge longitudinal study were found to prospectively predict depressive symptoms at 16 years (Murray, Halligan et al., 2010).

Social cognitions
Aside from physiological processes, certain patterns of social cognition regarding close relationships and emotions have been found to raise the risk for depression (Gjerde, 1995; Gore, Aseltine, & Colten, 1993). The question arises whether early relationships between PND mothers and their infants may set in train such biases in social cognition. In the Cambridge study, in interviews about friendship difficulties, girls of PND mothers showed substantially heightened sensitivity to negative social experience, which in turn was associated with their experience of depressive symptoms (Murray, Halligan, Adams, Patterson, & Goodyer, 2006). These social cognitions also showed continuity with both insecure attachment to the mother in infancy and with representations of family relationships at age 5 (Murray, Woolgar, Briers, & Hipwell, 1999).

Conclusion
Findings from both biophysiological and social–cognitive research suggest that the particularly difficult patterns of interaction in the early postpartum months that can occur in the context of PND may set in train developmental processes that confer increased risk for depressive disorder in adolescent offspring. Whether these are translated into actual disorder, however, is likely to depend upon subsequent adverse experience, most notably on further exposure to maternal depression. Further research is needed.

Treatment

Treatment studies

Given the evidence concerning the adverse impact of PND on mother–infant relationships and child development, the provision of effective interventions for the depression, and for the disturbances in mother–child relationships, is a priority. In the following, we review the evidence concerning psychological interventions.

Intervention effects on depression
Both a review of randomized control trials (Dennis & Hodnett, 2007) and a meta-analysis (Cuijpers, Brännmark, & van Straten, 2008) concluded that psychological interventions (cognitive behavior therapy (CBT) and interpersonal therapy (IPT)) and psychosocial interventions (primarily nondirective counseling) are moderately effective and similarly beneficial at alleviating maternal mood disorder. However, both reviews highlighted the short-term nature of most trials and their follow-ups, with a consequent lack of information about longer-term outcomes. In general, high-quality health economic data regarding these interventions is also lacking (e.g., see Stevenson et al., 2010).

Intervention effects on mother–infant relationships
A critical question regarding the treatment of PND concerns the extent to which treatment effects are reflected in improvements in mother–infant relationships and infant development. A few studies have addressed this issue, with mixed results. A large-scale randomized control trial comparing three forms of psychological intervention with a control group found that, while all active treatments were moderately effective in treating depression and brought about short-term benefits in the quality of the mother–infant relationship, there was no consistent improvement in infant outcomes and effects were generally not sustained at 18-month and 5-year follow-ups (Cooper, Murray, Wilson, & Romaniuk, 2003; Murray, Cooper, Wilson, & Romaniuk, 2003). Clark, Tluczek, and Wenzel (2003) conducted a pilot study comparing mother–infant therapy or IPT to a waiting list control condition. Although treatments were beneficial in improving depression, consistent effects on subsequent mother–child interactions or child outcome were not observed Finally, a study of IPT found that mother–infant dyads who received effective treatment for PND were no better than nontreated dyads in terms of observed mother–infant interactions, infant negative emotionality, and attachment security (Forman et al., 2007)—the same pattern of results held at a 4-year follow-up. This suggests that a major focus on treating maternal mood is insufficient and that programs addressing the mother–infant interaction may be necessary in order to yield benefits.

A related approach has been to directly focus on improving parenting and more specifically targeting the mother–infant interaction. Cicchetti, Rogosch, and Toth (2000) examined the impact in a depressed group of prolonged psychotherapy (average of 57 weeks) compared to nontreated depressed and nondepressed control groups. The intervention, which focused on promoting positive maternal attachment representations and mother–infant interactions, resulted in infant cognitive abilities that were comparable to control group levels at the end of treatment, whereas the untreated depressed group showed a relative decline over the same period. Several further studies focusing on improving mother–infant interactions have also indicated improvements, with interactive coaching (Horowitz et al., 2001), relationship facilitation based on maternal administrations of the

NBAS (Hart, Field, & Nearing, 1998), and infant massage (Glover, Onozawa, & Hodgkinson, 2002; Onozawa, Glover, Adams, Modi, & Kumar, 2001) all showing short-term benefits. Notably, a recent meta-analysis of 10 studies aiming to improve parenting sensitivity among depressed mothers (Kersten-Alvarez, Hosman, Riksen-Walraven, Van Doesum, & Hoefnagels, 2011) indicated that, overall, significant, albeit modest, improvements were achieved. However, there was also evidence of publication bias, and given the limited number of studies, the results should be treated with caution. Furthermore, few studies have assessed longer-term benefits or examined implications for infant development. One notable exception is that of van Doesum and colleagues (2008). This intervention for PND mothers combined home visiting with video feedback to promote mothers' sensitivity and responsiveness to infant cues, help broaden their repertoire of interactive behaviors, and challenge and modify negative thinking patterns. At posttest, the intervention showed robust effects on maternal sensitivity, relative to a control group, as well as improvements in infant attachment security and social competence. Nevertheless, in a follow-up at 5.5 years, Kersten-Alvarez et al. (2011) found little evidence of persistent benefits of the intervention for maternal behavior, child self-esteem, school adjustment, and behavior problems. Thus, it appears that while short-term effects may be demonstrated in improving parenting sensitivity, longer-term effects have yet to be further researched. It is possible that some of the outcome measures used in follow-up studies have not addressed the particular aspects of the parent–child interaction that has been protected or that over time other influences are powerful moderators of continuity. Further research of targeted tailored interventions with long-term outcomes is needed.

Provision of alternative care
Given the lack of evidence to date regarding the potential for preventing long-term adverse child outcome in the context of PND by altering difficulties in mother–infant relationships, it is also worth considering the possible role of alternative caregivers. Studies have shown that infants of PND mothers respond positively during interactions with their nondepressed fathers (Hossain et al., 1994), childminders, or day-care nurses (Pelaez-Nogueras, Field, Cigales, Gonzalez, & Clasky, 1994). Mother–infant relationships themselves were found in one study to be affected, with better engagement occurring in cases where the mother was not based at home full time (Cohn, Campbell, Matias, & Hopkins, 1990). Results from the early child care NICHD sample (SECC) showed that internalizing behavior problems were reduced at 24 and 36 months where the child received alternative care (Lee, Halpern, Hertz-Picciotto, Martin, & Suchindran, 2006). Provision of alternative caregivers may be important to institute in the first 6–9 months, before infants start to generalize the difficult behavior shown with their mother to interactions with other people. This would potentially provide the infant with additional attachment figures in the long term. Nevertheless, such strategies require considerable clinical sensitivity, since it is important not to increase depressed women's poor self-esteem, and therefore, ways of introducing additional caregivers need careful consideration.

Prospects for screening for mother–infant interactions difficulties
Despite the fact that evidence is not yet available showing that intervening early to promote the quality of mother–infant interactions in the context of PND has beneficial longer-term effects, given the powerful impact of PND on cognitive and behavioral outcomes, it may nevertheless be prudent to start interventions early when possible. Our view is that a standardized assessment of parent–child interactions should be a part of routine clinical

practice. There are several potential benefits. First, disturbances in parent–infant interactions often go unrecognized by practitioners, and so opportunities for appropriate intervention are commonly missed. Second, even where problems are identified, they may be assessed in highly inconsistent ways which is likely to lead to undermine the coherence of care for affected families. Third, successful interventions focused on parent–infant interactions depend critically on practitioners having a good level of understanding of the specific behavioral targets that require improvement. Thus, routine care will benefit from practitioners being trained in both observational measures of parent–child interactions and the fundamental concepts underpinning thinking within the field of infant mental health. Finally, clinical services need to be able to demonstrate that they are able to bring about positive changes in the quality of interactions; this necessitates access to measurement instruments that are well validated and robust, as well as the skills and experience to use them properly.

There are several measures that practitioners might use in clinical practice for the assessment of the mother–infant relationship. These vary in focus, length, and the degree of training (and cost) required to achieve adequate levels of reliability (Aspland & Gardner, 2003; Mesman & Emmen, 2013; Wolff & Van Ijzendoorn, 1997). The choice of observational measure is constrained by several practical and methodological issues. High inter-rater reliability is, of course, critical, as is predictive validity. Further, a single measurement in time, based on a limited sample of behavior (and in a particular context), inevitably does not capture all of what might be important in a parent–infant relationship. A recent study, for example, showed that repeated assessments of sensitivity (i.e., taken on more than one occasion) dramatically increased the predictive validity of the ratings (Lindhiem, Bernard, & Dozier, 2011). There are also good arguments for generally favoring home observations, as they probably provide a better gauge of a dyad's typical interactions.

Although it is important to consider measures that can capture some of the focal areas of parent–infant interaction discussed in this chapter (e.g., negative affect, withdrawn behavior, intrusiveness, and cognitive scaffolding), assessing overall sensitivity is clearly a key initial priority. In that regard, Mesman and colleagues (2013) identified 8 measures of sensitivity that had been validated in at least 10 studies (including our own Global Ratings of Mother–Infant Interaction (Murray, Fiori-Cowley et al., 1996)). Which measure one chooses will depend on the specific clinical focus and context. However, it must be noted that only five of them are free to use, and not all have been validated against attachment security and/or cognitive development (Mesman & Emmen, 2013).

The choice of measure and its implementation depend critically on a recognition of the specificity of effects highlighted earlier; that is, different kinds of parenting difficulty predict different kinds of child developmental difficulties, and this is best revealed in contexts that are directly relevant to the area of child development being considered. Thus, if the clinician is primarily concerned to identify the nature of *cognitive* support that the parent is able to provide, then it would make sense to assess the level of sensitivity (as well as specific behaviors that support cognitive development like facilitation of attention or scaffolding exploration of the environment) in a cognitive-relevant context—for example, during picture book sharing or helping the infant explore a new toy. Similarly, if the primary clinical focus is behavior problems such as aggression or poor emotion regulation, the interaction should be assessed in a context relevant to these behaviors, such as the frustration of the child's having an attractive toy removed from them. Finally, if the clinical focus is a parent's ability to provide support for the infant's attachment needs, such assessment should be made when attachment needs are challenged—as in when the infant is separated briefly from the parent or has to meet a stranger. A detailed description of observations of parenting in these different contexts is provided in *The Psychology of Babies: How Relationships Support Development from Birth to Two* (Murray, 2014).

Conclusions

A number of treatments have been shown to be effective in helping mothers recover from PND. Notably, however, more limited success has been achieved in improving mother–infant interactions and in preventing poor child outcome in the longer term. Interventions that are promising in this regard are ones that focus specifically on difficulties in mother–infant interactions. These may, however, need to be delivered beyond the early postpartum period. This is because many adverse child outcomes associated with PND are particularly likely to occur in the context of chronic, or recurrent, depression, and it is unsurprising that shortening the infant's initial exposure to depression is insufficient to prevent longer-term problems in child development. In high-risk contexts where depression is more likely to be prolonged or recurrent, it may be helpful to set up long-term monitoring of vulnerable families, so that support can be provided quickly if depression recurs. In addition, it would seem profitable for professionals working with parents to be trained in systematic identification of interaction difficulties in developmentally sensitive contexts. Finally, in addition to efforts to support mother–infant relationships, it may also be beneficial to give infants experience of positive interactions with additional caregivers.

Summary

PND is a common and disabling disorder associated with a range of adverse infant and child outcomes. These occur principally where the maternal depression is chronic or recurrent and in the presence of other background risks. Adverse patterns of parenting associated with PND are likely to play a major role in bringing about poor child outcome. Biological processes are also likely to be important in mediating effects of depression on the child but require further investigation. Attempts to change parental interactions in the postpartum period and thereby improve the longer-term outcome for children of PND mothers have met with only limited success. This is likely, in large measure, to be because chronic maternal depression and background difficulties are strongly linked to particularly poor child outcome. For these reasons, interventions that are restricted to the early postpartum period may be of limited use, and longer-term monitoring and support for families may be necessary; an additional therapeutic strategy could include enhancing the role of other caregivers. There is a need for further research on the impact of depression in the developing world and on deliverable screening for parenting difficulties, in particular general parental sensitivity, as well as interventions.

References

Achenbach, T. M. (1991). *Manual for the Child Behavior Checklist/4-18*. Burlington, VT: University of Vermont.

Alpern, L., & Lyons-Ruth, K. (1993). Preschool children at social risk: Chronicity and timing of maternal depressive symptoms and child behavior problems at school and at home. *Development and Psychopathology, 5*, 371–387. doi:10.1017/S0954579400004478.

Aspland, H., & Gardner, F. (2003). Observational measures of parent-child interaction: An introductory review. *Child and Adolescent Mental Health, 8,* 136–143. doi:10.1111/1475-3588.00061.

Atkinson, L., Paglia, A., Coolbear, J., Niccols, A., Parker, K. C. H., & Guger, S. (2000). Attachment security: A meta-analysis of maternal mental health correlates. *Clinical Psychology Review, 20,* 1019–1040. doi: 10.1016/S0272-7358(99)00023-9.

Avan, B., Richter, L. M., Ramchandani, P. G., Norris, S. A., & Stein, A. (2010). Maternal postnatal depression and children's growth and behaviour during the early years of life: Exploring the interaction between physical and mental health. *Archives of Disease in Childhood, 95,* 690–695. doi:10.1136/adc.2009.164848.

Bagner, D. M., Pettit, J. W., Lewinsohn, P. M., Seeley, J. R., & Jaccard, J. (2013). Disentangling the temporal relationship between parental depressive symptoms and early child behavior problems: A transactional framework. *Journal of Clinical Child & Adolescent Psychology, 42,* 78–90. doi:10.1080/15374416.2012.715368.

Bartels, M., Van den Berg, M., Sluyter, F., Boomsma, D. I., & de Geus, E. J. C. (2003). Heritability of cortisol levels: Review and simultaneous analysis of twin studies. *Psychoneuroendocrinology, 28,* 121–137. doi: 10.1016/S0306-4530(02)00003-3.

Beck, C. T. (2001). Predictors of postpartum depression: An update. *Nursing Research, 50,* 275–285.

Bekkhus, M., Rutter, M., Barker, E. D., & Borge, A. I. H. (2011). The role of pre- and postnatal timing of family risk factors on child behavior at 36 months. *Journal of Abnormal Child Psychology, 39,* 611–621. doi: 10.1007/s10802-010-9477-z.

Bettes, B. A. (1988). Maternal depression and motherese: Temporal and intonational features. *Child Development, 59,* 1089–1096. doi:10.2307/1130275.

Brazelton, T. B., Koslowski, B., & Main, M. (1974). The origins of reciprocity: The early mother-infant interaction. In M. Lewis, & L. A. Rosenblum (Eds.), *The effect of the infant on its caregiver.* New York, NY: Elsevier.

Brennan, P. A., Hammen, C., Andersen, M. J., Bor, W., Najman, J. M., & Williams, G. M. (2000). Chronicity, severity, and timing of maternal depressive symptoms: Relationships with child outcomes at age 5. *Developmental Psychology, 36,* 759–766. doi:10.1037/0012-1649.36.6.759.

Breznitz, Z., & Sherman, T. (1987). Speech patterning of natural discourse of well and depressed mothers and their young children. *Child Development, 58,* 395–400. doi:10.2307/1130516.

Brown, G. W., & Harris, T. O. (Eds.). (1978). *Social origins of depression: A study of depressive disorder in women.* New York, NY: The Free Press.

Bugental, D. B., Martorell, G. A., & Barraza, V. (2003). The hormonal costs of subtle forms of infant maltreatment. *Hormones and Behavior, 43,* 237–244. doi:10.1016/S0018-506X(02)00008-9.

Campbell, S. B., Brownell, C. A., Hungerford, A., Spieker, S. J., Mohan, R., & Blessing, J. S. (2004). The course of maternal depressive symptoms and maternal sensitivity as predictors of attachment security at 36 months. *Development and Psychopathology, 16,* 231–252. doi:10.1017/S0954579404044499.

Campbell, S. B., Cohn, J. F., & Meyers, T. (1995). Depression in first-time mothers: Mother-infant interaction and depression chronicity. *Developmental Psychology, 31,* 349–357. doi:10.1037/0012-1649.31.3.349.

Caplan, H. L., Cogill, S. R., Alexandra, H., Robson, K. M., Katz, R., & Kumar, R. (1989). Maternal depression and the emotional development of the child. *British Journal of Psychiatry, 154,* 818–822.

Cicchetti, D., Rogosch, F. A., & Toth, S. L. (1998). Maternal depressive disorder and contextual risk: Contributions to the development of attachment insecurity and behavior problems in toddlerhood. *Development and Psychopathology, 10,* 283–300.

Cicchetti, D., Rogosch, F. A., & Toth, S. L. (2000). The efficacy of toddler-parent psychotherapy for fostering cognitive development in offspring of depressed mothers. *Journal of Abnormal Child Psychology, 28,* 135–148. doi:10.1023/A:1005118713814.

Clark, R., Tluczek, A., & Wenzel, A. (2003). Psychotherapy for postpartum depression: A preliminary report. *American Journal of Orthopsychiatry, 73,* 441–454. doi:10.1037/0002-9432.73.4.441.

Cogill, S. R., Caplan, H. L., Alexandra, H., Robson, K. M., & Kumar, R.. (1986). Impact of maternal postnatal depression on cognitive development of young children. *British Medical Journal (Clinical Research Ed.), 292,* 1165–1167.

Cohn, J. F., Campbell, S. B., Matias, R., & Hopkins, J. (1990). Face-to-face interactions of postpartum depressed and nondepressed mother-infant pairs at 2 months. *Developmental Psychology, 26,* 15–23. doi:10.1037/0012-1649.26.1.15.

Cohn, J. F., Matias, R., Tronick, E. Z., Connell, D., & Lyons-Ruth, K. (1986). Face-to-face interactions of depressed mothers and their infants. *New Directions for Child and Adolescent Development, 34,* 31–45. doi:10.1002/cd.23219863405.

Cooper, P. J., Murray, L., Wilson, A., & Romaniuk, H. (2003). Controlled trial of the short-and long-term effect of psychological treatment of post-partum depression 1. Impact on maternal mood. *The British Journal of Psychiatry, 182,* 412–419. doi:10.1192/bjp.02.177.

Cooper, P. J., Tomlinson, M., Swartz, L., Woolgar, M., Murray, L., & Molteno, C. (1999). Post-partum depression and the mother-infant relationship in a South African peri-urban settlement. *The British Journal of Psychiatry, 175,* 554–558. doi:10.1192/bjp.175.6.554.

Coplan, J. D., Andrews, M. W., Rosenblum, L. A., Owens, M. J., Friedman, S., Gorman, J. M., & Nemeroff, C. B. (1996). Persistent elevations of cerebrospinal fluid concentrations of corticotropin-releasing factor in adult nonhuman primates exposed to early-life stressors: Implications for the pathophysiology of mood and anxiety disorders. *Proceedings of the National Academy of Sciences, 93,* 1619–1623.

Coplan, J. D., Eric L. P., Smith, M. A., Mathew, S. J., Perera, T., Kral, J. G., … Rosenblum, L. A., (2006). Maternal–infant response to variable foraging demand in nonhuman primates. *Annals of the New York Academy of Sciences, 1071,* 525–533. doi:10.1196/annals.1364.05.

Coplan, J. D., Smith, E. L. P., Altemus, M., Scharf, B. A., Owens, M. J., Nemeroff, C. B., … Rosenblum, L. A. (2001). Variable foraging demand rearing: sustained elevations in cisternal cerebrospinal fluid corticotropin-releasing factor concentrations in adult primates. *Biological Psychiatry, 50,* 200–204. doi:10.1016/S0006-3223(01)01175-1.

Cornish, A. M., McMahon, C. A., Ungerer, J. A., Barnett, B., Kowalenko, N., & Tennant, C. (2005). Postnatal depression and infant cognitive and motor development in the second postnatal year: The impact of depression chronicity and infant gender. *Infant Behavior and Development, 28,* 407–417. doi:10.1016/j.infbeh.2005.03.004.

Cuijpers, P., Brännmark, J. G., & van Straten, A. (2008). Psychological treatment of postpartum depression: A meta-analysis. *Journal of Clinical Psychology, 64,* 103–118. doi:10.1002/jclp.20432.

Davidson, R. J., Ekman, P., Saron, C. D., Senulis, J. A., & Friesen, W. V. (1990). Approach-withdrawal and cerebral asymmetry: Emotional expression and brain physiology: I. *Journal of Personality and Social Psychology, 58,* 330–341. doi:10.1037/0022-3514.58.2.330.

Dawson, G., Ashman, S. B., Panagiotides, H., Hessl, D., Self, J., Yamada, E., & Embry, L. (2003). Preschool outcomes of children of depressed mothers: Role of maternal behavior, contextual risk, and children's brain activity. *Child Development, 74,* 1158–1175. doi:10.1111/1467-8624.00599.

Dawson, G., Frey, K., Panagiotides, H., Osterling, J., & Hessl, D. (1997a). Infants of depressed mothers exhibit atypical frontal brain activity a replication and extension of previous findings. *Journal of Child Psychology and Psychiatry, 38,* 179–186. doi:10.1111/j.1469-7610.1997.tb01852.x.

Dawson, G., Frey, K., Panagiotides, H., Self, J., Hessl, D., & Yamada, E. (1997b). Atypical frontal brain activity in infants of depressed mothers: The role of maternal behavior. Poster presented at the Meeting of the Society for Research in Child Development as part of a symposium on The Impact of Trauma and Adversity on Behavioral and Physiological Development: Clarifying the Issues, Washington, DC.

Dawson, G., Frey, K., Panagiotides, H., Yamada, E., Hessl, D, & Osterling, J. (1999). Infants of depressed mothers exhibit atypical frontal electrical brain activity during interactions with mother and with a familiar, nondepressed adult. *Child Development, 70,* 1058–1066. doi:10.1111/1467-8624.00078.

DeGangi, G. A., Breinbauer, C., Roosevelt, J. D., Porges, S., & Greenspan, S. (2000). Prediction of childhood problems at three years in children experiencing disorders of regulation during infancy. *Infant Mental Health Journal, 21*, 156–175.

Dennis, C.-L., & Hodnett, E. (2007). Psychosocial and psychological interventions for treating post-partum depression. *Cochrane Database of Systematic Reviews*, CD006116. doi:10.1002/1465185.

Diego, M. A., Field, T., & Hernandez-Reif, M. (2001). BIS/BAS scores are correlated with frontal EEG asymmetry in intrusive and withdrawn depressed mothers. *Infant Mental Health Journal, 22*, 665–675. doi:10.1002/imhj.1025.

Eshel, N., Daelmans, B., Cabral De Mello, M., & Martines, J. (2006). Responsive parenting: Interventions and outcomes. *Bulletin of the World Health Organization, 84*(12), 992–998.

Essex, M. J., Klein, M. H., Cho, E., & Kalin, N. H. (2002). Maternal stress beginning in infancy may sensitize children to later stress exposure: Effects on cortisol and behavior. *Biological Psychiatry, 52*, 776–784. doi:10.1016/S0006-3223(02)01553-6.

Essex, M. J., Klein, M. H., Cho, E., & Kraemer, H. C. (2003). Exposure to maternal depression and marital conflict: Gender differences in children's later mental health symptoms. *Journal of the American Academy of Child & Adolescent Psychiatry, 42*, 728–737. doi:10.1097/01. CHI.0000046849.56865.1D.

Essex, M. J., Klein, M. H., Miech, R., & Smider, N. A. (2001). Timing of initial exposure to maternal major depression and children's mental health symptoms in kindergarten. *The British Journal of Psychiatry, 179*, 151–156. doi:10.1192/bjp.179.2.151.

Evans, J., Melotti, R., Heron, J., Ramchandani, P., Wiles, N., Murray, L., & Stein, A. (2012). The timing of maternal depressive symptoms and child cognitive development: A longitudinal study. *Journal of Child Psychology and Psychiatry, 53*, 632–640. doi:10.1111/j.1469-7610.2011.02513.x.

Fagen, J. W., Ohr, P. S., Fleckenstein, L. K., & Ribner, D. R. (1985). The effect of crying on long-term memory in infancy. *Child Development, 56*, 1584–1592. doi:10.2307/1130477.

Ferber, S. G., Feldman, R., & Makhoul, I. R. (2008). The development of maternal touch across the first year of life. *Early Human Development, 84*, 363–370. doi:10.1016/j.earlhumdev. 2007.09.019.

Fernald, A. (1989). Intonation and communicative intent in mothers' speech to infants: Is the melody the message? *Child Development, 60*, 1497–1510. doi:10.2307/1130938.

Field, T. M. (1984). Early interactions between infants and their postpartum depressed mothers. *Infant Behavior and Development, 7*, 517–522.

Field, T. (1995). Infants of depressed mothers. *Infant Behavior and Development, 18*, 1–13. doi:10.101 6/0163-6383(95)90003-9.

Field, T., Diego, M., Dieter, J., Hernandez-Reif, M., Schanberg, S., Kuhn, C., … Bendell, D. (2004). Prenatal depression effects on the fetus and the newborn. *Infant Behavior and Development, 27*, 216–229. doi:10.1016/j.infbeh.2003.09.010.

Field, T., Fox, N. A., Pickens, J., & Nawrocki, T. (1995). Relative right frontal EEG activation in 3-to 6-month-old infants of "depressed" mothers. *Developmental Psychology, 31*, 358–363. doi:10.1037/0012-1649.31.3.358.

Field, T., Healy, B. T., Goldstein, S., & Guthertz, M. (1990). Behavior-state matching and synchrony in mother-infant interactions of nondepressed versus depressed dyads. *Developmental Psychology, 26*, 7–14. doi:10.1037/0012-1649.26.1.7.

Field, T., Healy, B., Goldstein, S., Perry, S., Bendell, D., Schanberg, S., … Kuhn, C. (1988). Infants of depressed mothers show "depressed" behavior even with nondepressed adults. *Child Development, 59*, 1569–1579. doi:10.2307/1130671.

Field, T., Sandberg, D., Garcia, R., Vega-Lahr N., Goldstein, S., & Guy, L. (1985). Pregnancy problems, postpartum depression, and early mother–infant interactions. *Developmental Psychology, 21*, 1152–1156. doi:10.1037/0012-1649.21.6.1152.

Forbes, E. E., Shaw, D. S., Silk, J. S., Feng, X., Cohn, J F., Fox, N. A., & Kovacs, M. (2008). Children's affect expression and frontal EEG asymmetry: Transactional associations with mothers' depres-sive symptoms. *Journal of Abnormal Child Psychology, 36*, 207–221. doi:10.1007/s10802-007-9171-y.

Forman, D. R., O'Hara, M. W., Stuart, S., Gorman, L. L., Larsen, K E., & Coy, K. C. (2007). Effective treatment for postpartum depression is not sufficient to improve the developing mother–child relationship. *Development and Psychopathology, 19*, 585–602. doi:10.1017/S0954579407070289.

Ghodsian, M., Zajicek, E., & Wolkind, S. (1984). A longitudinal study of maternal depression and child behaviour problems. *Journal of Child Psychology and Psychiatry, 25*, 91–109. doi:10.1111/j.1469-7610.1984.tb01721.x.

Gjerde, P. F. (1995). Alternative pathways to chronic depressive symptoms in young adults: Gender differences in developmental trajectories. *Child Development, 66*(5), 1277–1300.

Glover, V., Onozawa, K., & Hodgkinson, A. (2002). Benefits of infant massage for mothers with post-natal depression. *Seminars in Neonatology, 7*, 495–500. doi:10.1053/siny.2002.0154.

Goodyer, I. M., Tamplin, A., Herbert J., & Altham, P. M. E. (2000). Recent life events, cortisol, dehy-droepiandrosterone and the onset of major depression in high-risk adolescents. *The British Journal of Psychiatry, 177*, 499–504. doi:10.1192/bjp.177.6.499.

Gore, S., Aseltine Jr R. H., & Colten, M. E. (1993). Gender, social-relationship involvement, and depression. *Journal of Research on Adolescence, 3*, 101–125. doi:10.1207/s15327795jra0302_1.

Halligan, S. L., Herbert, J., Goodyer, I. M., & Murray, L. (2004). Exposure to postnatal depression pre-dicts elevated cortisol in adolescent offspring. *Biological Psychiatry, 55*, 376–381. doi:10.1016/j.biopsych.2003.09.013.

Hammen, C., & Brennan, P. A. (2003). Severity, chronicity, and timing of maternal depression and risk for adolescent offspring diagnoses in a community sample. *Archives of General Psychiatry, 60*, 253–258. doi:10.1001/archpsyc.60.3.253.

Harris, T. O., Borsanyi, S., Messari, S., Stanford, K., Brown, G. W., Cleary, S. E., … Herbert, J. (2000). Morning cortisol as a risk factor for subsequent major depressive disorder in adult women. *The British Journal of Psychiatry, 177*, 505–510. doi:10.1192/bjp.177.6.505.

Hart, S., Field, T., & Nearing, G. (1998). Depressed mothers' neonates improve following the MABI and a Brazelton demonstration. *Journal of Pediatric Psychology, 23*, 351–356. doi:10.1093/jpepsy/23.6.351.

Hay, D. F., & Kumar, R. (1995). Interpreting the effects of mothers' postnatal depression on children's intelligence: A critique and re-analysis. *Child Psychiatry and Human Development, 25*, 165–181. doi:10.1007/BF02251301.

Hay, D. F., Pawlby, S., Angold, A., Harold, G. T., & Sharp, D. (2003). Pathways to violence in the chil-dren of mothers who were depressed postpartum. *Developmental Psychology, 39*, 1083–1094. doi:10.1037/0012-1649.39.6.1083.

Hay, D. F., Pawlby, S., Sharp, D., Asten, P., Mills, A., & Kumar, R. (2001). Intellectual problems shown by 11-year-old children whose mothers had postnatal depression. *Journal of Child Psychology and Psychiatry, 42*, 871–889. doi:10.1111/1469-7610.00784.

Henriques, J. B., & Davidson, R. J. (1990). Regional brain electrical asymmetries discriminate bet-ween previously depressed and healthy control subjects. *Journal of Abnormal Psychology, 99*, 22–31.

Herrera, E., Reissland, N., & Shepherd, J. (2004). Maternal touch and maternal child-directed speech: Effects of depressed mood in the postnatal period. *Journal of Affective Disorders, 81*, 29–39. doi:10.1016/j.jad.2003.07.001.

Hessl, D., Dawson, G., Frey, K., Panagiotides, H., Self, J., Yamada, E., & Osterling, J. (1998). A longitudinal study of children of depressed mothers: Psychobiological findings related to stress. In D. M. Hann, L. C. Huffman, K. K. Lederhendler, & D. Minecke (Eds.), *Advancing research on developmental plasticity: Integrating the behavioral sciences and the neurosciences of mental health* (pp. 256–265). Bethseda, MD: National Institutes of Mental Health.

Hill, J. (2002). Biological, psychological and social processes in the conduct disorders. *Journal of Child Psychology and Psychiatry and Allied Disciplines, 43*(1), 133–164.

Hipwell, A. E., Murray, L., Ducournau, P., & Stein, A. (2005). The effects of maternal depression and parental conflict on children's peer play. *Child: Care, Health and Development, 31*, 11–23. doi:10.1111/j.1365-2214.2005.00448.x.

Horowitz, J. A., Bell, M., Trybulski, J., Munro, B. H., Moser, D., Hartz, S. A., … Sokol, E. S. (2001). Promoting responsiveness between mothers with depressive symptoms and their infants. *Journal of Nursing Scholarship, 33*, 323–329. doi:10.1111/j.1547-5069.2001.00323.x.

Hossain, Z., Field, T., Gonzalez, J., Malphurs, J., Del Valle, C., & Pickens, J. (1994). Infants of "depressed" mothers interact better with their nondepressed fathers. *Infant Mental Health Journal, 15*, 348–357.

Isabella, R. A., & Belsky, J. (1991). Interactional synchrony and the origins of infant-mother attachment: A replication study. *Child Development, 62*, 373–384. doi:10.1111/j.1467-8624.1991.tb01538.x.

Jaffe, J., Beebe, B., Feldstein, S., Crown, C. L., & Jasnow, M. D. (2001). Rhythms of dialogue in infancy. *Monographs of the Society for Research in Child Development, 66*, 1–151.

Jameson, P. B., Gelfand, D. M., Kulcsar, E., & Teti, D. M. (1997). Mother-toddler interaction patterns associated with maternal depression. *Development and Psychopathology, 9*, 537–550.

James-Roberts, I., & Plewis, I. (1996). Individual differences, daily fluctuations, and developmental changes in amounts of infant waking, fussing, crying, feeding, and sleeping. *Child Development, 67*, 2527–2540. doi:10.1111/j.1467-8624.1996.tb01872.x.

Jones, N. A., Field, T., Davalos, M., & Pickens, J. (1997a). EEG stability in infants/children of depressed mothers. *Child Psychiatry and Human Development, 28*, 59–70. doi:10.1023/A:1025197101496.

Jones, N. A., Field, T., Fox, N. A., Lundy, B., & Davalos, M. (1997b). EEG activation in 1-month-old infants of depressed mothers. *Development and Psychopathology, 9*, 491–505.

Joormann, J., Talbot, L., & Gotlib, I. H. (2007). Biased processing of emotional information in girls at risk for depression. *Journal of Abnormal Psychology, 116*, 135–143. doi:10.1037/0021-843X.116.1.135.

Kaffman, A., & Meaney, M. J. (2007). Neurodevelopmental sequelae of postnatal maternal care in rodents: Clinical and research implications of molecular insights. *Journal of Child Psychology and Psychiatry, 48*, 224–244. doi:10.1111/j.1469-7610.2007.01730.x.

Kaplan, P. S., Bachorowski, J.-A., Smoski, M. J., & Hudenko, W. J. (2002). Infants of depressed mothers, although competent learners, fail to learn in response to their own mothers' infant-directed speech. *Psychological Science, 13*, 268–271. doi:10.1111/1467-9280.00449.

Kaplan, P. S., Bachorowski, J.-A., Smoski, M. J., & Zinser, M. (2001). Role of clinical diagnosis and medication use in effects of maternal depression on infant-directed speech. *Infancy, 2*, 537–548. doi:10.1207/S15327078IN0204_08.

Kaplan, P. S., Bachorowski, J.-A., & Zarlengo-Strouse, P. (1999). Child-directed speech produced by mothers with symptoms of depression fails to promote associative learning in 4-month-old infants. *Child Development, 70*, 560–570. doi:10.1111/1467-8624.00041.

Kendler, K. S. (1996). Major depression and generalised anxiety disorder. Same genes, (partly) different environments—revisited. *British Journal of Psychiatry, 168*(Suppl 30), 68–75.

Kersten-Alvarez, L. E., Hosman, C. M. H., Riksen-Walraven, J. M., Van Doesum, K., & Hoefnagels, C. (2011). Which preventive interventions effectively enhance depressed mothers' sensitivity? A meta-analysis. *Infant Mental Health Journal, 32*, 362–376. doi:10.1002/imhj.20301.

Kochanska, G., Murray, K. T., & Harlan, E. T. (2000). Effortful control in early childhood: Continuity and change, antecedents, and implications for social development. *Developmental Psychology, 36*, 220. doi:10.1037/0012-1649.36.2.220.

Kochanska, G., Tjebkes, J. L., & Forman, D. R. (1998). Children's emerging regulation of conduct: Restraint, compliance, and internalization from infancy to the second year. *Child Development, 69*, 1378–1389. doi:10.1111/j.1467-8624.1998.tb06218.x.

Kurstjens, S., & Wolke, D. (2001). Effects of maternal depression on cognitive development of children over the first 7 years of life. *Journal of Child Psychology and Psychiatry, 42*, 623–636. doi:10.1111/1469-7610.00758.

Lee, L.-C., Halpern, C. T., Hertz-Picciotto, I., Martin, S. L., & Suchindran, C. M. (2006). Child care and social support modify the association between maternal depressive symptoms and early childhood behaviour problems: A US national study. *Journal of Epidemiology and Community Health, 60*, 305–310. doi:10.1136/jech.2005.040956.

Lindhiem, O., Bernard, K., & Dozier, M. (2011). Maternal sensitivity: Within-person variability and the utility of multiple assessments. *Child Maltreatment, 16,* 41–50. doi:10.1177/1077559510387662.

Mannie, Z., Harmer, C., & Cowen, P. (2007). Increased waking salivary cortisol levels in young people at familial risk of depression. *American Journal of Psychiatry, 164,* 617–621. doi:10.1176/appi.ajp.164.4.617.

Martins, C., & Gaffan, E. A. (2000). Effects of early maternal depression on patterns of infant-mother attachment: A meta-analytic investigation. *Journal of Child Psychology and Psychiatry, 41,* 737–746. doi:10.1111/1469-7610.00661.

Maughan, A., Cicchetti, D., Toth, S L., & Rogosch, F. A. (2007). Early-occurring maternal depression and maternal negativity in predicting young children's emotion regulation and socioemotional difficulties. *Journal of Abnormal Child Psychology, 35,* 685–703. doi:10.1007/s10802-007-9129-0.

McMahon, C. A., Barnett, B., Kowalenko, N. M., & Tennant, C. C. (2006). Maternal attachment state of mind moderates the impact of postnatal depression on infant attachment. *Journal of Child Psychology and Psychiatry, 47,* 660–669. doi:10.1111/j.1469-7610.2005.01547.x.

Mesman, J., & Emmen, R. A. G. (2013). Mary Ainsworth's legacy: A systematic review of observational instruments measuring parental sensitivity. *Attachment & Human Development, 15,* 485–506. doi:10.1080/14616734.2013.820900.

Milgrom, J., Westley, D. T., & Gemmill, A. W. (2004). The mediating role of maternal responsiveness in some longer term effects of postnatal depression on infant development. *Infant Behavior and Development, 27,* 443–454. doi:10.1016/j.infbeh.2004.03.003.

Monk, C., Klein, R., Telzer, E., Schroth, E., Mannuzza, S., Moulton, J., … Ernst, M. (2008). Amygdala and nucleus accumbens activation to emotional facial expressions in children and adolescents at risk for major depression. *American Journal of Psychiatry, 165,* 90–98. doi:10.1176/appi.ajp.2007.06111917.

Morrell, J., & Murray, L. (2003). Parenting and the development of conduct disorder and hyperactive symptoms in childhood: A prospective longitudinal study from 2 months to 8 years. *Journal of Child Psychology and Psychiatry, 44,* 489–508. doi:10.1111/1469-7610.t01-1-00139.

Murray, L. (1992). The impact of postnatal depression on infant development. *Journal of Child Psychology and Psychiatry, 33,* 543–561. doi:10.1111/j.1469-7610.1992.tb00890.x.

Murray, L. (2014). *The psychology of babies: How relationships support development from birth to two.* London, UK: Constable & Robinson.

Murray, L., Arteche, A., Fearon, P., Halligan, S., Croudace, T., & Cooper, P. (2010a). The effects of maternal postnatal depression and child sex on academic performance at age 16 years: A developmental approach. *Journal of Child Psychology and Psychiatry, 51,* 1150–1159. doi:10.1111/j.1469-7610.2010.02259.x.

Murray, L., Arteche, A., Fearon, P., Halligan, S., Goodyer, I., & Cooper, P. (2011). Maternal postnatal depression and the development of depression in offspring up to 16 years of age. *Journal of the American Academy of Child & Adolescent Psychiatry, 50,* 460–470. doi:10.1016/j.jaac.2011.02.001.

Murray, L., Cooper, P. J., Wilson, A., & Romaniuk, H. (2003). Controlled trial of the short-and long-term effect of psychological treatment of post-partum depression 2. Impact on the mother-child relationship and child outcome. *The British Journal of Psychiatry, 182,* 420–427. doi:10.1192/bjp.02.178.

Murray, L., Fiori-Cowley, A., Hooper, R., & Cooper, P. (1996a). The impact of postnatal depression and associated adversity on early mother-infant interactions and later infant outcome. *Child Development, 67,* 2512–2526. doi:10.1111/j.1467-8624.1996.tb01871.x.

Murray, L., Halligan, S. L., Adams, G., Patterson, P., & Goodyer, I. M. (2006). Socioemotional development in adolescents at risk for depression: The role of maternal depression and attachment style. *Development and Psychopathology, 18,* 489–516. doi:10.1017/S0954579406060263.

Murray, L., Halligan, S. L., Goodyer, I., & Herbert, J. (2010b). Disturbances in early parenting of depressed mothers and cortisol secretion in offspring: A preliminary study. *Journal of Affective Disorders, 122,* 218–223. doi:10.1016/j.jad.2009.06.034.

Murray, L., Hipwell, A., Hooper, R., Stein, A., & Cooper, P. (1996b). The cognitive development of 5-year-old children of postnatally depressed mothers. *Journal of Child Psychology and Psychiatry*, *37*, 927–935. doi:10.1111/j.1469-7610.1996.tb01490.x.

Murray, L., Kempton, C., Woolgar, M., & Hooper, R. (1993). Depressed mothers' speech to their infants and its relation to infant gender and cognitive development. *Journal of Child Psychology and Psychiatry*, *34*, 1083–1101. doi:10.1111/j.1469-7610.1993.tb01775.x.

Murray, L., Marwick, H., & Arteche, A. (2010c). Sadness in mothers' 'baby-talk' predicts affective disorder in adolescent offspring. *Infant Behavior and Development*, *33*, 361–364. doi:10.1016/j.infbeh.2010.03.009.

Murray, L., & Ramchandani, P. (2007). Might prevention be better than cure? A perspective on improving infant sleep and maternal mental health: A cluster randomized trial. *Archives of Disease in Childhood*, *92*, 943–944. doi:10.1136/adc.2007.124628.

Murray, L., Sinclair, D., Cooper, P., Ducournau, P., Turner, P., & Stein, A. (1999a). The socioemotional development of 5-year-old children of postnatally depressed mothers. *Journal of Child Psychology and Psychiatry*, *40*, 1259–1271. doi:10.1111/1469-7610.00542.

Murray, L., Stanley, C., Hooper, R., King, F., & Fiori-Cowley, A. (1996c). The role of infant factors in postnatal depression and mother-infant interactions. *Developmental Medicine & Child Neurology*, *38*, 109–119. doi:10.1111/j.1469-8749.1996.tb12082.x.

Murray, L., Woolgar, M., Briers, S., & Hipwell, A. (1999b). Children's social representations in dolls' house play and theory of mind tasks, and their relation to family adversity and child disturbance. *Social Development*, *8*, 179–200. doi:10.1111/1467-9507.00090.

Murray, L., Woolgar, M., Cooper, P., & Hipwell, A. (2001). Cognitive vulnerability to depression in 5-year-old children of depressed mothers. *Journal of Child Psychology and Psychiatry*, *42*, 891–899. doi:10.1111/1469-7610.00785.

NICHD, Early Child Care Research Network. (1999). Chronicity of maternal depressive symptoms, maternal sensitivity, and child functioning at 36 months. *Developmental Psychology*, *35*, 1297–1310.

O'Connor, T. G., Ben-Shlomo, Y., Heron, J., Golding, J., Adams, D., & Glover, V. (2005). Prenatal anxiety predicts individual differences in cortisol in pre-adolescent children. *Biological Psychiatry*, *58*, 211–217. doi:10.1016/j.biopsych.2005.03.032.

O'Hara, M. W., & Swain, A. M. (1996). Rates and risk of postpartum depression-a meta-analysis. *International Review of Psychiatry*, *8*, 37–54. doi:10.3109/09540269609037816.

Onozawa, K., Glover, V., Adams, D., Modi, N., & Kumar, R. C. (2001). Infant massage improves mother–infant interaction for mothers with postnatal depression. *Journal of Affective Disorders*, *63*, 201–207. doi:10.1016/S0165-0327(00)00198-1.

Papoušek, H., & Papoušek, M. (1987). Intuitive parenting: A dialectic counterpart to the infant's integrative competence. In Joy Doniger Osofsky, J. D. (Ed.), *Handbook of infant development* (2nd ed., pp. 669–720). New York, NY: John Wiley & Sons, Inc.

Parsons, C. E., Young, K. S., Rochat, T. J., Kringelbach, M., & Stein, A. (2012). Postnatal depression and its effects on child development: A review of evidence from low-and middle-income countries. *British Medical Bulletin*, *101*, 57–79.

Pawlby, S., Hay, D. F., Sharp, D., Waters, C. S., & O'Keane, V. (2009). Antenatal depression predicts depression in adolescent offspring: Prospective longitudinal community-based study. *Journal of Affective Disorders*, *113*, 236–243. doi:10.1016/j.jad.2008.05.018.

Pelaez-Nogueras, M., Field, T., Cigales, M., Gonzalez, A., & Clasky, S. (1994). Infants of depressed mothers show less "depressed" behavior with their nursery teachers. *Infant Mental Health Journal*, *15*, 358–367.

Petterson, S. M., & Albers, A. B. (2001). Effects of poverty and maternal depression on early child development. *Child Development*, *72*, 1794–1813. doi:10.1111/1467-8624.00379.

Philipps, L. H., & O'Hara, M. W. (1991). Prospective study of postpartum depression: 4½-year follow-up of women and children. *Journal of Abnormal Psychology*, *100*, 151–155. doi:10.1037/0021-843X.100.2.151.

Posner, M. I., & Rothbart, M. K. (2000). Developing mechanisms of self-regulation. *Development and Psychopathology, 12,* 427–441.

Richman, N., & Graham, P. J. (1971). A behavioural screening questionnaire for use with three-year-old Children. Preliminary findings. *Journal of Child Psychology and Psychiatry, 12,* 5–33. doi:10.1111/j.1469-7610.1971.tb01047.x.

Robertson, E., Grace, S., Wallington, T., & Stewart, D. E. (2004). Antenatal risk factors for postpartum depression: A synthesis of recent literature. *General Hospital Psychiatry, 26,* 289–295. doi:10.1016/j.genhosppsych.2004.02.006.

Rosenblum, L. A., Coplan, J. D., Friedman, S., Bassoff, T., Gorman, J. M., & Andrews, M. W. (1994). Adverse early experiences affect noradrenergic and serotonergic functioning in adult primates. *Biological Psychiatry, 35,* 221–227. doi:10.1016/0006-3223(94)91252-1.

Sameroff, A. J., Emde, R. N. (Eds.). (1989). *Relationship disturbances in early childhood.* New York, NY: Basic Books.

Schaffer, C. E., Davidson, R. J., & Saron, C. (1983). Frontal and parietal electroencephalogram asymmetry in depressed and nondepressed subjects. *Biological Psychiatry, 18,* 753–762.

Sharp, D., Hay, D. F., Pawlby, S., Schmücker, G., Allen, H., & Kumar, R. (1995). The impact of postnatal depression on boys' intellectual development. *Journal of Child Psychology and Psychiatry, 36,* 1315–1336. doi:10.1111/j.1469-7610.1995.tb01666.x.

Silberg, J. L., Maes, H., & Eaves, L. J. (2010). Genetic and environmental influences on the transmission of parental depression to children's depression and conduct disturbance: An extended Children of Twins study. *Journal of Child Psychology and Psychiatry, 51,* 734–744. doi:10.1111/j.1469-7610.2010.02205.x.

Sinclair, D., & Murray, L. (1998). Effects of postnatal depression on children's adjustment to school. Teacher's reports. *The British Journal of Psychiatry, 172,* 58–63. doi:10.1192/bjp.172.1.58.

Slater, A. (1995). Individual differences in infancy and later IQ. *Journal of Child Psychology and Psychiatry, 36,* 69–112. doi:10.1111/j.1469-7610.1995.tb01656.x.

Southwick, S. M., Vythilingam, M., & Charney, D. S. (2005). The psychobiology of depression and resilience to stress: Implications for prevention and treatment. *Annual Review of Clinical Psychology, 1,* 255–291. doi:10.1146/annurev.clinpsy.1.102803.143948.

Stanley, C., Murray, L., & Stein, A. (2004). The effect of postnatal depression on mother-infant interaction, infant response to the still-face perturbation, and performance on an instrumental learning task. *Development and Psychopathology, 16,* 1–18.

Stein, A., Gath, D. H., Bucher, J., Bond, A., Day, A., & Cooper, P. J. (1991). The relationship between post-natal depression and mother-child interaction. *The British Journal of Psychiatry, 158,* 46–52. doi:10.1192/bjp.158.1.46.

Stern, D. N., Beebe, B., Jaffe, J., & Bennett, S. L. (1977). The infant's stimulus world during social interaction: A study of caregiver behaviors with particular reference to repetition and timing. In H. R. Schaffer (Ed.), *Studies in mother-infant interaction* (pp. 177–202). New York, NY: Academic Press.

Stern, D. N., Spieker, S., & MacKain, K. (1982). Intonation contours as signals in maternal speech to prelinguistic infants. *Developmental Psychology, 18,* 727–735. doi:10.1037/0012-1649.18.5.727.

Stevenson, M., Scope, A., Sutcliffe, P. A., Booth, A., Slade, P., Parry, G., … Kalthenthaler, E. (2010). Group cognitive behavioural therapy for postnatal depression: A systematic review of clinical effectiveness, cost effectiveness and value of information analyses. *Health Technology Assessment, 14,* 1–135. doi:10.3310/hta14440.

Sutter-Dallay, A.-L., Murray, L., Dequae-Merchadou, L., Glatigny-Dallay, E., Bourgeois, M.-L., & Verdoux, H. (2011). A prospective longitudinal study of the impact of early postnatal vs. chronic maternal depressive symptoms on child development. *European Psychiatry, 26,* 484–489. doi:10.1016/j.eurpsy.2010.05.004.

Thibodeau, R., Jorgensen, R. S., & Kim, S. (2006). Depression, anxiety, and resting frontal EEG asymmetry: A meta-analytic review. *Journal of Abnormal Psychology, 115,* 715–729. doi:10.1037/0021-843X.115.4.715.

Tomarken, A. J., Davidson, R. J., & Henriques, J. B. (1990). Resting frontal brain asymmetry predicts affective responses to films. *Journal of Personality and Social Psychology*, *59*, 791–801. doi:10.1037/0022-3514.59.4.791.

Trevarthen, C. (1979). Communication and cooperation in early infancy: A description of primary intersubjectivity. In M. Bullowa (Ed.), *Before speech: The beginning of interpersonal communication* (pp. 321–347). New York, NY: Cambridge University Press.

Tronick, E. Z. (1989). Emotions and emotional communication in infants. *American Psychologist*, *44*, 112–119. doi:10.1037/0003-066X.44.2.112.

Tronick, E. Z., & Gianino, A. F. (1986). The transmission of maternal disturbance to the infant. *New Directions for Child and Adolescent Development*, *34*, 5–11. doi:10.1002/cd.23219863403.

Tronick, E. Z., & Weinberg, M. K. (1999). Depressed mothers and infants: Failure to form. In L. Murray, & P. Cooper (Eds.), *Postpartum depression and child development* (p. 54). New York, NY: Guilford Press.

Van Doesum, K., Riksen-Walraven, J. M., Hosman, C. M. H., & Hoefnagels, C. (2008). A randomized controlled trial of a home-visiting intervention aimed at preventing relationship problems in depressed mothers and their infants. *Child Development*, *79*, 547–561. doi:10.1111/j.1467-8624.2008.01142.x.

Wachs, T. D., Black, M. M., & Engle, P. L. (2009). Maternal depression: A global threat to children's health, development, and behavior and to human rights. *Child Development Perspectives*, *3*, 51–59. doi:10.1111/j.1750-8606.2008.00077.x.

Waters, C., Van Goozen, S., Phillips, R., Swift, N., Hurst, S., Mundy, L., … Hay, D. (2013). Infants at familial risk for depression show a distinct pattern of cortisol response to experimental challenge. *Journal of Affective Disorders*, *150*(3), 955–960.

Weaver, I. C. G., Cervoni, N., Champagne, F. A., D'Alessio, A. C., Sharma, S., Seckl, J. R., … Meaney, M. J. (2004). Epigenetic programming by maternal behavior. *Nature Neuroscience*, *7*, 847–854. doi:10.1038/nn1276.

Weinberg, K. M., Olson, K. L., Beeghly, M., & Tronick, E. Z. (2006). Making up is hard to do, especially for mothers with high levels of depressive symptoms and their infant sons. *Journal of Child Psychology and Psychiatry*, *47*, 670–683. doi:10.1111/j.1469-7610.2005.01545.x.

Weissman, M. M., Warner, V., Wickramaratne, P., & Prusoff, B. A. (1988). Early-onset major depression in parents and their children. *Journal of Affective Disorders*, *15*, 269–277. doi:10.1016/0165-0327(88)90024-9.

Weissman, M., Wickramaratne, P., Nomura, Y., Warner, V., Pilowsky, D., & Verdeli, H. (2006). Offspring of depressed parents: 20 years later. *American Journal of Psychiatry*, *163*, 1001–1008. doi:10.1176/appi.ajp.163.6.1001.

Wolff, M. S., & Ijzendoorn, M. H. (1997). Sensitivity and attachment: A meta-analysis on parental antecedents of infant attachment. *Child Development*, *68*, 571–591. doi:10.1111/j.1467-8624.1997. tb04218.x.

Wrate, R. M., Rooney, A. C., Thomas, P. F., & Cox, J. L. (1985). Postnatal depression and child development. A three-year follow-up study. *The British Journal of Psychiatry*, *146*, 622–627. doi:10.1192/bjp.146.6.622.

Wright, C. A., George, T. P., Burke, R., Gelfand, D. M., & Teti, D. M. (2000). Early maternal depression and children's adjustment to school. *Child Study Journal*, *30*, 153–168.

Young, E. A., Vazquez, D., Jiang, H., & Pfeffer, C. R. (2006). Saliva cortisol and response to dexamethasone in children of depressed parents. *Biological Psychiatry*, *60*, 831–836. doi:10.1016/j.biopsych.2006.03.077.

Zlochower, A. J., & Cohn, J. F. (1996). Vocal timing in face-to-face interaction of clinically depressed and nondepressed mothers and their 4-month-old infants. *Infant Behavior and Development*, *19*, 371–374. doi:10.1016/S0163-6383(96)90035-1.

10

Fathers' Perinatal Mental Health

Richard Fletcher, Craig F. Garfield, and Stephen Matthey

Introduction

The birth of a child can change a man forever. His relationships with his partner and his view of himself are permanently altered. So too are his status and level of social obligation. Through fathering relationships, men "grow up" their children, contributing to the well-being of the entire society. For many men, these changes are welcome and enhancing to their emotional and psychological well-being. For some, the inevitable stresses and adjustments of parenthood can overwhelm their coping ability, and as a result, their mental health suffers.

Early detection of mental health disorders among fathers and the provision of support are important for the well-being of fathers, their families, and the wider community. Depression and anxiety can be crippling for the father and can impair his relationships and adversely affect his children's successful development. Maladaptive behaviors such as drug use and relationship conflict can result from and can worsen his mental state. The costs to society are enormous as they impact the father, the children, and the family (Deloitte Access Economics, 2012; Hanington, Heron, Stein, & Ramchandani, 2012; Ramchandani, Stein, Evans, & O'Connor, 2005). However, conditions such as depression and anxiety are common, and there are known treatments that have been shown to be effective. What has been lacking is a way to identify fathers in need and provide them with appropriate levels of support.

The recognition of the importance of maternal mental health disorders and the possible deleterious effects on children's development has spurred the development of comprehensive programs of screening and treatment (e.g., Buist, 2005). While models of detection of depression and the provision of pathways to care for mothers can provide a broad template for imagining how fathers may be supported, it would be mistaken to simply mimic mothers' services in designing services for fathers. The research evidence for proposing appropriate

Identifying Perinatal Depression and Anxiety: Evidence-Based Practice in Screening, Psychosocial Assessment, and Management, First Edition. Edited by Jeannette Milgrom and Alan W. Gemmill.
© 2015 John Wiley & Sons, Ltd. Published 2015 by John Wiley & Sons, Ltd.

screening and treatments for fathers is underdeveloped compared to that for mothers. As well, a father's role, particularly in terms of his readiness to engage with health services due to time, familiarity, and social context, may necessitate a different style of support.

In this chapter, the emerging evidence for assessing fathers' mental health, including its connection with infant and mothers' well-being, is described. The application of screening tools, in particular the widely used Edinburgh Postnatal Depression Scale (EPDS) (Cox, Holden, & Sagovsky, 1987) for detecting depression in fathers, is discussed, and recently proposed alternative measures are described. Finally, a scenario is presented offering a hypothetical model of perinatal mental health care for fathers.

Depression in Fathers

Evidence regarding new fathers' mental health status has followed from the recognition of the effects of postnatal depression among mothers. Harvey and McGrath (1988) examined the partners of mothers admitted with a postnatal psychiatric illness and found that 42% had a diagnosis according to the Diagnostic and Statistical Manual of Mental Disorders (DSM). Lovestone and Kumar (1993) reported that 12 of the 24 men whose partners were admitted to a mother and baby unit with severe puerperal psychiatric illness were found to be "cases" judged from their Schedule for Affective Disorders and Schizophrenia (SADS) assessment interview. While it is unsurprising that partners of mothers with a psychiatric illness show signs of depression, studies with nonclinical samples have also reported concordant mood disturbances in mothers and fathers. For example, Deater-Deckard and colleagues (1998) measured depression in 7108 women and their partners using the EPDS at 18 weeks' gestation and 8 weeks' postpartum. Partners' scores were significantly correlated with the women's depression both before ($r = 0.24$, $p < 0.001$) and after the birth ($r = 0.26$, $p < 0.001$) (Deater-Deckard et al., 1998) though it should be noted that these are quite low correlations. A meta-analysis of 43 studies of perinatal depression involving 28,004 participants' reported a moderate ($r = 0.308$; 95% confidence interval [CI], 0.228–0.384) correlation between paternal and maternal depression (Paulson & Bazemore, 2010). In examining possible contributors to new fathers' depression, Zelkowitz and Milet (1997) compared stresses and supports among 50 fathers whose partners had been diagnosed with postnatal depression and among 50 fathers whose partners had no such disorder. Fathers with depressed partners had significantly higher stress from work and economic pressures and significantly lower support from in-laws, other relatives, and friends than fathers without depressed partners.

Fathers may also be depressed irrespective of their partner's assessed mood. In a review of the published literature on fathers and depression over a 22-year span, Goodman (2004) found, in line with the evidence presented earlier, that the incidence of paternal depression ranged from 24 to 50% among those with depressed partners, while for community samples, the reported rates were 1.2–25.5%. More recently, a meta-analysis of 43 studies originating in 16 countries estimated the overall rate for paternal depression at 10.4% (95% CI, 8.5–12.7%) with higher rates during the 3- to 6-month postnatal period (25.6%; 95% CI, 17.3–36.1%) and the lowest rates (7.7%; 95% CI, 5.3–11.1%) occurring in the first 3 postpartum months (Paulson & Bazemore, 2010). In a 23-year longitudinal study from adolescence through young adulthood, Garfield et al. (2014) found that across the first 5 years of their child's life, depression symptom scores for fathers who lived with their children rose by an average of 68%.

A consistent finding of studies estimating the rates of depression among parents over the perinatal period is that rates for mothers are approximately twice that found for fathers. In the Paulson and Bazemore study cited earlier, for example, the overall rate for mothers was 23.8% (95% CI, 18.7–29.7%) with rates of 41.6% reported during the 3- to 6-month postpartum period. As scholarship on men's mental health has expanded however, it has been suggested that the divergent rates for men and women may be artifacts of the way that depression is conceived and measured (Cochran & Rabinowitz, 2003). The possibility that men's expression of depression differs from that of women's, by resorting to alcohol or by becoming aggressive, for example, has found support from researchers and clinicians. When depressed patients were asked to describe their most recent depressed episode, males reported more irritability and almost four times the number of anger attacks compared to females. The results were suggested as evidence for a "male depressive syndrome" (Winkler, Pjrek, & Kasper, 2005). Therapists treating men for depression have also argued, based on their clinical experience, for recognizing men's tendency to externalize their distress and provoke interpersonal conflict as "masculine-specific manifestations of depression" (Cochran & Rabinowitz, 2003).

Men also differ from women in that men are widely considered to be reluctant to access mental health and counseling services (Addis & Mahalik, 2003; McCarthy & Holliday, 2004) and those adhering to more traditional values of male identity are less likely to seek or accept psychological help (Berger, Levant, McMillan, Kelleher, & Sellers, 2005). However, males' reluctance to disclose their distress has not been shown to explain the gender difference in community depression rates. Weissman et al. (1997) reanalyzed data on depression from two large cross-national surveys—the National Comorbidity Survey ($N = 8000$) and the Epidemiologic Catchment Area Study ($N = 18,000$)—to remove from the counts of depressed individuals those who had "told the doctor or another health professional about the depressive episode." They found the female-to-male ratio of depression virtually unchanged and pointed to males' use of alcohol as a more likely factor influencing the masking of male depression.

The possibility of a male-specific type of depression suggests a need for both gender-sensitive screening tools and treatment options tailored to fathers. The general argument for gender-sensitive screening can be put as follows: if men either have different symptoms of depression or they express their emotions less openly compared to women, then depression assessment scales may need to include different items for men and women and possibly have gender-specific cutoff scores to identify, for example, "possible depression." Yet commonly used self-assessment scales, including those used for perinatal depression, usually have identical items for males and females. It should be noted that this argument also applies to the way that depression scales are validated, even if the scales have gender-specific items or gender-specific cut-off scores. When participants are interviewed to decide if their self-report score truly indicates depression, researchers utilize the DSM diagnostic criteria of five or more symptoms from the list of nine possible symptoms for depression (APA, 1994, 2013). These symptoms are the same for both men and women. Thus, there is no acknowledgement in this diagnostic system that the two genders may experience, or exhibit, depression differently.

One alternative instrument for assessing depression, based on the experience of researchers in Sweden, is the Gotland Male Depression Scale (GMDS) (Zierau, Bille, Rutz, & Bech, 2002). In this scale, standard depression indicators such as sleep, anxiety, and difficulty making decisions are included. However, changes in irritability and aggression, substance use, and overwork are also assessed. To address the possibility that men will fail to

Table 10.1   Comparison of EPDS and GMDS questionnaire items

Question focus in GMDS	Question focus in EPDS
1. Stress	1. Ability to laugh
2. Aggression	2. Enjoyment
3. Feelings of emptiness	3. Self-blame
4. Inexplicable tiredness	4. Anxiety
5. Irritability	5. Panic
6. Difficulty with everyday decisions	6. Feeling overwhelmed
7. Sleep problems	7. Sleep problems
8. Morning anxiety	8. Sadness
9. Alcohol use or hyperactivity	9. Tearfulness
10. Family history of depression	10. Self-harm
11. Others perceive you as difficult	
12. Others perceive you as gloomy	
13. Others perceive you as complaining	

recognize their behaviors as symptoms, questions also relate to other people's views as in "Have you or others noticed that you have a greater tendency to self-pity, to be complaining or to seem 'pathetic'?" (Zierau et al., 2002). Comparing the GMDS to the EPDS illustrates the different approaches to conceptualizing depression (Table 10.1).

In a study of Danish fathers completing both the GMDS and the EPDS 6 weeks post birth, 5.0% had depression symptom scores that resulted in a positive depression symptom screen using an EPDS cutoff ≥10 and 3.4% with GMDS cutoff ≥13. While 2.1% of the fathers had scores above the cutoff on both scales, 3.1% were identified only by the EPDS and 1.3% only with GMDS (Madsen & Juhl, 2007). Clearly, the widespread use of the GMDS would not lead to a large increase in the numbers of fathers with positive screening results for depression, and early results suggest it may be an equally valid measurement tool for depression in men.

Fathers' Anxiety

As with research into maternal perinatal mental health, there is an increasing recognition that depression is not the only important dimension of men's mental health. Matthey, Barnett, Kavanagh, and Howie (2001) have argued that equating depression with distressed mood is unnecessarily narrow and suggested the criteria for "caseness" be expanded to include anxiety alongside depression to better capture the experience of fathers. In their assessment of 356 first-time fathers at 6 weeks' postpartum (using the Diagnostic Interview Schedule), the inclusion of panic disorder and acute adjustment disorder with anxiety increased the rates of caseness by between 31 and 130%. As a result, the authors suggested the term "postnatal mood disorder" instead of "postnatal depression" to capture the significant adjustment difficulties experienced by men and women in the perinatal period, though this concept has subsequently been expanded to that of "postnatal distress" (e.g., Matthey & Ross-Hamid, 2012).

Support for this approach has come from a recent factor analysis of new parents' responses on the EPDS at three months postnatally from a population-based sample of 1014 couples (Massoudi, Hwang, & Wickberg, 2013). For fathers, the first factor, explaining 35.8% of the variance, included the self-blame item and the two anxiety items as well as three items assessing unhappiness. The second factor, including other depression items, explained only 7.4% of the variance. The authors conclude that among fathers the EPDS is a better measure of distress than depression (Massoudi et al., 2013). Thus, while much of the extant literature focuses on the serious health problem of depression, clearly, distress and anxiety are also issues for fathers and require attention (Matthey, Barnett, & Kavanagh, 2002).

Sad Dads: Influence on Children and Families

Effects on children

In the case of depression, it will be important to assess how a father's lowered affect or intrusive thoughts may impact on his children's development or his partner's well-being. In a study utilizing over 1000 new parents, Ramchandani and colleagues (2005) measured fathers' and mothers' symptoms of postnatal depression at 8 weeks' postpartum and then had teachers assess their children's emotional and behavioral development using validated instruments at 3 and a half years of age. Children of fathers who had scored 13 or more on the EPDS had twice the risk of behavioral and emotional problems compared to children from nondepressed fathers. This association remained after controlling for social class, degree of education, maternal depression, and fathers' later (21-month) depression. Analysis of data from an Australian cohort ($n = 2620$), using the Kessler Psychological Distress Scale (K6: Kessler et al., 2002) to indicate possible depression also found highly elevated behavior problems in preschool children whose fathers had shown signs of depression in the first year (Fletcher, Freeman, Garfield, & Vimpani, 2011). A meta-analysis of 21 studies examining the effect of paternal depression found a moderate effect size for the impact of paternal depression on children's internalizing and externalizing symptoms or diagnoses, similar to the effect size reported for maternal depression (Kane & Garber, 2004).

Some indications of how fathers' depression might impact on the development of infants are now emerging in the literature. In a nationally representative, longitudinal birth cohort study of US children, born from 1998 to 2000, and their parents, Davis, Davis, Freed, and Clark (2011) examined four fathering behaviors: three positive behaviors (playing games, singing songs, and reading) and one negative behavior (spanking). Of the 1746 fathers in the sample, 7% reported a major depressive episode in the previous year. These depressed fathers were only half as likely to read to their children but 4 times more likely to spank their 1-year-old as nondepressed dads.

Effects on partners

Fathers also influence children's development through their relationship with the child's mother. Marital conflict or relationship difficulty has been consistently linked to maternal postnatal depression (Burke, 2003; Cummings, Keller, & Davies, 2005; Gross, Wells, Radigan-Garcia, & Dietz, 2002) although causality may be bidirectional (Karney, 2001). Among new mothers, the degree of partner support has been identified as a key factor in the development of postnatal depression. Canadian researchers assessed the influence of mothers' perceptions of support from the partner on the development of depressive symptoms in the first 8 weeks' postpartum (Dennis & Ross, 2006). Mothers with depressive symptoms at 8 weeks had significantly lower partner support than nondepressed mothers. Two specific areas of support, "partner encouragement to obtain help when needed' and "partner agrees with how I am taking care of the baby" explained 10% of the variance in EPDS scores at 8 weeks' postpartum ($p < 0.001$).

Fathers' poor mental health can also add to the deleterious effects of mothers' depression to increase children's risk of emotional and behavioral disorder (Dierker, Merikangas, & Szatmari, 1999; Kahn, Brandt, & Whitaker, 2004). Conversely, fathers' support of mothers may reduce the development of depression (Morgan, Matthey, Barnett, & Richardson, 1997) or improve treatment outcomes for mothers with depression (Grube, 2005; Misri, Kostaras, Fox, & Kostaras, 2000). Fathers' positive involvement can also buffer the impact of poor maternal mental health on children's outcomes (Bifulco, Brown, Moran, Ball, & Campbell, 1998; Burke, 2003), particularly if fathers are involved in the care of their infant (Chang, Halpern, & Kaufman, 2007; Mezulis, Hyde, & Clark, 2004).

Screening Fathers for Depression and Anxiety

Given the widespread use of the EPDS for detecting probable depression among mothers, screening for paternal perinatal depression with the EPDS would seem to offer a starting point. However, as discussed earlier, the reliance on traditional depression questions in the EPDS may need to be addressed.

In order to incorporate gender awareness into the use of the EPDS, further research would be required to explore the validity of the scale in men, to establish suitable cutoff scores for detecting depression, and to understand male-specific reactions to particular items. In a validation study comparing the EPDS responses for 208 fathers and 230 mothers who were interviewed using the Diagnostic Interview Schedule (Robins, Helzer, Croughan, & Ratcliff, 1981), Matthey and colleagues (2001) found that fathers endorsed 7 of the 10 EPDS questions at lower rates than mothers, the largest difference being for the question on crying ("I have been so unhappy that I have been crying"). Matthey et al. (2001) suggested a cutoff score of 6 or more to detect depression or anxiety in new fathers—and that this cutoff score, and the optimal scores for major or minor depression were indeed different for the two genders.

It is also important to consider the debate surrounding the screening of mothers for depression, which is focused on the question of whether the benefits of screening outweigh the costs. The UK National Screening Committee, for example, have commissioned reviews of screening tools and found there to be insufficient evidence to justify universal screening for mothers using any instrument, including the EPDS (Hill, 2010). Nevertheless, they recommend using two questions developed by Spitzer et al. (1994): "During the past month, have you often been bothered by feeling down, depressed, or hopeless?" and "During the past month, have you often been bothered by little interest or pleasure in doing things?" If a parent (in the UK case, a mother) answers "yes" to either question, then a third question (Arroll, Goodyear-Smith, Kerse, Fishman, & Gunn, 2005), "Is this something you feel you need or want help with?," is recommended (National Institute for Clinical Excellence, 2007). In the United States, a similar two-question screener has been employed with mothers (Beck, Gable, Sakala, & Declercq, 2011) and in one study with fathers (Rosenthal, Learned, Liu, & Weitzman, 2013). However, these questions only inquire about symptoms related to depression and thus are not adequate for services wishing to broaden this to include anxiety or even stress. A generic mood question, developed by Matthey (see Chapter 6) which is being trialed with women and is planned to be trialed with men, may prove to be more useful than brief questions simply focusing on a single mood difficulty.

Acceptability and Engagement

The acceptability of any screening instrument to the fathers to be screened and the quality of the referral pathways for those identified as depressed or anxious/stressed are also crucial questions. For example, while the EPDS has been validated for fathers in populations including Chinese (Hong Kong) and Vietnamese (Lai, Tang, Lee, Yip, & Chung, 2010; Tran, Tran, & Fisher, 2012), no studies have evaluated the acceptability of the items in the EPDS to fathers.

While identifying what tools are useful in screening receives attention by researchers and clinicians, where to screen and how to make services available and insure uptake by fathers is an area where much work remains. Mothers historically have benefited from serial antenatal and postnatal health-care encounters wherein depression screenings have become part of the standard of care in many places; no corollary exists for fathers. While father-specific programs are being offered as part of antenatal care in some regions (Friedewald, Fletcher, & Fairbairn, 2005) and fathers in many countries regularly attend the birth, clearly fathers' contact with the health system in the perinatal period is minimal compared to that of mothers. Opportunities to engage with fathers in a primary health-care setting where their mental health could be assessed remain to be fully identified.

One avenue for connecting with fathers to assess their mental health and offer support or treatment is via the new communication technologies. With the increased use of the Internet for health- and parenting-related information and the rapid increase in mobile phone ownership, the possibility arises of developing screening and support processes which do not require the father to attend a clinic.

Innovations for Addressing Fathers with Perinatal Depression

Designing an effective perinatal service for fathers to address their mental health issues and maximize their positive contribution to family well-being will need to confront the stark differences between fathers' and mothers' access to perinatal health services. In a father-inclusive model (FIM) of perinatal mental health services, fathers would be enrolled in the existing schedule of health-care encounters as full partners with the mothers. They would be assessed for depression and anxiety and for psychosocial risk factors alongside the mother (although separately in reference to family violence). The FIM approach would require small but significant changes to the administrative arrangements, clinic protocols, and clinicians' skills. A hypothetical scenario is presented below.

The Father-Inclusive Model

When the mother rings to make an appointment for her visit to the antenatal clinic, the administration clerk (who has received father-inclusive model (FIM)-specific training) determines whether she has a partner and advises her that the clinic operates on a family-based care model and that she will receive a package in the mail explaining that the health and well-being of both parents is important to the baby's well-being. The administration clerk explains the main idea of father inclusion and the need to have an appointment time convenient for both mother and father. Possible barriers including work schedules, family separation, and intimate partner violence are discussed. The mother's wishes in regard to the father's presence at the clinic are accepted. The package mailed to the family is addressed to the mother. A letter and brochures included explain the rationale, based on research, for focusing on both mothers and fathers. In the material, situations where there may be no father available or where the mothers does not wish to have the father involved are acknowledged, but the policy position of the clinic to ensure fathers are included wherever possible, in the interests of the health of the mother and infant, is clearly stated. A separate letter addressed to the father (which the mother can choose not to hand on) explains the recent evidence linking a father's health and parenting to infant well-being and the importance of a father's support for the mother. When the couple arrive at the clinic, they are met by a clinician who has received FIM-specific training. The father is asked to complete a male-adapted depression and anxiety screening tool and asked relevant psychosocial questions. While the mother is assessed for depression and anxiety and for psychosocial vulnerability (including for family violence), the father is interviewed separately to evaluate his mental health and to identify any psychosocial needs. In the event of mother or father identifying significant need, they are seen separately by a mental health clinician (the fathers' clinician has received FIM-specific training) to review their responses and discuss any further action.

There are plusses and minuses in the FIM approach. Including the father in the processes of care for the mother reinforces the value of both parents' involvement with the care of young infants, a value which accords with gender-equity policies and with community beliefs supporting fathers' involvement in child rearing. This approach also finds support in recent research identifying coparenting as a key factor in infant well-being apart from dyadic, infant–parent factors (Teubert & Pinquart, 2010). The idea of including fathers as full partners in the birth process however will face the difficulty of engaging both parents while sensitively assessing the risk of intimate partner violence (Gartland, Hemphill, Hegarty, & Brown, 2011). In addition, the FIM approach requires that staff are competent to assess fathers' mental health and psychosocial needs and both parents must attend clinics.

Conclusions

Screening tools for detecting fathers' depression and anxiety are being trialed (Massoudi et al., 2013), and validation of further tools which assess broader areas of distress may be relevant. While an FIM approach requires evidence of successful implementation, elements of the approach have already been described in the literature. For example, psychosocial questions for fathers, modeled on those used for mothers, have been reported (Fletcher, Vimpani, Russell, & Sibbritt, 2008), and father-inclusive practices have been reported in several health and welfare services (Ferguson & Gates, 2013; May et al., 2013). Professionals' competencies in engaging fathers have been described (Fletcher, 2008; Fletcher, Freeman, Ross, & St George, 2013).

Considerable promise for addressing the issue of fathers' attendance at clinics or parenting programs may lie in the widespread adoption of mobile phones with Internet capability. New communication modes, including text, apps, and web-based programs, have the advantage of national coverage which can help to bridge urban–rural differences as well as the more general issues of access to care for lower socioeconomic status populations (Fox & Duggan, 2012). Web-based treatments for depression and anxiety are now accepted as effective (Andrews, Cuijpers, Craske, McEvoy, & Titov, 2010) and online therapy tailored for postnatal depression in mothers has been developed (Danaher et al., 2013). New fathers could be linked to mobile phone and Internet support to provide tailored assessment and treatment for both parents during the perinatal period. Training of staff in father-inclusive practice will be extremely important.

References

Addis, M. E., & Mahalik, J. R. (2003). Men, masculinity, and the contexts of help seeking. *American Psychologist*, *58*, 5–14.

American Psychiatric Association and American Psychiatric Association. Task Force on DSM-IV. (1994). *Diagnostic and statistical manual of mental disorders: DSM-IV*. Washington, DC: American Psychiatric Pub Inc.

American Psychiatric Association, and American Psychiatric Association. DSM-5 Task Force. (2013). *Diagnostic and statistical manual of mental disorders: DSM-5* (5th ed.). Washington, DC: American Psychiatric Association.

Andrews, G., Cuijpers, P., Craske, M. G., McEvoy, P., & Titov, N. (2010). Computer therapy for the anxiety and depressive disorders is effective, acceptable and practical health care: A meta-analysis. *PLoS One*, *5*, e13196. doi:10.1371/journal.pone.0013196.

Arroll, B., Goodyear-Smith, F., Kerse, N., Fishman, T., & Gunn, J. (2005). Effect of the addition of a "help" question to two screening questions on specificity for diagnosis of depression in general practice: Diagnostic validity study. *BMJ: British Medical Journal*, *331*(7521), 884.

Beck, C. T., Gable, R. K., Sakala, C., & Declercq, E. R. (2011). Posttraumatic stress disorder in new mothers: Results from a two-stage US National Survey. *Birth*, *38*(3), 216–227.

Berger, J. M., Levant, R., McMillan, K. K., Kelleher, W., & Sellers, A. (2005). Impact of gender role conflict, traditional masculinity ideology, alexithymia, and age on men's attitudes toward psychological help seeking. *Psychology of Men & Masculinity*, *6*, 73–78.

Bifulco, A., Brown, G. W., Moran, P., Ball, C., & Campbell, C. (1998). Predicting depression in women: The role of past and present vulnerability. *Psychological Medicine*, *28*, 39–50.

Buist, A. E. (2005). The BeyondBlue National Postnatal Depression Program. Prevention and early intervention 2001–2005 (Final Report). National Screening Program (Vol. 1). Melbourne, Australia: BeyondBlue.

Burke, L. (2003). The impact of maternal depression on familial relationships. *International Review of Psychiatry*, *15*, 243–255.

Chang, J. J., Halpern, C. T., & Kaufman, J. S. (2007). Maternal depressive symptoms, father's involvement, and the trajectories of child problem behaviors in a US national sample. *Archives of Pediatrics & Adolescent Medicine*, *161*, 697. doi:10.1001/archpedi.161.7.697.

Cochran, S. V., & Rabinowitz, F. E. (2003). Gender-sensitive recommendations for assessment and treatment of depression in men. *Professional Psychology: Research and Practice*, *34*, 132.

Cox, J. L., Holden, J. M., & Sagovsky, R. (1987). Detection of postnatal depression. Development of the 10-item Edinburgh Postnatal Depression Scale. *The British Journal of Psychiatry*, *150*(6), 782–786.

Cummings, M. E., Keller, P. S., & Davies, P. T. (2005). Towards a family process model of maternal and paternal depressive symptoms: Exploring multiple relations with child and family functioning. *Journal of Child Psychology and Psychiatry*, *46*, 479–489.

Danaher, B. G., Milgrom, J., Seeley, J. R., Stuart, S., Schembri, C., Tyler, M. S., … Kosty, D. B. (2013). MomMoodBooster web-based intervention for postpartum depression: Feasibility trial results. *Journal of Medical Internet Research, 15*, e242. doi:10.2196/jmir.2876.

Davis, R. N., Davis, M. M., Freed, G. L., & Clark, S. J. (2011). Fathers' depression related to positive and negative parenting behaviors with 1-year-old children. *Pediatrics, 127*(4), 612–618.

Deater-Deckard, K., Pickering, K., Dunn, J. F., & Golding, J. (1998). Family structure and depressive symptoms in men preceding and following the birth of a child. *American Journal of Psychiatry, 155*, 818–823.

Deloitte Access Economics. (2012). The cost of perinatal depression in Australia (Final report). Melbourne, Australia: Post and Antenatal Depression Association.

Dennis, C.-L., & Ross, L. (2006). Women's perceptions of partner support and conflict in the development of postpartum depressive symptoms. *Journal of Advanced Nursing, 56*, 588–599.

Dierker, L. C., Merikangas, K. R., & Szatmari, P. (1999). Influence of parental concordance for psychiatric disorders on psychopathology in offspring. *Journal of the American Academy of Child & Adolescent Psychiatry, 38*, 280–288. doi:10.1097/00004583-199903000-0001.

Ferguson, H., & Gates, P. (2013). Early intervention and holistic, relationship-based practice with fathers: Evidence from the work of the family nurse partnership. *Child & Family Social Work.* doi:10.1111/cfs.12059.

Fletcher, R. (2008). *Father-inclusive practice and associated professional competencies.* Melbourne, Australia: Australian Institute of Family Studies.

Fletcher, R. J., Freeman, E., Garfield, C., & Vimpani, G. (2011). The effects of early paternal depression on children's development. *Medical Journal of Australia, 195*, 685–689. doi:10.5694/mja11.10192.

Fletcher, R., Freeman, E., Ross, N., & St George, J. (2013). A quantitative analysis of practitioners' knowledge of fathers and fathers' engagement in family relationship services. *Australian Dispute Resolution Journal, 24*, 270–277.

Fletcher, R., Vimpani, G., Russell, G., & Sibbritt, D. (2008). Psychosocial assessment of expectant fathers. *Archives of Women's Mental Health, 11*, 27–32. doi:10.1007/s00737-008-0211-6.

Fox, S., & Duggan, M. (2012). Mobile health 2012. *Pew Internet and American Life Project, 8*. Retrieved from http://www.pewinternet.org/Reports/2012/Mobile-Health.aspx. Accessed December 17, 2014.

Friedewald, M., Fletcher, R., & Fairbairn, H. (2005). All-male discussion forums for expectant fathers: Evaluation of a model. *The Journal of Perinatal Education, 14*, 8. doi:10.1624/105812405X44673.

Garfield, C. F., Duncan, G., Rutsohn, J., McDade, T. W., Adam, E. K., Coley, R. L., & Chase-Lansdale, P. L. (2014). A longitudinal study of paternal mental health during transition to fatherhood as young adults. *Pediatrics, 133*(5), 836–843.

Gartland, D., Hemphill, S. A., Hegarty, K., & Brown, S. J. (2011). Intimate partner violence during pregnancy and the first year postpartum in an Australian Pregnancy Cohort Study. *Maternal and Child Health Journal, 15*, 570–578. doi:10.1007/s10995-010-0638-z.

Goodman, J. H. (2004). Paternal postpartum depression, its relationship to maternal postpartum depression, and implications for family health. *Journal of Advanced Nursing, 45*, 26–35.

Gross, K. H., Wells, C. S., Radigan-Garcia, A., & Dietz, P. M. (2002). Correlates of self-reports of being very depressed in the months after delivery: Results from the Pregnancy Risk Assessment Monitoring System. *Maternal and Child Health Journal, 6*, 247–253.

Grube, M. (2005). Inpatient treatment of women with postpartum psychiatric disorders: The role of the male partners. *Archives of Women's Mental Health, 8*, 163–170. doi:10.1007/s00737-005-0087-7.

Hanington, L., Heron, J., Stein, A., & Ramchandani, P. (2012). Parental depression and child outcomes: Is marital conflict the missing link?. *Child: Care, Health and Development, 38*, 520–529.

Harvey, I., & McGrath, G. (1988). Psychiatric morbidity in spouses of women admitted to a mother and baby unit. *The British Journal of Psychiatry, 152*, 506–510.

Hill, C. (2010). *An Evaluation of Screening for Postnatal Depression against NSC Criteria.* London, England: UK National Screening Committee.

Kahn, R. S., Brandt, D., & Whitaker, R. C. (2004). Combined effect of mothers' and fathers' mental health symptoms on children's behavioral and emotional well-being. *Archives of Pediatrics & Adolescent Medicine, 158*, 721. doi:10.1001/archpedi.158.8.721.

Kane, P., & Garber, J. (2004). The relations among depression in fathers, children's psychopathology, and father–child conflict: A meta-analysis. *Clinical Psychology Review, 24,* 339–360. doi:10.1016/j.cpr.2004.03.004.

Karney, B. R. (2001). Depressive symptoms and marital satisfaction in the early years of marriage: Narrowing the gap between theory and research. In S. R. H. Beach (Ed.), *Marital and family processes in depression: A Scientific Foundation for Clinical Practice* (pp. 45–68). Washington, DC: American Psychological Association. doi:10.1037/10350-003.

Kessler, R. C., Andrews, G., Colpe, L. J., Hiripi, E., Mroczek, D. K., Normand, S. L., … Zaslavsky, A. M. (2002). Short screening scales to monitor population prevalences and trends in non-specific psychological distress. *Psychological Medicine, 32*(06), 959–976.

Lai, B. P. Y., Tang, A. K. L., Lee, D. T. S., Yip, A. S. K., & Chung, T. K. H. (2010). Detecting postnatal depression in Chinese men: A comparison of three instruments. *Psychiatry Research, 180*(2–3), 80–85. doi:10.1016/j.psychres.2009.07.015.

Lovestone, S., & Kumar, R. (1993). Postnatal psychiatric illness: The impact on partners. *The British Journal of Psychiatry, 163,* 210–216. doi:10.1192/bjp.163.2.210.

Madsen, S. A., & Juhl, T. (2007). Paternal depression in the postnatal period. *Journal of Men's Health & Gender, 4*(1), 26–31.

Massoudi, P., Hwang, C. P., & Wickberg, B. (2013). How well does the Edinburgh Postnatal Depression Scale identify depression and anxiety in fathers? A validation study in a population based Swedish sample. *Journal of Affective Disorders, 149*(1), 67–74.

Matthey, S., Barnett, B., Howie, P., & Kavanagh, D. J. (2002). Diagnosing postpartum depression in mothers and fathers: Whatever happened to anxiety? *Journal of Affective Disorders, 74,* 139–147.

Matthey, S., Barnett, B., Kavanagh, D. J., & Howie, P. (2001). Validation of the Edinburgh Postnatal Depression scale for men, and comparison of item endorsement with their partners. *Journal of Affective Disorders, 64,* 175–184.

Matthey, S., & Ross-Hamid, C. (2012). Repeat testing on the Edinburgh Depression Scale and the HADS-A in pregnancy: Differentiating between transient and enduring distress. *Journal of Affective Disorders, 141,* 213–221. doi:10.1016/j.jad.2012.02.037.

May, F. S., Mclean, L. A., Anderson, A., Hudson, A., Cameron, C., & Matthews, J. (2013). Father participation with mothers in the signposts program: An initial investigation. *Journal of Intellectual and Developmental Disability, 38,* 39–47. doi:10.3109/13668250.2012.748184.

McCarthy, J., & Holliday, E. L. (2004). Help-seeking and counseling within a traditional male gender role: An examination from a multicultural perspective. *Journal of Counseling & Development, 82,* 25–30.

Mezulis, A. H., Hyde, J. S., & Clark, R. (2004). Father involvement moderates the effect of maternal depression during a child's infancy on child behavior problems in kindergarten. *Journal of Family Psychology, 18,* 575. doi:10.1037/0893-3200.18.4.575.

Misri, S., Kostaras, X., Fox, D., & Kostaras, D. (2000). The impact of partner support in the treatment of postpartum depression. *The Canadian Journal of Psychiatry/La Revue canadienne de psychiatrie, 45*(6), 554–558.

Morgan, M., Matthey, S., Barnett, B., & Richardson, C. (1997). A group programme for postnatally distressed women and their partners. *Journal of Advanced Nursing, 26,* 913–920.

National Institute for Clinical Excellence [NICE]. (2007). *Antenatal and postnatal mental health: Clinical management and service guidance guidelines* (NICE Clinical Guideline 45). London, England: National Institute for Health and Clinical Excellence.

Paulson, J. F., & Bazemore, S. D. (2010). Prenatal and postpartum depression in fathers and its association with maternal depression. *JAMA: The Journal of the American Medical Association, 303,* 1961–1969. doi:10.1001/jama.2010.605.

Ramchandani, P., Stein, A., Evans, J., & O'Connor, T. G. (2005). Paternal depression in the postnatal period and child development: A prospective population study. *The Lancet, 365,* 2201–2205. doi:10.1016/S0140-6736(05)66778-5.

Robins, L. N., Helzer, J. E., Croughan, J., Ratcliff, K. S. (1981). National Institute of Mental Health Diagnostic Interview Schedule: Its history, characteristics and validity. *Archives of General Psychiatry, 38,* 381–389.

Rosenthal, D. G., Learned, N., Liu, Y.-H., & Weitzman, M. (2013). Characteristics of mothers with depressive symptoms outside the postpartum period. *Maternal and Child Health Journal, 17,* 1030–1037. doi:10.1007/s10995-012-1084-x.

Spitzer, R. L., Williams, J. B. W., Kroenke, K., Linzer, M., deGruy, F. V., Hahn, S. R., … Johnson, J. G. (1994). Utility of a new procedure for diagnosing mental disorders in primary care: The PRIME-MD 1000 study. *JAMA, 272*(22), 1749–1756.

Teubert, D., & Pinquart, M. (2010). The association between coparenting and child adjustment: A meta-analysis. *Parenting: Science and Practice, 10,* 286–307. doi:10.1080/15295192.2010.492040.

Tran, T. D., Tran, T., & Fisher, J. (2012). Validation of three psychometric instruments for screening for perinatal common mental disorders in men in the north of Vietnam. *Journal of Affective Disorders, 136,* 104–109. doi:10.1016/j.jad.2011.08.012.

Weissman, M. M., Greenwald, S., Wickramaratne, P., Bland, R. C., Newman, S. C., Canino, G. J., … Wells, J. E. (1997). What happens to depressed men? Application of the Stirling County criteria. *Harvard Review of Psychiatry, 5,* 1–6.

Winkler, D., Pjrek, E., & Kasper, S. (2005). Anger attacks in depression: Evidence for a male depressive syndrome. *Psychotherapy and Psychosomatics, 74,* 303–307. doi:10.1159/000086321.

Zelkowitz, P., & Milet, T. H. (1997). Stress and support as related to postpartum paternal mental health and perceptions of the infant. *Infant Mental Health Journal, 18,* 424–435.

Zierau, F., Bille, A., Rutz, W., & Bech, P. (2002). The Gotland male depression scale: A validity study in patients with alcohol use disorder. *Nordic Journal of Psychiatry, 56,* 265–271. doi:10.1080/08039480260242750.

11

Evidence-Based Treatments and Pathways to Care

Michael W. O'Hara, Cindy-Lee Dennis, Jennifer E. McCabe, and Megan Galbally

Over the past three decades, there has been an exponential rise in reports of clinical trials evaluating psychological and pharmacological treatments for perinatal depression. These trials have been conducted in a variety of health-care settings and university-based centers, mainly in developed countries but increasingly in developing countries around the world (e.g., Rahman et al., 2013; Sockol, Epperson, & Barber, 2011). Depending upon the nature of a country's health-care system, pathways to care vary considerably, ranging from complete integration with maternity care to a referral-based system that relies on community practitioners specializing in perinatal mental health to provide care. Unfortunately, in many developing countries, there are few resources to provide any perinatal mental health care. Mental health care is a multidisciplinary undertaking. Effective care can be provided by psychiatrists, psychologists, social workers, advanced practice nurses, counselors, and increasingly by nonmental health professionals who are trained in basic counseling skills to deliver brief interventions to mildly to moderately depressed perinatal women (e.g., Cooper et al., 2009; O'Hara, Stuart, Gorman, & Wenzel, 2000; Segre, Stasik, O'Hara, & Arndt, 2010). In addition to more established interventions, women are increasingly turning to complementary and alternative medicine (CAM), which is delivered by mental health and nonmental health providers (Deligiannidis & Freeman, 2014). As well, there are many self-help organizations around the world that provide support to struggling pregnant and postpartum women, sometimes as a complement to professional care and sometimes as the sole provider of support. The variety of settings and providers and the complex relation between perinatal health care and mental health care serve as the context for this brief review that will assess the current state of the literature regarding psychological, pharmacological, and complementary treatments and effective pathways to care.

Identifying Perinatal Depression and Anxiety: Evidence-Based Practice in Screening, Psychosocial Assessment, and Management, First Edition. Edited by Jeannette Milgrom and Alan W. Gemmill.
© 2015 John Wiley & Sons, Ltd. Published 2015 by John Wiley & Sons, Ltd.

Psychological Interventions

Postnatal depression

Numerous psychosocial and psychological treatment options have been evaluated as interventions for postnatal depression, including nondirective counseling, professional and lay home visits, telephone-based peer support, cognitive behavioral therapy (CBT), and interpersonal psychotherapy (IPT). Several quantitative reviews in recent years have documented the efficacy of these psychological treatments for postnatal depression (Cuijpers, Brännmark, & van Straten, 2008; Dennis & Hodnett, 2007; Sockol, Epperson, & Barber, 2011). The effect size estimates that these reviews have yielded are "medium," similar to the results obtained in the general depression treatment literature (Cuijpers, Brannmark, & van Straten, 2008). In some distinction to treatment trials with general depression, these studies often use "cutoff" scores on self-report measures such as the Edinburgh Postnatal Depression Scale as an entry criterion. As a consequence, many of the women in these trials may not have been suffering from a depressive disorder. Another limitation of this research is that studies have been underpowered to detect predicted treatment effects (O'Hara & McCabe, 2013). Finally, Cuijpers et al. (2008) noted the lack of long-term follow-up.

Despite the limitations in this area of research, there are a select few randomized controlled trials (RCTs) that include large samples of perinatal women with diagnosed major depression and follow-up outcome data. For example, two such RCTs found evidence in support of CBT-based interventions compared to routine primary care in the treatment of postnatal depression (Cooper, Murray, Wilson, & Romaniuk, 2003; Milgrom, Negri, Gemmill, McNeil, & Martin, 2005). Both of these RCTs included other treatment conditions. Cooper et al. included psychodynamic therapy, nondirective counseling, and CBT counseling. Milgrom et al. included group counseling, individual counseling, and CBT-based group therapy. Interestingly, both studies found a significant effect for treatment versus routine care, but no differences among the various interventions at posttreatment or follow-up. Another of these RCTs examined the use of IPT for the treatment of postnatal depression (O'Hara et al., 2000). In this trial, women diagnosed with postnatal depression who were randomized to the IPT condition demonstrated higher rates of recovery and decreased symptoms of depression compared to the waitlist control condition. Furthermore, the proportion of time these women spent in a major depressive episode following treatment continued to decline across an 18-month follow-up period (Nylen et al., 2010).

Antenatal depression

Due to maternal treatment preferences related to potential concerns about fetal and infant health outcomes, there is a need for diverse nonpharmacological treatment options. Interestingly, very few trials have targeted the treatment of antenatal depression. IPT has been validated for the treatment of antenatal depression in two trials undertaken by Spinelli and colleagues (Spinelli & Endicott, 2003; Spinelli et al., 2013). The more recent study was a large controlled study comparing 12 sessions of IPT and a parenting education group. The interventions were conducted in English and Spanish at three different settings in New York City. Both conditions resulted in significant improvement in depressive symptoms, but there were no differences in efficacy. Other recent trials have evaluated a culturally relevant brief IPT (Grote et al., 2009) and CBT (Burns et al., 2013; McGregor, Coghlan, & Dennis, 2013;

O'Mahen, Himle, Fedock, Henshaw, & Flynn, 2013; Milgrom, Gemmill, Ericksen et al., in Press) for antenatal depression. The results of these studies were encouraging, but clearly, this is an area that warrants additional research.

Perinatal anxiety

Significantly less research has been conducted related to the prevention and treatment of perinatal anxiety. Two trials have evaluated group CBT with pregnant women. One trial recruited women with subclinically elevated stress and anxiety levels (Richter et al., 2012), while the other trial recruited women with mild to moderate symptoms in pregnancy and/ or at risk of developing depression or anxiety in the perinatal period (Austin et al., 2008). The effects were modest in the former trial and nonexistent in the latter trial. An antenatal intervention that included a self-guided workbook with weekly telephone support was evaluated with the intent to reduce postnatal depression, anxiety, and parenting difficulties and resulted in fewer cases of above the threshold for mild to moderate depression/anxiety symptoms (Milgrom, Schembri, Ericksen, Ross, & Gemmill, 2011).

A Cochrane review has evaluated mind–body interventions during pregnancy for preventing or treating anxiety (Marc et al., 2011). The review included eight trials (556 women) evaluating hypnotherapy (one trial), imagery (five trials), autogenic training (one trial), and yoga (one trial). The review found limited evidence for the effectiveness of mind–body interventions for the management of anxiety during pregnancy. The effects of acute relaxation (Bastani, Hidarnia, Kazemnejad, Vafaei, & Kashanian, 2005; Teixeira, Martin, Prendiville, & Glover, 2005) and music therapy (Chang, Chen, & Huang, 2008) on indices of anxiety during pregnancy also have been examined. These individual trials do not provide strong evidence for the prevention and treatment of anxiety across the perinatal period. Given the growing suggestion that prenatal exposure to maternal stress/ anxiety can have lasting effects on infant development with risk of psychopathology (Monk, Spicer, & Champagne, 2012), this is an important area of focus which warrants further investigation.

Prevention of Postnatal Depression

Results of recent meta-analysis

The majority of research on the prevention of common perinatal mental disorders has focused on depression in the postnatal period. A recently updated Cochrane systematic review (Dennis & Dowswell, 2013) suggests that preventing postnatal depression is an important public health approach that holds much promise. The objective of this review was to assess the preventive effect of diverse psychosocial and psychological interventions. Twenty-eight RCTs of acceptable quality were included in the review. These trials included ones that began in pregnancy or early in the postnatal period. Some of them targeted low- and high-risk women and others were limited to high-risk women. Overall, women who received a psychosocial or psychological intervention were significantly less likely to develop postnatal depression compared with those receiving standard care (relative risk (RR) 0.78, 95% confidence interval (CI) 0.66–0.93).

Effective approaches

Several promising interventions identified in the Dennis and Dowswell review included (i) the provision of intensive, individualized postnatal home visits provided by public health nurses (Armstrong, Fraser, Dadds, & Morris, 1999) or midwives (MacArthur et al., 2002) (RR 0.56, 95% CI 0.43–0.73), (ii) lay (peer)-based postnatal telephone support (Dennis et al., 2009) (RR 0.54, 95% CI 0.38–0.77), and (iii) IPT (Zlotnick, Miller, Pearlstein, Howard, & Sweeney, 2006) (standardized mean difference −0.27, 95% CI −0.52 to −0.01). There was no clear evidence to recommend that the following interventions be implemented into practice in order to prevent postnatal depression: antenatal classes and postnatal classes, early postnatal follow-up, continuity of care models, and in-hospital psychological debriefing. Although these interventions may be beneficial for other maternal outcomes, at this time there is no evidence that they may prevent postnatal depression. The effectiveness of postnatal lay-based home visits (Morrell, Spiby, Stewart, Walters, & Morgan, 2000) and CBT (Le, Perry, & Stuart, 2011) remains uncertain.

Moderator analyses

The Cochrane review also found professional- and lay-based interventions were both effective in reducing the risk to develop postnatal depression. Individually based interventions were beneficial at final assessment (RR 0.75, 95% CI 0.61–0.92) as were multiple-contact interventions (RR 0.78, 95% CI 0.66–0.93). Prevention trials can be further classified into different categories depending on the target population: universal interventions are designed to be offered to all women, selective interventions are designed to be offered to women at increased risk of developing depression, and indicated interventions are designed to be offered to women who have been identified as depressed or probably depressed (Mrazek & Haggerty, 1994). Although no trial that evaluated an indicated intervention was included in the Cochrane review, to examine the effects of universal and selective interventions, subgroup analyses were conducted. The results suggested identifying mothers "at risk" may assist in the prevention of postnatal depression (RR 0.66, 95% CI 0.50–0.88). However, currently, there is no consistency in the identification of women "at risk," and there is no measure with acceptable predictive validity to accurately identify asymptomatic women who will later develop postnatal depression (Austin & Lumley, 2003). This may partially explain why interventions initiated postnatally rather than antenatally had a more beneficial effect (RR 0.73, 95% CI 0.59–0.90).

Depression treatment during pregnancy as a prevention strategy

Treating depression in pregnancy may also be an important postnatal depression prevention strategy. A review of antenatal interventions for high-risk women found interventions were most likely to be effective when (a) delivered to women who were depressed during pregnancy, (b) incorporated evidence-based psychological treatments, and (c) address interpersonal difficulties (Clatworthy, 2012).

Other approaches to prevention   Aside from psychosocial and psychological approaches, enhanced education, sleep strategies, and exercise have also been evaluated for the prevention of postnatal depression (Dennis & Dowswell, 2013). While the preventive effects of educational strategies appear equivocal, there is some evidence to suggest an association between maternal mood and physical exercise (Nascimento, Surita, & Cecatti, 2012; Norman, Sherburn, Osborne, & Galea, 2010). An RCT of insomnia treatment during pregnancy demonstrated that treatment with trazodone and diphenhydramine during the third trimester resulted in lower depressive symptoms at 2 and 6 weeks postpartum compared to a control group (Khazaie, Ghadami, Knight, Emamian, & Tahmasian, 2013). There is little support for the use of estrogens and progestins for preventing postnatal depression (Dennis, Ross, & Herxheimer, 2008).

Pharmacological Treatment

Mental illness has been a leading indirect cause of maternal mortality in Australia, the United Kingdom, and elsewhere; hence, adequate treatment to ensure a resolution of symptoms, particularly suicidal ideation, is essential (Austin, Kildea, & Sullivan, 2007; Oates, 2003). Within general adult mental health, antidepressants have been found to be effective in the treatment of more severe depressive disorders (Fournier et al., 2010). The current recommendation regarding any decision to start, continue, or cease antidepressant treatment in pregnancy is an individual one, given there are clear documented risks and benefits inherent in each of these choices (Galbally, Snellen, & Lewis, 2011). As a result, several countries, including the United States, the United Kingdom, and Australia, have developed national guidelines to assist clinicians, women, and their families with this process. All three guidelines agree that antidepressants may be a warranted treatment option for some women with depression in pregnancy and the postpartum period.

Pregnancy

There have been no controlled trials of antidepressant medication use in pregnant women despite the fact that antidepressants are commonly prescribed for these women. The major barrier to research in this area has been reluctance on the part of investigators, institutional review boards, drug companies, and governments to undertake studies that would deliberately expose pregnant women to drugs that might cause harm to the fetus/child. As a consequence, almost all reports on the efficacy of antidepressant medications come from case reports or case series. These observational studies are quite valuable in providing some guidance to the clinician but do not provide definitive findings in the same way as RCTs. At the present time, the official policy of the American Psychiatric Association and the American College of Obstetricians and Gynecologists is that clinicians should collaborate with patients and make decisions regarding medication use based on the woman's clinical state, past history, and her treatment preferences (Yonkers et al., 2009). Given the documented deleterious effects of untreated major depression and the risks of relapse among women who stop taking antidepressant medication during pregnancy, refraining from treatment altogether is unwise and may lead to adverse outcomes for the mother and fetus.

Despite the obvious need to treat antenatal depression, there is a very large literature emerging on the potential teratogenic effects of antidepressant medication on the developing fetus and the child after delivery (Galbally, Lewis, & Buist, 2011; Galbally, Snellen et al., 2011). The effects include structural teratogenicity (malformations), pregnancy complications (such as miscarriage, gestational diabetes, pregnancy outcomes of gestation at delivery), neonatal complications (such as persistent pulmonary hypertension of the newborn, neonatal abstinence syndrome), and neurodevelopmental teratogenicity and outcomes for offspring. Antidepressant medications have been linked to all of these types of adverse outcomes in some studies but not in others. Overall, there is still a lack of consensus regarding specific links between most types of antidepressants and adverse neonatal outcomes.

Postpartum

In contrast to the case for pregnancy, there have been several controlled trials of antidepressant medication with postnatally depressed women, although in almost all cases study subjects were not breastfeeding. Outcomes reported in open trials have largely been positive (e.g., Cohen et al., 2001; Pearlstein et al., 2006). Findings from controlled trials have not been as consistent. An early trial found that fluoxetine outperformed placebo in a double-blind controlled trial (Appleby, Warner, Whitton, & Faragher, 1997). In another double-blind clinical trial, there were no differences in clinical response among women treated with sertraline (56% response rate) or nortriptyline (69% response rate), but both groups showed a good clinical response (Wisner et al., 2006). A more recent placebo-controlled trial evaluated paroxetine and found mixed evidence for its efficacy (Yonkers, Lin, Howell, Heath, & Cohen, 2008). There were no differences between groups on clinical and self-report measures of depression; however, the Clinical Global Improvement Severity of Illness Scale did show a significant effect in favor of the paroxetine condition. A significant limitation of this study was the very high attrition rate in both groups (paroxetine = 51%; placebo = 60%). Finally, two add-on treatment trials have been conducted, one in which CBT was added to paroxetine (randomized but not placebo controlled) and one in which sertraline (placebo controlled) was added to brief dynamic psychotherapy (Bloch et al., 2012; Misri, Reebye, Corral, & Mills, 2004); however, in neither case did the added treatment (either medicine or psychotherapy) add benefit to the base treatment.

   At the present time, there is little evidence from randomized trials that antidepressant medication outperforms placebo or psychotherapy (Milgrom, Gemmill, Ericksen, Burrows, Buist, & Reece, 2015). Nevertheless, it is likely that the positive effects observed for antidepressant medication in trials including depressed nonpostnatal women would be observed in depressed postnatal women. Antidepressant medication use with depressed breastfeeding women is generally viewed as a reasonable treatment option and widely used (Davanzo, Copertino, De Cunto, Minen, & Amaddeo, 2011; di Scalea & Wisner, 2009) despite the lack of definitive studies on short- and long-term effects of antidepressant medication exposure in infants.

CAM

Despite empirical support for the efficacy of psychosocial treatments for perinatal depression and the widespread use of pharmacological treatments, pregnant and postnatal women demonstrate low rates of help-seeking and treatment engagement (Kim et al., 2010; Liberto, 2012; Whitton, Warner, & Appleby, 1996). Low rates of treatment utilization by perinatal women are due to a variety of barriers including stigma associated with mental health, costs of treatment, and the perceived risks of antidepressant use while pregnant or breastfeeding (Bilszta, Ericksen, Buist, & Milgrom, 2010; Goodman, 2009; Kim et al., 2010).

CAM therapy provides a treatment alternative for perinatal women who do not prefer traditional psychosocial or pharmacological treatment options.

CAM therapy refers to treatments that are not standard practice in Western medicine. Studies suggest that the use of CAM therapy is high among both pregnant women and women with depression in general (Frawley et al., 2013; Wu et al., 2007), making CAM therapy for perinatal depression an important area of research. There is a growing evidence base for the treatment of depression with CAM therapy in the general population (Qureshi & Al-Bedah, 2013), and much of this work has carried over into the study of perinatal women. In particular, RCTs of bright light therapy, omega-3 fatty acid supplements, exercise, and massage have been conducted in perinatal populations.

Limited evidence suggests that bright light therapy may be an effective treatment option for antenatal depression. Bright light therapy involves exposure to a light source of a specified intensity (e.g., 7000 lux) for a limited period of time (e.g., 60 min). At least two RCTs of bright light therapy for antenatal depression have been published, providing evidence for effective treatment of depression during pregnancy (Epperson et al., 2004; Wirz-Justice et al., 2011). In contrast, the only RCT of this modality that included a postnatal sample of depressed women did not find significant differences in depression between the treatment and control group following bright light therapy (Corral, Wardrop, Zhang, Grewal, & Patton, 2007). Thus, it seems that there are preliminary evidence for bright light therapy as a treatment for antenatal depression and no empirical support for bright light therapy in the treatment of postnatal depression.

Regardless of a woman's depression status, omega-3 fatty acid supplements are recommended for pregnant and postnatal women because of their established health benefits (Dunstand, Simmer, Dixon, & Prescott, 2008; McGregor et al., 2001). A number of studies have examined omega-3 fatty acid supplements as a prevention or treatment for both antenatal and postnatal depressions. Findings in this area have demonstrated inconsistent results, with most RCTs of omega-3 fatty acid for perinatal depression not finding a significant effect (Doornbos et al., 2009; Freeman et al., 2008; Makrides et al., 2010; Rees, Austin, & Parker, 2008) and at least one small trial ($N = 24$) demonstrating a significant benefit of the supplement (Su et al., 2008).

Exercise as a CAM therapy for depression in the general population has received significant support (Brosse, Sheets, Lett, & Blumenthal, 2002), making it a promising treatment option to test in perinatal women. Further, the American College of Obstetricians and Gynecologists (ACOG) recommend that in the absence of medical or obstetric complications, pregnant women engage in 30 min of moderate physical activity per day (ACOG, 2002). Despite these recommendations and the empirical support for exercise as a treatment for depression in the general population, few RCTs of exercise for perinatal women have been conducted. With regard to pregnant women, no RCT has examined the efficacy of exercise for the treatment of depression. In contrast, there is limited empirical support for exercise as a treatment of postnatal depression (Armstrong & Edwards, 2003; Heh, Huang, Ho, Fu, & Wang, 2008). For example, Armstrong and Edwards (2004) randomized 19 women with postnatal depression to 12 weeks of either a pram walking intervention or a social support group. Women in the pram walking condition demonstrated a significantly higher reduction in depression symptoms than women in the social support group (Armstrong & Edwards, 2004). In combination with its general health benefits, this limited empirical support makes exercise a reasonable consideration for women experiencing depression symptoms in the postnatal period. Future work is needed to examine the efficacy of exercise for treating antenatal depression.

Another promising CAM therapy candidate for treating perinatal depression is massage. Massage has shown to be effective in decreasing depression symptoms in the general population (Hou, Chiang, Hsu, Chiu, & Yen, 2010), and these findings appear to generalize to perinatal samples as well. Tiffany Field and her colleagues have conducted a number of RCTs that have provided support for the positive effects of massage on women with perinatal depression, including lower levels of prenatal depression, lower levels of postnatal depression, lower rates of premature birth, and higher infant scores on the Brazelton Neonatal Behavioral Assessment Scales (e.g., Field, Diego, Hernandez-Reif, Deeds, & Figueiredo, 2009; Field, Diego, Hernandez-Reif, Schanberg, & Kuhn, 2004; Field et al., 2008).

Although results from RCTs are promising, studies of CAM therapy for perinatal depression are limited by small sample sizes, few RCTs, and lack of long-term follow-up. In addition to future studies that utilize a more rigorous methodology, the area of research may benefit from testing additional CAM therapies for both depression and anxiety in pregnant and postnatal women. For example, Field and colleagues have demonstrated that a yoga intervention during pregnancy is effective in decreasing prenatal depression and anxiety symptoms (Field et al., 2012). Increased research regarding CAM therapy for perinatal depression and anxiety is critical to increase options for perinatal women and, ultimately, increase treatment seeking and utilization among pregnant and postnatal women.

Pathways to Care

Collaborative care

To address the gap between the existence of effective perinatal mental health interventions and the uptake of these interventions, new treatment approaches are needed. "Collaborative care" is an approach to treatment that is highly effective for the management of depression in primary care settings (Archer et al., 2012). In a collaborative care model, case identification occurs at the primary care level, and a depression care manager works in collaboration with a mental health specialist to direct individuals to appropriate treatment and monitors progress. Part of the success of this approach is that it actively promotes treatment initiation and adherence while addressing patient preferences and perceived barriers. Several studies have reported on the implementation of programs that incorporate components of collaborative care for postnatal depression (Davies, Howells, & Jenkins, 2003; Gjerdingen, Crow, McGovern, Miner, & Center, 2009; Honikman, van Heyningen, Field, Baron, & Tomlinson, 2012; Kuosmanen, Vuorilehto, Kumpuniemi, & Melartin, 2010; Logsdon, Foltz, Stein, Usui, & Josephson, 2010). Although most of these programs have not been rigorously evaluated, they do provide evidence for acceptability and feasibility of the collaborative care approach adapted for this population. In the largest trial, 28 primary care practices in the United States were randomized to usual care ($n=14$) or intervention ($n=14$) (Yawn et al., 2012). The intervention sites received education and tools for postnatal depression screening, diagnosis, initiation of therapy, and follow-up within their practices. Usual-care practices received a 30-min presentation about postnatal depression. Of 1897 women who provided outcome information, 654 (34.5%) women had elevated screening scores indicative of depression, with comparable rates in the intervention and usual-care groups. Among the 654 women with elevated postnatal depression screening scores, those in the intervention practices were more likely to receive treatment for postnatal depression, and they had lower depressive symptom levels at 6 and 12 months postpartum. The results from this trial suggest primary care-based screening, diagnosis, and management may significantly improve maternal depression outcomes at 12 months. This is an important area of research that requires further investigation.

Home visiting and nontraditional providers

High-income countries Given the low rates of treatment utilization by women with perinatal depression (e.g., Watt, Sword, Krueger, & Sheehan, 2002), one critical question pertains to how the various perinatal treatment recommendations can be carried out. In other words, once perinatal depression has been detected, what programs are in place to provide women treatment? A number of efficacious treatments for perinatal depression have been carried out by practitioners with advanced degrees, such as psychologists and psychiatrists, who provide individual psychotherapy (e.g., IPT, CBT) or pharmacotherapy (Sockol, Epperson, & Barber, 2011). However, a growing body of research has demonstrated that there are other avenues through which perinatal depression and anxiety may be addressed, including home visitors and peer support models of care.

One of the most widely explored pathways of care for the treatment of perinatal depression and anxiety is the use of home visitors (nurses and nonnurses). Having a health visitor provide services in the home of a pregnant or postnatal woman circumvents a number of previously recognized barriers to care (e.g., childcare, stigma; Dennis & Chung-Lee, 2006; Goodman, 2009). In the United Kingdom, health visitors are in place to provide families support from pregnancy through early childhood. Health visitors provide perinatal women services within the home, including screening and treatment of depression. The National Institute for Health and Care Excellence (NICE) guidelines recommend Listening Visits, a nondirective form of counseling, as a treatment option for women with mild to moderate depression during the perinatal period (National Institute for Health and Care Excellence, 2007). Listening Visits were designed to be a depression intervention administered by health visitors with little or no prior training in mental health. There are a number of studies that have supported the efficacy of Listening Visits and other nurse-delivered counseling for the short-term improvement of postnatal depression (Cooper, Murray, Wilson, & Romaniuk, 2003; Holden, Sagovsky, & Cox, 1989; Milgrom, Holt et al., 2011; Morrell et al., 2009).

Similar to the health visitor program in the United Kingdom, a program called Healthy Start exists in the United States to prevent poor outcomes for infants of low-income families. As with the UK health visitors, Healthy Start case managers (who are not usually nurses) provide care services that include screening and referral for maternal depression. In addition to screening and treatment referral, Healthy Start case managers are in the ideal position to provide counseling for mildly to moderately depressed women. Preliminary evidence has suggested that Listening Visits may also be effective in the context of Healthy Start case management (Segre, Stasik, O'Hara, & Arndt, 2010).

Peer support models of care are another way in which perinatal depression and anxiety may be treated. There has been support for a telephone-based intervention provided by women who have previously experienced postnatal depression (Dennis, 2003) and for a weekly social support group in decreasing depression symptoms (Chen, Tseng, Chou, & Wang, 2000). In contrast, other studies have not found support for weekly social support groups (Fleming, Klein, & Corter, 1992) or home visits from women who previously experienced postnatal depression (Letourneau et al., 2011). Presently, findings in the literature are equivocal as to whether a peer support model of care may be effective in improving maternal depressive symptoms.

Low- and middle-income countries A recent systematic review assessed the effectiveness of interventions to improve the mental health of women in the perinatal period in low- and middle-income (LAMI) countries (Rahman et al., 2013). In all but one of the 13 studies, nonspecialist health and community workers (who were supervised) delivered the interventions, which proved more beneficial than routine care. The pooled effect size for maternal depression was −0.38 (95% CI −0.56 to −0.21).

To make depression interventions more accessible to perinatal women, researchers have focused their efforts on developing and testing interventions delivered by nonprofessionals (i.e., lay community workers or peer volunteers). In their RCT (*N* = 449), Cooper et al. (2009) demonstrated significant improvements in maternal mental health and mother–child interactions following an intervention conducted by lay community volunteers near Cape Town, South Africa. The home visitors in the study were four female residents of the local community with no specialized training prior to the training they received for this study. Although the intervention group demonstrated significantly better parenting and child outcomes compared to the control group, the prevalence of depression did not differ between groups. Despite this null finding regarding improvements in maternal depression, Cooper et al.'s results are promising in that they demonstrate the effectiveness of lay community workers in improving mother–child outcomes during the first 2 years postpartum.

With respect to interventions in LAMI countries, Rahman et al. (2013) in their review argued that (i) it is feasible to train nonspecialist workers to deliver mental health interventions effectively, (ii) interventions must be adapted to the circumstances of women in LAMI countries, (iii) integration of mental health interventions into regular work activities may be less stigmatizing to women, and (iv) community-based approaches are beneficial and may be preferable to stand-alone vertical programs.

In the context of high-income countries, studies of treatment delivery by both professionals and lay volunteers have demonstrated that women with postnatal depression may benefit from treatment by nonmental health specialists. Health visitors and support groups may be viable treatment options for women without access to or interest in traditional pharmacotherapy or psychotherapy for postnatal depression. However, it is important that there be a provision for referral to professional mental health services in cases of more severe depressions or when women do not respond to an intervention provided by a nonmental health professional. Overall, research in this area is limited by a number of factors including lack of a control group, nonrandomization, small sample sizes, and nongeneralizable findings. Another limitation in this area of study is the specific focus on postnatal depression with little examination of pathways to care for antenatal depression or perinatal anxiety. Expanding the variety of pathways to care as well as improving upon existing pathways is critical to increasing the proportion of women receiving treatment for perinatal depression and anxiety.

Conclusions

Much progress has been made over the past three decades in developing and disseminating evidence-based treatments for perinatal depression. There is good evidence that psychological treatments are efficacious when delivered by mental health professionals. The evidence is somewhat less compelling for pharmacological treatments; however, it is clear from the general depression literature that antidepressants are very efficacious for more severe depression (Fournier et al., 2010). More controlled studies are needed with respect to antidepressant use, particularly during pregnancy. There is also good evidence that health professionals and well-trained laypersons can deliver efficacious interventions to postnatal women with mild to moderate severity depression. Preventive approaches may be more efficacious when delivered postnatally. However, treatment of depression during pregnancy can have immediate benefits for women, and it can also diminish the likelihood of postnatal depression (prevention).

Progress is being made in deploying psychological interventions to benefit postnatal depressed women in LAMI countries. These interventions are often based on established treatments but are adapted for the particular circumstances of providers and intervention recipients (for example online treatment - see Chapter 15). Complementary and alternative treatments are increasingly popular, and early work suggests that they may offer an effective alternative to traditional psychological and pharmacological treatments. All of these areas are subject of ongoing research and development. The major challenge ahead will be to make effective interventions available to perinatal women who need them around the world.

References

American College of Obstetricians and Gynecologists Committee on Obstetric Practice. (2002). Committee opinion No. 267: Exercise during pregnancy and the postpartum period. *Obstetrics & Gynecology, 99*(1), 171–173.

Appleby, L., Warner, R., Whitton, A., & Faragher, B. (1997). A controlled study of fluoxetine and cognitive-behavioural counselling in the treatment of postnatal depression. *BMJ (Clinical Research Ed.), 314*(7085), 932–936.

Archer, J., Bower, P., Gilbody, S., Lovell, K., Richards, D., Gask, L., … Coventry, P. (2012). Collaborative care for depression and anxiety problems. *Cochrane Database of Systematic Reviews, 10*, CD006525.

Armstrong, K., & Edwards, H. (2003). The effects of exercise and social support on mothers reporting depressive symptoms: A pilot randomized controlled trial. *International Journal of Mental Health Nursing, 12*(2), 130–138. doi:10.1046/j.1440-0979.2003.00229.x

Armstrong, K., & Edwards, H. (2004). The effectiveness of a pram walking exercise program in reducing depressive symptomatology for postnatal women. *International Journal of Nursing Practice, 10*, 177–194. doi:10.1111/j.1440-172X.2004.00478.x

Armstrong, K. L., Fraser, J. A., Dadds, M. R., & Morris, J. (1999). A randomized, controlled trial of nurse home visiting to vulnerable families with newborns. *Journal of Paediatrics & Child Health, 35*(3), 237–244.

Austin, M. P., Frilingos, M., Lumley, J., Hadzi-Pavlovic, D., Roncolato, W., Acland, S., … Parker, G. (2008). Brief antenatal cognitive behaviour therapy group intervention for the prevention of postnatal depression and anxiety: A randomised controlled trial. *Journal of Affective Disorders, 105*(1–3), 35–44.

Austin, M., Kildea, S., & Sullivan, E. (2007). Maternal mortality and psychiatric morbidity in the perinatal period: Challenges and opportunities for prevention in the Australian setting. *Medical Journal of Australia, 186*(7), 364.

Austin, M., & Lumley, J. (2003). Antenatal screening for postnatal depression: A systematic review. *Acta Psychiatrica Scandinavica, 107*(1), 10–17.

Bastani, F., Hidarnia, A., Kazemnejad, A., Vafaei, M., & Kashanian, M. (2005). A randomized controlled trial of the effects of applied relaxation training on reducing anxiety and perceived stress in pregnant women. *Journal of Midwifery & Women's Health, 50*(4), e36–e40.

Bilszta, J., Ericksen, J., Buist, A., & Milgrom, J. (2010). Women's experience of postnatal depression— Beliefs and attitudes as barriers to care. *Australian Journal of Advanced Nursing, 27*(3), 44–54.

Bloch, M., Meiboom, H., Lorberblatt, M., Bluvstein, I., Aharonov, I., & Schreiber, S. (2012). The effect of sertraline add-on to brief dynamic psychotherapy for the treatment of postpartum depression: A randomized, double-blind, placebo-controlled study. *Journal of Clinical Psychiatry, 73*, 235–241.

Brosse, A. L., Sheets, E. S., Lett, H. S., & Blumenthal, J. A. (2002). Exercise and the treatment of clinical depression in adults. *Sports Medicine, 32*(12), 741–760.

Burns, A., O'Mahen, H., Baxter, H., Bennert, K., Wiles, N., Ramchandani, P., … Evans, J. (2013). A pilot randomised controlled trial of cognitive behavioural therapy for antenatal depression. *BMC Psychiatry, 13*(1), 33.

Chang, M. Y., Chen, C. H., & Huang, K. F. (2008). Effects of music therapy on psychological health of women during pregnancy. *Journal of Clinical Nursing, 17*(19), 2580–2587.

Chen, C., Tseng, Y., Chou, F., & Wang, S. (2000). Effects of support group intervention in the postnatally distressed women: A controlled study in Taiwan. *Journal of Psychosomatic Research, 49*, 395–399.

Clatworthy, J. (2012). The effectiveness of antenatal interventions to prevent postnatal depression in high-risk women. *Journal of Affective Disorders, 137*(1–3), 25–34.

Cohen, L. S., Viguera, A. C., Bouffard, S. M., Nonacs, R. M., Morabito, C., Collins, M. H., … Ablon, J. S. (2001). Venlafaxine in the treatment of postpartum depression. *Journal of Clinical Psychiatry, 62*, 592–596.

Cooper, P. J., Murray, L., Wilson, A., & Romaniuk, H. (2003). Controlled trial of the short- and long-term effect of psychological treatment of post-partum depression: 1. Impact on maternal mood. *The British Journal of Psychiatry, 182*, 412–419. doi:10.1192/bjp.02.177.

Cooper, P. J., Tomlinson, M., Swartz, L., Landman, M., Molteno, C., Stein, A., … Murray, L. (2009). Improving quality of mother-infant relationship and infant attachment in socioeconomically deprived community in South Africa: Randomized controlled trial. *The British Medical Journal, 338*, b974. doi:10.1136/bmj.b974

Corral, M., Wardrop, A. A., Zhang, H., Grewal, A. K., & Patton, S. (2007). Morning light therapy for postpartum depression. *Archives of Women's Mental Health, 10*, 221–224. doi:10.1007/s00737-007-0200-1

Cuijpers, P., Brännmark, J. G., & van Straten, A. (2008). Psychological treatment of postpartum depression: A meta-analysis. *Journal of Clinical Psychology, 64*, 103–118.

Davanzo, R., Copertino, M., De Cunto, A., Minen, F., & Amaddeo, A. (2011). Antidepressant drugs and breastfeeding: A review of the literature. *Breastfeeding Medicine, 6*, 89–98.

Davies, B. R., Howells, S., & Jenkins, M. (2003). Early detection and treatment of postnatal depression in primary care. *Journal of Advanced Nursing, 44*(3), 248–255.

Deligiannidis, K. M., & Freeman, M. P. (2014). Complementary and alternative medicine therapies for perinatal depression. *Best Practice & Research Clinical Obstetrics and Gynaecology, 28*, 85–95.

Dennis, C. L. (2003). The effect of peer support on postpartum depression: A pilot randomized controlled trial. *Canadian Journal of Psychiatry, 48*(2), 115–124.

Dennis, C., & Chung-Lee, L. (2006). Postpartum depression help-seeking barriers and maternal treatment preferences: A qualitative systematic review. *Birth, 33*(4), 323–331. doi: 10.1111/j.1523-536X.2006.00130.x

Dennis, C., & Dowswell, T. (2013). Psychosocial and psychological interventions for preventing postpartum depression. *Cochrane Database of Systematic Reviews, 2*(4), CD001134. doi:10.1002/14651858.CD001134.pub2.

Dennis, C. L., & Hodnett, E. (2007). Psychosocial and psychological interventions for treating postpartum depression. *Cochrane Database of Systematic Reviews, 4*, CD006116.

Dennis, C.-L., Hodnett, E. D., Kenton, L., Weston, J., Zupancic, J., Stewart, D. E., … Kiss, A. (2009). Effect of peer support on prevention of postnatal depression among high risk women: Multisite randomised controlled trial. *British Medical Journal, 338*, a3064.

Dennis, C. L., Ross, L. E., & Herxheimer, A. (2008). Oestrogens and progestins for preventing and treating postpartum depression. *Cochrane Database of Systematic Reviews (Online), 4*, CD001690.

di Scalea, T. L., & Wisner, K. L. (2009). Antidepressant medication use during breastfeeding. *Clinical Obstetrics and Gynecology, 52*, 483–497

Doornbos, B., van Goor, S. A., Dijck-Brouwer, D. A. J., Schaafsma, A., Korf, J., & Muskiet, F. A. J. (2009). Supplementation of a low dose of DHA or DHA + AA does not prevent peripartum depressive symptoms in a small population based sample. *Progress in Neuro-Psychopharmacology & Biological Psychiatry, 33*, 49–52. doi:10.1016/j.pnpbp.2008.10.003

Dunstan, J. A., Simmer, K., Dixon, G., & Prescott, S. L. (2008). Cognitive assessment of children at age 2½ years after maternal fish oil supplementation in pregnancy: A randomized controlled trial.

Archives of Disease in Childhood: Fetal & Neonatal Edition, *93*, F45–F50. doi:10.1136/adc.2006.099085

Epperson, C. N., Terman, M., Terman, J. S., Hanusa, B. H., Oren, D. A., Peindl, K. S., & Wisner, K. L. (2004). Randomized clinical trial of bright light therapy for antepartum depression: Preliminary findings. *The Journal of Clinical Psychiatry*, *65*(3), 421–425.

Field, T., Diego, M., Hernandez-Reif, M., Deeds, O., & Figueiredo, B. (2009). Pregnancy massage reduces prematurity, low birthweight, and postpartum depression. *Infant Behavior and Development*, *32*(4), 454–460. doi:10.1016/j.infbeh.2009.07.001

Field, T., Diego, M., Hernandez-Reif, M., Medina, L., Delgado, J., & Gernandez, A. (2012). Yoga and massage therapy reduce prenatal depression and prematurity. *Journal of Bodywork and Movement Therapies*, *16*(2), 204–209. doi:10.1016/j.jbmt.2011.08.002

Field, T., Diego, M. A., Hernandez-Reif, M., Schanberg, S., & Kuhn, C. (2004). Massage therapy effects on depressed pregnant women. *Journal of Psychosomatic Obstetrics and Gynecology*, *25*, 115–122. doi:10.1080/01674820412331282231

Field, T., Figueiredo, B., Hernandez-Reif, M., Diego, M., Deeds, O., & Ascensio, A. (2008). Massage therapy reduces pain in pregnant women, alleviates prenatal depression in both parents and improves their relationships. *Journal of Bodywork and Movement Therapies*, *12*, 146–150. doi:10.1016/j.jbmt.2007.06.003

Fleming, A. S., Klein, E., & Corter, C. (1992). The effects of a social support group on depression, maternal attitudes and behavior in new mothers. *Journal of Child Psychology and Psychiatry*, *33*(4), 685–698. doi:10.1111/j.1469-7610.1992.tb00905.x

Fournier, J. C., DeRubeis, R. J., Hollon, S. D., Dimidjian, S., Amsterdam, J. D., Shelton, R. C., & Fawcett, J. (2010). Antidepressant drug effects and depression severity: A patient-level meta-analysis. *JAMA*, *303*(1), 47–53.

Frawley, J., Adams, J., Sibbritt, D., Steel, A., Broom, A., & Gallois, C. (2013). Prevalence and determinants of complementary and alternative medicine use during pregnancy: Results from a nationally representative sample of Australian pregnant women. *Australian and New Zealand Journal of Obstetrics and Gynaecology*, *53*(4), 347–352. doi:10.1111/ajo.12056

Freeman, M. P., Davis, M., Sinha, P., Wisner, K. L., Hibbeln, J. R., & Gelenberg, A. J. (2008). Omega-3 fatty acids and supportive psychotherapy for perinatal depression: A randomized placebo-controlled study. *Journal of Affective Disorders*, *110*, 142–148. doi:10.1016/j.jad.2007.12.228

Galbally, M., Lewis, A. J., & Buist, A. (2011a) Developmental outcomes of children exposed to antidepressants in pregnancy. *The Australian and New Zealand Journal of Psychiatry*, *45*, 393–399.

Galbally, M., Snellen, M., & Lewis, A. J. (2011b). A review of the use of psychotropic medication in pregnancy. *Current Opinion in Obstetrics and Gynecology*, *23*(6), 408–414.

Gjerdingen, D., Crow, S., McGovern, P., Miner, M., & Center, B.. (2009). Stepped care treatment of postpartum depression: Impact on treatment, health, and work outcomes. *Journal of the American Board of Family Medicine: JABFM*, *22*(5), 473–482.

Goodman, J. H. (2009). Women's attitudes, preferences, and perceived barriers to treatment for perinatal depression. *Birth*, *36*(1), 60–69. doi:10.1111/j.1523-536X.2008.00296.x

Grote, N. K., Swartz, H. A., Geibel, S. L., Zuckoff, A., Houck, P. R., & Frank, E. (2009). A randomized controlled trial of culturally relevant, brief interpersonal psychotherapy for perinatal depression. *Psychiatric Services*, *60*(3), 313–321.

Heh, S., Huang, L., Ho, S., Fu, Y., & Wang, L. (2008). Effectiveness of an exercise support program in reducing the severity of postnatal depression in Taiwanese women. *Birth*, *35*(1), 60–65. doi:10.1111/j.1523-536X.2007.00192.x

Holden, J. M., Sagovsky, R., & Cox, J. L. (1989). Counselling in a general practice setting: Controlled study of health visitor intervention in treatment of postnatal depression. *British Medical Journal*, *298*, 223–226.

Honikman, S., van Heyningen, T., Field, S., Baron, E., & Tomlinson, M. (2012). Stepped care for maternal mental health: A case study of the perinatal mental health project in South Africa. *PLoS Medicine*, *9*(5), e1001222.

Hou, W. H., Chiang, P. T., Hsu, T. Y., Chiu, S. Y., & Yen, Y. C. (2010). Treatment effects of massage therapy in depressed people: A meta-analysis. *The Journal of Clinical Psychiatry*, *71*(7), 894–901. doi:10.4088/JCP.09r05009blu

Khazaie, H., Ghadami, M. R., Knight, D. C., Emamian, F., & Tahmasian, M. (2013). Insomnia treatment in the third trimester of pregnancy reduces postpartum depression symptoms: A randomized clinical trial. *Psychiatry Research*, *210*, 901–905.

Kim, J. J., La Porte, L. M., Corcoran, M., Magasi, S., Batza, J., & Silver, R. K. (2010). Barriers to mental health treatment among obstetric patients at risk for depression. *American Journal of Obstetrics and Gynecology*, *202*, 312.e1–312.e5. doi:10.1016/j.ajog.2010.01.004

Kuosmanen, L., Vuorilehto, M., Kumpuniemi, S., & Melartin, T. (2010). Post-natal depression screening and treatment in maternity and child health clinics. *Journal of Psychiatric and Mental Health Nursing*, *17*(6), 554–557.

Le, H. N., Perry, D. F., & Stuart, E. A. (2011). Randomized controlled trial of a preventive intervention for perinatal depression in high-risk Latinas. *Journal of Consulting & Clinical Psychology*, *79*(2), 135–141.

Letourneau, N., Stewart, M., Dennis, C., Hegadoren, K., Duffett-Leger, L., & Watson, B. (2011). Effect of home-based peer support on maternal-infant interactions among women with postpartum depression: A randomized, controlled trial. *International Journal of Mental Health Nursing*, *20*, 345–357. doi:10.1111/j.1447-0349.2010.00736.x

Liberto, T. L. (2012). Screening for depression and help-seeking in postpartum women during well-baby pediatric visits: An integrated review. *Journal of Pediatric Health Care*, *26*(2), 109–117. doi:10.1016/j.pedhc.2010.06.012

Logsdon, M. C., Foltz, M. P., Stein, B., & Usui, W., Josephson, A. (2010). Adapting and testing telephone-based depression care management intervention for adolescent mothers. *Archives of Women's Mental Health*, *13*(4), 307–317.

MacArthur, C., Winter, H. R., Bick, D. E., Knowles, H., Lilford, R., Henderson, C., … Gee, H. (2002). Effects of redesigned community postnatal care on women's health 4 months after birth: A cluster randomised controlled trial. *Lancet*, *359*(9304), 378–385.

Makrides, M., Gibson, R. A., McPhee, A. J., Yelland, L., Quinlivan, J., Ryan, P., & DOMInO Investigative Team. (2010). Effect of DHA supplementation during pregnancy on maternal depression and neurodevelopment of young children: A randomized controlled trial. *The Journal of the American Medical Association*, *304*(15), 1675–1683. doi:10.1001/jama.2010.1507

Marc, I., Toureche, N., Ernst, E., Hodnett, E. D., Blanchet, C., Dodin, S., … Njoya, M. M. (2011). Mind-body interventions during pregnancy for preventing or treating women's anxiety. *The Cochrane Database of Systematic Reviews*, *7*, CD007559.

McGregor, J. A., Allen, K. G. D., Harris, M. A., Reece, M., Wheeler, M., French, J. I., & Morrison, J. (2001). The omega-3 story: Nutritional prevention of preterm birth and other adverse pregnancy outcomes. *Obstetrical and Gynecological Survey*, *56*(5), S1–S13.

McGregor, M., Coghlan, M., & Dennis, C. L. (2013). The effect of physician-based cognitive behavioural therapy among pregnant women with depressive symptomatology: A pilot quasi-experimental trial. *Early Intervention in Psychiatry*, *8*(4), 348–357.

Milgrom, J., Gemmill, A.W., Ericksen, J., Burrows, G., Buist, A., & Reece, J. (2015). Treatment of Postnatal Depression with Cognitive Behavioural Therapy, Sertraline and Combination Therapy: A Randomised Controlled Trial. *Australian and New Zealand Journal of Psychiatry*. [E-Pub ahead of print] doi: 10.1177/0004867414565474.

Milgrom, J., Gemmill, A.W., Ericksen, J., Ross, J., Holt, C., & Holt, C.J. (in Press). Feasibility Study and Pilot Randomised Trial of an Antenatal Depression Treatment with Infant Follow-up. *Archive of Women's Mental Health*. Accepted for Publication February 9, 2015.

Milgrom, J., Holt, C. J., Gemmill, A. W., Ericksen, J., Leigh, B., Buist, A., & Schembri, C. (2011a). Treating postnatal depressive symptoms in primary care: A randomized controlled trial of GP management, with and without adjunctive counselling. *BMC Psychiatry*, *11*, 95. doi:10.1186/1471-244X-11-95.

Milgrom, J., Negri, L. M., Gemmill, A. W., McNeil, M., & Martin, P. R. (2005). A randomized controlled trial of psychological interventions for postnatal depression. *British Journal of Clinical Psychology, 44*, 529–542.

Milgrom, J., Schembri, C., Ericksen, J., Ross, J., & Gemmill, A. W. (2011b). Towards parenthood: An antenatal intervention to reduce depression, anxiety and parenting difficulties. *Journal of Affective Disorders, 130*(3), 385–394.

Misri, S., Reebye, P., Corral, M., & Mills, L. (2004). The use of paroxetine and cognitive-behavioral therapy in postpartum depression and anxiety: A randomized controlled trial. *Journal of Clinical Psychiatry, 65*, 1236–1241.

Monk, C., Spicer, J., & Champagne, F. A. (2012). Linking prenatal maternal adversity to developmental outcomes in infants: The role of epigenetic pathways. *Development and Psychopathology, 24*(4), 1361–1376.

Morrell, C. J., Slad, P., Warner, R., Paley, G., Dixon, S., Walters, S. J., … Nicholl, J. (2009). Clinical effectiveness of health visitor training in psychologically informed approaches for depression in postnatal women: Pragmatic cluster randomised trial in primary care. *British Medical Journal, 338*, a3045. doi:10.1136/bmj.a3045

Morrell, C. J., Spiby, H., Stewart, P., Walters, S., & Morgan, A. (2000). Costs and effectiveness of community postnatal support workers: Randomised controlled trial. *British Medical Journal, 321*(7261), 593–598.

Mrazek, P. J., & Haggerty, R. J. (1994). *Reducing risks for mental disorders—Frontiers for prevention intervention research.* Washington, DC: National Academy Press.

Nascimento, S. L., Surita, F. G., & Cecatti, J. G. (2012). Physical exercise during pregnancy: A systematic review. *Current Opinion in Obstetrics & Gynecology, 24*(6), 387–394.

National Institute for Health and Care Excellence. (2007). *Antenatal and postnatal mental health: The NICE guideline on clinical management and service guidance.* London, UK: The British Psychological Society.

Norman, E., Sherburn, M., Osborne, R. H., & Galea, M. P. (2010). An exercise and education program improves well-being of new mothers: A randomized controlled trial. *Physical Therapy, 90*(3), 348–355.

Nylen, K. J., O'Hara, M. W., Brock, R., Moel, J., Gorman, L., & Stuart, S. (2010). Predictors of the longitudinal course of postpartum depression following interpersonal psychotherapy. *Journal of Consulting and Clinical Psychology, 78*(5), 757.

O'Hara, M. W., & McCabe, J. E. (2013). Postpartum depression: Current status and future directions. *Annual Review of Clinical Psychology, 9*, 379–407. doi:10.1146/annurev-clinpsy-050212-185612.

O'Hara, M. W., Stuart, S., Gorman, L. L., & Wenzel, A. (2000). Efficacy of interpersonal psychotherapy for postpartum depression. *Archives of General Psychiatry, 57*, 1039–1045.

O'Mahen, H., Himle, J. A., Fedock, G., Henshaw, E., & Flynn, H. (2013). A pilot randomized controlled trial of cognitive behavioral therapy for perinatal depression adapted for women with low incomes. *Depression and Anxiety, 30*, 679–687.

Oates, M. (2003). Perinatal psychiatric disorders: A leading cause of maternal morbidity and mortality. *British Medical Bulletin, 67*, 219–229.

Pearlstein, T. B., Zlotnick, C., Battle, C. L., Stuart, S., O'Hara, M. W., Price, A. B., … Howard, M. (2006). Patient choice of treatment for postpartum depression: A pilot study. *Archives of Women's Mental Health, 9*, 303–308

Qureshi, N. A., & Al-Bedah, A. M. (2013). Mood disorders and complementary and alternative medicine: A literature review. *Neuropsychiatric Disease and Treatment, 9*, 639–658. doi:10.2147/NDT. S43419

Rahman, R., Fisher, J., Bower, P., Luchters, S., Tran, T., Yasamy, T., … Waheed, W. (2013). Interventions for common perinatal mental disorders in women in low- and middle-income countries: A systematic review and meta-analysis. *Bulletin of the World Health Organization, 91*(8), 593–601.

Rees, A., Austin, M., & Parker, G. B. (2008). Omega-3 fatty acids as a treatment for perinatal depression: Randomized double-blind placebo-controlled trial. *Australian and New Zealand Journal of Psychiatry, 42*, 199–205. doi:10.1080/00048670701827267

Richter, J., Bittner, A., Petrowski, K., Junge-Hoffmeister, J., Bergmann, S., Joraschky, P., & Weidner, K. (2012). Effects of an early intervention on perceived stress and diurnal cortisol in pregnant women with elevated stress, anxiety, and depressive symptomatology. *Journal of Psychosomatic Obstetrics & Gynecology*, *33*(4), 162–170.

Segre, L. S., Stasik, S. M., O'Hara, M. W., & Arndt, S. (2010). Listening visits: An evaluation of the effectiveness and acceptability of a home-based depression treatment. *Psychotherapy Research*, *20*(6), 712–721. doi:10.1080/10503307.2010.518636

Sockol, L. E., Epperson, C. N., & Barber, J. P. (2011). A meta-analysis of treatments for perinatal depression. *Clinical Psychology Review*, *31*(5), 839–849. doi:10.1016/j.cpr.2011.03.009

Spinelli, M. G., & Endicott, J. (2003). Controlled clinical trial of interpersonal psychotherapy versus parenting education program for depressed pregnant women. *The American Journal of Psychiatry*, *160*(3), 555–562.

Spinelli, M. G., Endicott, J., Leon, A. C., Goetz, R. R., Kalish, R. B., Brustman, L. E., ... Schulick, J. L. (2013). Controlled clinical treatment trial of interpersonal psychotherapy for depressed pregnant women at 3 New York City sites. *Journal of Clinical Psychiatry*, *74*(4), 393–399.

Su, K., Huang, S., Chiu, T., Huang, K., Huang, C., Chang, H., & Pariante, C. M. (2008). Omega-3 fatty acids for major depressive disorder during pregnancy: Results from a randomized, double-blind, placebo-controlled trial. *The Journal of Clinical Psychiatry*, *69*, 644–651. doi:10.1016/S0924-977X(03)00032-4

Teixeira, J., Martin, D., Prendiville, O., & Glover, V. (2005). The effects of acute relaxation on indices of anxiety during pregnancy. *Journal of Psychosomatic Obstetrics and Gynaecology*, *26*(4), 271–276.

Watt, S., Sword, W., Krueger, P., & Sheehan, D. (2002). A cross-sectional study of early identification of postpartum depression: Implications for primary care providers from The Ontario Mother & Infant Survey. *BMC Family Practice*, *3*, 5. doi:10.1186/1471-2296-3-5

Whitton, A., Warner, R., & Appleby, L. (1996). The pathway to care in post-natal depression: Women's attitudes to post-natal depression and its treatment. *British Journal of General Practice*, *46*(408), 427–428.

Wirz-Justice, A., Bader, A., Frisch, U., Stieglitz, R., Alder, J., Bitzer, J., ... Riecher-Rossler, A. (2011). A randomized, double-blind, placebo-controlled study of light therapy for antepartum depression. *The Journal of Clinical Psychiatry*, *72*(7), 986–993. doi:10.4088/JCP.10m06188blu

Wisner, K. L., Hanusa, B. H., Perel, J. M., Peindl, K. S., Piontek, C. M., Sit, D. K., ... Moses-Kolko, E. L. (2006). Postpartum depression: A randomized trial of sertraline versus nortriptyline. *Journal of Clinical Psychopharmacology*, *26*, 353–360.

Wu, P., Fuller, C., Liu, X., Lee, H., Fan, B., Hoven, C. W., ... Kronenberg, F. (2007). Use of complementary and alternative medicine among women with depression: Results of a national survey. *Psychiatric Services*, *58*(3), 349–356. doi:10.1176/appi.ps.58.3.349

Yawn, B. P., Dietrich, A. J., Wollan, P., Bertram, S., Graham, D., Huff, J., ... TRIPPD Practices. (2012). TRIPPD: A practice-based network effectiveness study of postpartum depression screening and management. *Annals of Family Medicine*, *10*(4), 320–329.

Yonkers, K. A., Lin, H., Howell, H. B., Heath, A. C., Cohen, & L. S. (2008). Pharmacologic treatment of postpartum women with new-onset major depressive disorder: A randomized controlled trial with paroxetine. *Journal of Clinical Psychiatry*, *69*, 659–665.

Yonkers, K. A., Wisner, K. L., Stewart, D. E., Oberlander, T. F., Dell, D. L., Stotland, N., ... Lockwood, C. (2009). The management of depression during pregnancy: A report from the American Psychiatric Association and the American College of Obstetricians and Gynecologists. *Obstetrics & Gynecology*, *114*, 703–713.

Zlotnick, C., Miller, I. W., Pearlstein, T., Howard, M., & Sweeney, P. (2006). A preventive intervention for pregnant women on public assistance at risk for postpartum depression. *American Journal of Psychiatry*, *163*(8), 1443–1445.

12

International Approaches to Perinatal Mental Health Screening as a Public Health Priority

Katherine L. Wisner, Marie-Paule Austin,
Angela Bowen, Roch Cantwell, and
Nine M.-C. Glangeaud-Freudenthal

Introduction

The perinatal period is a uniquely opportune time for health-care interventions. Focusing on childbearing, we can build upon women's interest in embracing positive health behaviors to invest in the welfare of their offspring (Wisner et al., 2007). Moreover, successful interventions have the potential to reduce maternal disability as well as mitigate negative impacts upon the children and family. Within a lifespan approach that recognizes multiple determinants of reproductive health, Misra, Guyer, and Allston (2003) devised a perinatal health framework, which was adapted to focus on mental health (Wisner, Scholle, & Stein, 2008). This model places childbearing in perspective as a critical biopsychosocial life event with major health impact. A woman's health immediately prior to conception affects her and her fetus/infant's short- and long-term disease risk, health, and functioning. Alterations in the intrauterine climate associated with maternal mental illness affect the offspring's neurobehavioral function and overall health into adulthood, termed "fetal programming" (Gluckman, Hanson, Cooper, & Thornburg, 2008; Kaplan, Evans, & Monk, 2008). The pairing of psychiatric illness with the rapid development of the infant creates a new generation at risk (Murray & Cooper, 1997). Therefore, screening followed by early intervention for psychiatric illnesses and maladaptive parenting behaviors holds great promise to prevent negative sequelae for families. To the extent that negative biopsychosocial exposures (including stress and mental illness) can be diminished, eliminated, or replaced with positive factors, health outcomes in pregnancy and later can be improved.

Health-care organizations in various countries have addressed maternal mental health and illness differently (Chisholm et al., 2004). The evolution of approaches to screening across countries provides the opportunity to compare and contrast them and thereby

Identifying Perinatal Depression and Anxiety: Evidence-Based Practice in Screening, Psychosocial Assessment, and Management, First Edition. Edited by Jeannette Milgrom and Alan W. Gemmill.
© 2015 John Wiley & Sons, Ltd. Published 2015 by John Wiley & Sons, Ltd.

understand the different views of mental health assessment and treatment, impact of social values and societal acceptability, resource investments, support for the tasks of motherhood, and, more broadly, parenthood. In this chapter, investigators from Australia, the United Kingdom, Canada, France, and the United States provide commentary for their respective countries. We defined screening as a complex process that includes detection, evaluation, engagement, intervention, reduction of symptoms or risk, and achievement of functional improvements. The goal was to discuss and synthesize the observations on differing international approaches to support moving forward on behalf of women to identify, support, and treat affected women and families. The key questions were:

In your country, do guidelines for screening for perinatal mental disorders exist?

Is the screening undertaken for perinatal mental *health*, psychiatric *disorders* or depression?

Who are the screeners?

Is the screening incorporated into the health-care system?

Do women and health-care professionals expect to screen as part of maternity care?

Are screening guidelines enforced?

What are barriers to screening?

What is the "culture" of maternity care that supported (or not) the development of perinatal screening guidelines?

What happens to women who screen positive?

Is the mental health care integrated with maternity or primary care?

How are the health-care costs for the evaluations of positively screened women paid?

Australia

Australia is at the forefront of developing national public health policy for women with high levels of psychosocial risk and emergent perinatal mental illness. For the last two decades, a core group of influential mental health clinicians and researchers have been strong advocates. Perinatal psychiatrists and psychologists joined forces with maternity care clinicians (midwives, early childhood nurses, family physicians, general practitioners, and obstetricians), public health administrators, and policy makers. They developed guidelines aimed at primary care health professionals and emphasized the need to provide a broad assessment (as well as depression screening) to identify psychosocial risk factors for poor mental health across childbearing. In Australia and increasingly around the world, the conceptualization has moved from a limited focus on identifying postnatal depression to encompass (i) the full perinatal period, (ii) inclusion of both frequent disorders (depression and anxiety) and low-prevalence disorders (acute puerperal psychoses, mania), and (iii) the impact of mental health and social problems on the woman's function with respect to self-care, infant attachment, parenting, and interpersonal relationships. To emphasize evaluation for distress, symptoms, diagnoses, maladaptive coping styles, and social problems that arise during the perinatal period, the phrase psychosocial assessment is preferred.

The Australian guidelines utilize accessible language. Careful use of words and phrasing was crucial because the guidelines were targeted for primary care clinicians; therefore, less medical- and psychiatric-specific terminology was used. Examples are the terms "mental health problems" or "conditions" rather than "psychiatric disorders." The term perinatal has a narrower meaning in obstetrics; therefore, it was operationalized to include the period from conception through the first postnatal year. A summary of the Australian guidelines is shown in Table 12.1.

Table 12.1 Current clinical practice guidelines: approach, main elements of care models and psychosocial assessment

Guidelines and methodology	*Australian Clinical Practice Guidelines for Perinatal Depression and Related Disorders* (Beyondblue, 2011b). A multidisciplinary advisory formulated these guidelines. Includes a systematic literature review which informs graded recommendations based on the evidence base (e.g., for psychosocial assessment, EPDS, and treatment modality) and good practice points
Overall approach	Aim is to provide integrated perinatal care (IPC: (Barnett, Glossop, Matthey, & Stewart, 2005)), which is integrated with holistic maternity care according to the woman's level of need from mild or "at-risk cases" needing monitoring to severe mental health illness (MHI) requiring psychiatric care and/or complex comorbidity, with a family-/woman-centered approach
Main guideline elements	• Clear criteria for management within primary care and for referral to psychosocial services • Most care provided through primary health care; supported by mental health services • Case plans for women with severe mental illness • Multidisciplinary case conferences for Same • Model supported by staff education and ongoing clinical supervision • Secondary and tertiary treatment options (stepped care based on clinical presentation/level of risk) also available • Clear criteria for management within primary care and for referral to psychosocial services • Most care provided through primary health care; supported by mental health services
Psychosocial assessment recommendations	• Routine psychosocial assessment using structured questions covering broad risk factors for psychosocial morbidity and EPDS (for symptoms of depression and anxiety) in pregnancy and at 6–12 weeks postnatally • Identify both MHI and risk for poor adjustment to parenting • Specific focus on mother–infant interaction, parenting, and impact on family • The guidelines recommend psychosocial assessment be undertaken at first antenatal visit and again at 2–3 months postpartum

The well-developed perinatal assessment framework is paralleled by formal training programs available to clinicians who function as perinatal psychosocial assessors. Key to the success of this public health model is the role of psychiatric services in providing assessment for high-risk women and being available to primary care colleagues for both clinical supervision and consultation. The implementation of training programs varies across Australia. However, many states provide at least brief education in the use of the Edinburgh Postnatal Depression Scale (EPDS; (Cox, Holden, & Sagovsky, 1987)) and psychosocial assessment, and some offer multiday training programs. Online training is also available (Beyondblue, 2011a).

As part of their core curriculum, the College of Midwives has endorsed perinatal mental health training, including routine psychosocial assessment.

In some parts of Australia informal surveys suggest that up to 80% of women receive a depression screen at least once in the perinatal period. The majority of urban public maternity hospitals also provide psychosocial assessments (past psychiatric history, substance use, and domestic violence). This practice is less common in smaller rural and remote centers where appropriate referral pathways are less available. For the ~30% of women who choose to deliver in the private maternity sector in which obstetricians provide the antenatal care, the rates of assessment are lower.

Survey studies demonstrated that women have the expectation of undergoing a psychosocial assessment and accept it as routine. Primary health-care professionals incorporate this evaluation into routine maternity care. The success of the uptake of perinatal psychosocial assessment has been through education and culture change. Barriers to assessments exist in some settings and include clinician time pressures, lack of referral pathways, lack of support for primary care by psychiatric services, and practitioner resistance to psychosocial assessment of patients. There has been no systematic national evaluation of practice to date.

Women who screen positive for depression or who are at high psychosocial risk can access a well-developed intervention infrastructure. The Medicare system provides universal medical care to all Australians including subsidies for psychiatric services. Special mental health legislation was introduced in 2006 to allow women with a formal diagnosis to receive a heavily subsidized set of psychologically focused treatments that use an evidence-based mental health approach. In 2009, following the Perinatal Mental Health National Action Plan (BeyondBlue, 2008), specific perinatal mental health support was added. The national government funds these services through taxes, and at the state level, maternity hospitals fund services such as specialist perinatal psychiatry clinics and maternal and child health services where many of these women are initially screened. General (or family) medical practitioners (funded nationally) provide most of the mental health care, especially medication, for women with moderate to severe episodes. Women who need admission may have access to public mother–baby units in some states or else rely on private health insurance where such public units are not available. Guidelines for referral pathways are locally tailored to the available resources. In Australia, the well-developed system of care provides an opportunity to collect data to define the benefits of screening and psychosocial assessment as well as the costs (see Chapter 16 for some history and ongoing challenges of The National Perinatal Depression Initiative).

United Kingdom

The United Kingdom has provided international leadership in perinatal psychiatry and is the birthplace of the EPDS. Evidence-based national guidelines derived from systematic literature reviews include the National Institute for Health and Care Excellence (NICE) Antenatal and Postnatal Mental Health Guideline (National Institute for Clinical Excellence, 2007) and the Scottish Intercollegiate Guidelines Network (SIGN) Management of Perinatal Mood Disorders (2012). In addition, the Royal College of Obstetricians and Gynaecologists (RCOG) has produced a Good Practice Guideline on Management of Women with Mental Health Issues during Pregnancy and the Postnatal Period (Royal College of Obstetricians and Gynaecologists, 2011). Further exploration of the impact of perinatal mental illness is included in the triennial UK National Confidential Enquiries into Maternal Deaths (Cantwell et al., 2011).

The NICE guideline (2007) was developed for the UK National Health Service (NHS). Recommendations are made for a wide range of psychiatric disorders, including existing depression and psychosis or new psychiatric episodes arising during pregnancy or after childbirth. Recommendations include information on the prediction of risk, early detection of existing illness, and prevention of illness progression in women with subthreshold disorders. The guideline also addresses service organization to meet demands of identification and management. The NICE guideline is under revision and due for publication in 2014/2015.

The SIGN guideline (2012) was developed for the NHS in Scotland. Recommendations are made for the prevention, detection, and management of mood (psychotic and nonpsychotic) disorders during pregnancy and after birth. Prediction and reduction of risk, prevention, and early detection are included. The guideline also makes recommendations on the organization of services to meet clinical need.

The RCOG Good Practice Guideline (2011) was derived from evidence-based UK guidelines focused on the role of maternity staff in the identification of high-risk status, prevention and early detection of perinatal mental disorder, and appropriate liaison with mental health services. Saving Mothers' Lives (Cantwell et al., 2011) is a triennial report on all deaths occurring in the United Kingdom in pregnant and postnatal women, including lessons learned and recommendations for changes in practice. The last four reports have included recommendations on screening for high risk of severe perinatal mental illness and service organization to meet that need.

The UK guidances are broadly based on and address prevalent psychiatric disorders in the perinatal period, that is, preexisting or beginning in pregnancy or the first postpartum year. The emphasis is on identification of women at high risk for severe peripartum mental illness, such as psychosis. A shift away from using the term "screening" in relation to perinatal depression has occurred due to the finding that insufficient evidence is available to recommend universal screening for postnatal depression using UK National Screening Committee criteria (Hewitt et al., 2009). The language more commonly used is risk reduction and early identification.

Identification of risk is integrated into the universal health care that all women in the United Kingdom receive across childbearing. Midwives and health visitors (HV) have the primary role in delivering the first stage of risk reduction strategies recommended by NICE and SIGN. However, both guidelines place a duty of care on all professionals to inquire about risk factors for severe postnatal mental illness and depressive symptoms. No specific training curriculum exists but education on perinatal mental health is included in many undergraduate and postgraduate training programs for HV, midwives, obstetricians, and psychiatrists.

Questions are included in the baseline information obtained at the booking appointment, which marks the woman's first contact with maternity services. Those for depression are based on the Whooley questions (Whooley, Avins, & Browner, 1997) or the EPDS. Examples of the questions routinely asked, taken from the National Scottish Woman-Held Maternity Record (Healthcare Improvement Scotland, 2011), are shown in Table 12.2. Similar documents are used throughout the United Kingdom.

No screening incentives or sanctions exist, but the explicit expectation that risk reduction will occur imposes an obligation on health-care workers. Time pressures on maternity and primary care services may result in initial questions being asked without follow-up inquiry. Specialist perinatal mental health services are present in many areas across the United Kingdom, and they provide education, liaison, and support for maternity and primary care services in their localities. However, large gaps in the availability of specialists are a concern (National Institute for Clinical Excellence, 2007), and maternity and primary care professionals may be reluctant to make detailed queries because they do not have adequate skills to address mental health needs.

In the United Kingdom, the value assigned to keeping mother and infant together resulted in the early development of inpatient mother–baby joint admission units and the

Table 12.2   Extract from the Woman-Held Maternity Record (Scotland)

Your mental health	*No*	*Yes*
1. Do you have a close family member (parent or sibling) with a history of bipolar disorder (manic depression) or any other serious mental illness? Details_____		
2. Do you have a history of bipolar disorder (manic depression), puerperal psychosis, schizophrenia or other serious mental illness?		
3. During the past month, have you often been bothered by feeling down, depressed or hopeless?		
4. During the past month, have you often been bothered by having little interest of pleasure in doing things?		
5. If "yes" to question 3 or 4 then ask: Is this something you feel you need or want help with?		*
*If yes refer to GP for ongoing support		
Are any of the problems ongoing at the moment?		
Are you getting any help with the problems at the moment?		
Details of any agency providing mental health support		
Are they aware of current pregnancy?		
Referral needed details _____		

recognition of perinatal psychiatry as a distinct branch of adult psychiatry, with specific training needs. The stark findings of the last four confidential inquiries into maternal deaths in the United Kingdom have fostered a highly receptive culture for embracing perinatal mental health guidelines. However, the stigma of mental illness remains a barrier to women seeking help for high-risk psychosocial situations or for mental illness.

Screening for high risk of early severe postpartum mental illness is a relatively simple yet highly effective measure that identifies a small number of women at markedly elevated risk for progression to serious mental illness. Interventions are readily available, and there is evidence for preventative interventions (Bergink et al., 2012; Stewart, Klompenhouwer, Kendell, & Van Hulst, 1991). The benefits of screening for mild to moderate disorders are not as robustly established; however, Morrell and colleagues (2009) studied detection and intervention for depressive symptoms by HV and demonstrated that HV training was effective compared to HV usual care in reducing the proportion of women with a 6-month EPDS score ≥ 12. The effect remained for 1 year. The economic evaluation demonstrated that the HV intervention was highly likely to be cost-effective compared with the control condition. A study evaluating the likelihood of screening implementation following the first SIGN guideline (2002) demonstrated that health boards were more likely to implement screening recommendations for postnatal depression rather than psychosis, though the reasons for this are not clear (Alder et al., 2008).

After screening, referral to mental health services (ideally specialist perinatal services) for high-risk women is recommended. High risk is defined as being at risk for severe early postpartum illness. Women with subthreshold or mild to moderate depression are followed regularly throughout pregnancy and postnatally by their general practitioner. For more significant depressive disorders, referrals are ideally made directly to mental health services. The NICE guidelines provide a stepped-care model (National Institute for Clinical Excellence, 2007). In general, mental health, maternity, and primary care are integrated although the confidential inquiries into maternal death reports have identified poor communication among care providers as a recurring factor among women who die by suicide.

The well-developed structure in the United Kingdom also provides an opportunity to collect adequate data for cost–benefit analyses (Hewitt et al., 2009), which are currently underway.

Canada

Canada's Medicare program offers universal free health care; however, attention to perinatal health, as with other health services, is the responsibility of the provinces and territories and often depends upon policy decisions at the regional level (Ministry of the Attorney General, 1985). There is no national policy for screening or treatment for perinatal mental disorders. Two provinces, British Columbia (BC Reproductive Mental Health Program, 2006) and Saskatchewan (Bruce, Béland, & Bowen, 2012; MotherFirst, 2010), have developed guidelines. Both include screening with the EPDS twice during pregnancy, within a few weeks of giving birth, and at the infants' 2- and 6-month immunization visits. The province of Alberta is developing policy, and Ontario held a campaign to increase screening for postpartum depression in select communities (Best Start and Ontario Prevention Clearinghouse, 2007). Local screening programs are embedded in public health and early childhood programs and in some indigenous communities.

The government provides 1 year of maternity leave with limited financial benefits after periods of employment during pregnancy. Some employers provide additional funds up to full income, and others allow an additional year of unpaid leave. These options should promote positive maternal mental health. However, because disability insurance usually begins after 90 days of sick time, a mentally ill pregnant woman may run out of sick time and have no paid time to count toward maternity benefits.

There is minimal incorporation of perinatal mental health risk assessment into the overall health-care system. Screening usually occurs in doctors' offices and health clinics by outreach workers, social workers, physicians, midwives, or public health nurses. A two-question version of the PHQ-9, the PHQ-2 (Kroenke, Spitzer, & Williams, 2001), is included on one province's prenatal record, but there is no requirement for completion. In most provinces, the routine 6-week postpartum check does not include formal screening or systematic psychosocial assessment.

No national training or certification programs are available, so education must be locally initiated. For example, Best Start in Ontario offers a workshop kit on postpartum major depression for health-care providers and patients (Best Start, 2013), and a maternal mental health training program is anticipated from Health Canada.

The culture of maternity care in Canada values the physical health of mother and baby, while mental health remains stigmatized. Other barriers to screening and care include lack of time and resources, limited or no remuneration for screening, lack of specialized referral services if the screen is positive, and privacy legislation that limits communication between care providers. There is growing interest in creating guidelines and developing specialized services, especially following tragedies such as maternal suicide and infanticide (Hildebrandt, 2013).

A recent report by the Canadian Task Force on Preventive Health Care recommended against routine depression screening, citing low quality of evidence to support routine screening, including for perinatal women (Joffres et al., 2013), which raised concern among maternal mental health advocates. The Canadian Mental Health Association, the Canadian Psychiatric Association, and the Society of Obstetricians and Gynaecologists of Canada do not specifically address perinatal mood disorders.

Aboriginal, newcomer, and refugee populations are rapidly growing groups of childbearing women who are at increased risk for mental and perinatal problems due to psychosocial adversity (Bowen, Baetz, McKee, & Klebaum, 2008; Bowen et al., 2013; Fung & Dennis, 2010; Ross et al., 2011). Quality care for women is dependent on translation, and culturally aware assessments and services are emerging (Best Start, 2013; British Colombia Perinatal Health Program, 2013). The EPDS has been validated for use with urban Aboriginal postpartum women (Clarke, 2008).

Treatment options and access vary greatly. Local communities offer postpartum depression support groups run by health-care workers or consumers. Primary health-care providers differ in their expertise and commitment to treat perinatal psychiatric illness. Some mental health practitioners are practicing shared care approaches with specialized reproductive psychiatry and maternal mental health clinics to better utilize scarce tertiary perinatal mental health services (BC Reproductive Mental Health Program, 2006; Bowen, Baetz, et al., 2008; University Health Network, 2013). No joint admission mother–baby units exist.

Canada is a vast country, with large urban as well as rural and remote communities, which has stimulated the development of novel interventions such as telephone-based health services, peer telephone support (Dennis, 2010), and online cognitive behavioral therapy for women with postpartum depression (Pugh, 2012). Despite promising innovations for perinatal mental health treatment, a thorough evaluation of the implementation of existing policy guidelines has not been conducted, and there is no enforcement. Guidelines that promote education and advocacy are increasing awareness, but despite these efforts, a recent environmental scan of policy across Canada revealed there is much to be done to improve maternal mental health (MotherFirst, 2010).

France

In France, all pregnant women have access to national health insurance, which routinely covers medical costs related to pregnancy from discovery through day 12 after birth. The 2010 National Perinatal Report showed that 81.5% of women had additional private insurance that reimbursed fees not covered by the national insurance program (Blondel & Kermarrec, 2011). There is no "gatekeeper" approval to access psychiatric care, which is fully supported by national insurance.

The maternity stay is usually 3–4 days after a vaginal delivery and longer for surgical deliveries or maternal/newborn complications. Women have a medical appointment at 8 weeks post birth. Two additional postpartum visits with a midwife can be arranged for vulnerable families or those who request assistance. The goals of these visits are to (i) assess maternal competence in infant care and feeding, (ii) enhance the mother–child interactional quality, (iii) assess the infant's development and (iv) screen for postpartum psychological problems and depression. However, this service is rarely utilized, and only about 6% of postpartum women received additional appointments (Blondel & Kermarrec, 2011).

The national insurance system also recommends medical checkups for the child within the first 8 days of birth, every month during the 6 first months, at 9 and 12 months, and twice a year until 6 years of age. These appointments are free in maternal and child protection centers (PMI) and 100% covered at public institutions.

The National Guidelines (2005–2007) recommended a medical psychosocial interview with both parents during early pregnancy, with continuity of care through pregnancy and postpartum, in collaboration with regional perinatal networks (La Société Marcé Francophone, 2011). This interview was intended to allow future parents to meet with a midwife or doctor in early pregnancy to identify problems and provide interventions to optimize health and function and prepare for childbirth (Isserlis, Sutter-Dallay, Dugnat, & Glangeaud-Freudenthal, 2008). The inclusion of mother and father underscores the importance of both parents and their relationship.

The National Guidelines also advised increasing the number of mother–baby units to support early mother–infant attachment. There are presently 19 mother–baby units in France (Glangeaud-Freudenthal et al., 2011; Glangeaud-Freudenthal, Howard, & Sutter-Dallay, 2013; La Société Marcé Francophone 2011). The guidelines also recommended development of a regional network of psychiatric units, maternity units, PMI, and psycho-social and medical community care centered on the child and parents. In PMI, there is a systematic primary care follow-up evaluation specifically for vulnerable families and for women detected to be at risk for postpartum depression or under psychosocial duress. Assessments are done by health-care professionals who refer the family to mental health professionals when appropriate. Regional perinatal multidisciplinary staff meetings are held to discuss case studies and improve communication.

National psychiatric and mental health guidelines stress the importance of training of maternity staff and all perinatal primary caregivers about mental disorders and perinatal health-care networks. Training of all maternity care professionals is reinforced with a program of clinical practice assessments for institutions and for individual health professionals. In France, the Société Marcé Francophone (SMF) is contributing to such training by editing guidebooks (Isserlis et al., 2008) and recommending that mental health be included in perinatal training topics for professionals and caregivers.

Despite societal support for perinatal mental health, some barriers persist. The early prenatal psychosocial interview is not yet integrated into all regional prenatal care systems. The National Perinatal 2010 Report found that only 21% of pregnant women, predominantly those with high educational levels, had this interview (Blondel & Kermarrec, 2011). Moreover, training of midwives to conduct this interview is not organized everywhere in France. Currently, the Perinatal Health Networks are not fully operational in all French regions, which is a barrier to a continuity of care through childbearing and for coordination between community primary care, maternity staff, and mental health professionals. The postpartum visits include a medical check, but mental health screens are not routinely done for all postpartum women. Coordination of care is further complicated by widely varied intervention approaches (Oates et al., 2004).

A large-scale national cohort project l'Enfance (Etude Longitudinale Francais depuis l'Enfance; Bales et al., 2014) is following 18,000 children after childbirth (recruited at maternity units in 2011) to evaluate the impact of early biological–social–somatic environment, as well as early parental mental health, on child development. Their results may provide data to support the long-term benefits of early perinatal mental health screening and prevention for the child and his/her parents.

United States

The United States is one of the few countries with no nationally mandated maternity leave, and women with uncomplicated vaginal deliveries are hospitalized for 48 h. It is not surprising that screening for perinatal mental illness has received less policy attention compared to other industrialized countries. No national guidelines for maternal depression have been implemented (National Institute for Health Care Management, 2010). However, individual states have advanced perinatal depression policies. In 2001, Representative Bobby Rush (Illinois) introduced the Melanie Blocker Stokes Postpartum Depression Research and Care Act, with the goal of preventing postpartum suicide, which took the life of the bill's namesake. New Jersey was the first state to pass a law mandating education and screening, due to advocacy provided by State Senate President Richard Codey's wife, Mary Jo, who experienced perinatal depression. The majority of states offer coverage of psychosocial assessments and depression screening and treatment for pregnant women enrolled in the public Medicaid program (National Institute for Health Care Management, 2010).

The Melanie Blocker Stokes Act was the basis for the Mom's Opportunity To Access Help, Education, Research, and Support for Postpartum Depression Act (MOTHERS), and sections of this act were incorporated into the Patient Protection and Affordable Care Act that Barack Obama signed into law in March 2010. This legislation requires coverage for perinatal depression screening and provides grants to states to provide services to women. The Affordable Care Act's health reform provisions may improve access to insurance and result in support for screening and treatment among the childbearing women enrolled in their maternity programs (National Institute for Health Care Management, 2010).

The first major report on perinatal mental health was commissioned by the Agency for Healthcare Research and Quality and published in 2005 (Agency for Healthcare Research and Quality, 2005). The US Preventive Services Task Force recommended screening of all adults for depression with the caveat that "staff-assisted depression care supports are in place to assure accurate diagnosis, effective treatment and follow-up" (U.S. Preventative Services Task Force, 2009). The American Congress of Obstetricians and Gynecologists (ACOG) (2010) concluded that insufficient evidence was available to support universal screening; however, they suggested that screening be strongly considered due to the potential benefit for a woman and her family. The Joint American Academy of Pediatrics/ACOG Guidelines for Perinatal Care recommended that psychosocial assessments be conducted across childbearing (American Academy of Pediatrics and American College of Obstetricians and Gynecologists, 2007). They suggested that pregnant women be monitored for negative feelings and symptoms of severe postpartum depression and offered culturally appropriate treatment or referral to community resources.

Recently, the government Agency for Healthcare Research and Quality reported that current evidence supports screening for depression in the postpartum period only when resources are available to ensure appropriate diagnosis and treatment. They identified many of the same uncertainties noted in previous reviews, including a lack of evidence that screening and treatment for depression directly improve maternal–infant functioning (Agency for Healthcare Research and Quality, 2013).

Although minimal attention has been paid to postscreening models of care in the United States, model development has been published by Miller and colleagues (2009). To be coupled with effective treatment, screening must be linked with diagnostic assessment strategies. The disease management model facilitated identification of women with major depressive disorder, eliminated referral of women with false-positive screens to specialty services, and provided on-site treatment of women with mild to moderate unipolar depression. This stepped-care depression management model increased the rate of pregnant women identified as having significant depressive symptoms from 0.4 to 17.1%. Yawn et al. (2012) also showed that screening and intervention were effective when delivered within a primary care practice. Practices were randomized for postpartum depression treatment training or usual care. Intervention tools included repeated use of the PHQ-9 to monitor response to therapy and a format for nursing follow-up telephone calls to address medication initiation, adherence, and side effects. Among women with elevated depression screening scores, those in the intervention practices were more likely to receive both a diagnosis and treatment for postpartum depression. They also had lower depressive symptom levels at 6 and 12 months postpartum.

An increasing practice in the United States is the collaboration between mental health professionals and caregivers within home visiting programs (Every Child Succeeds, 2013). Home visitation combines psychosocial support and evidence-based psychotherapy for depression treatment. The goal is to strengthen individual and family protective factors and mitigate risks. Frequent contact between community-based home visitors and families and extended program duration ensure that home visitors are present during developmental transitions (Ammerman et al., 2013). This practice may represent an early pathway toward the more established screening and referral infrastructures that exist in other countries. Although there is interest on the part of perinatal mental health advocates and professionals, no joint admission mother–baby inpatient hospital units exist in the United States. Day hospital and inpatient admission of the mother combined with baby day visitation programs are early efforts toward specialized programming (Battle & Howard, 2014; University of North Carolina, 2014).

Synthesis and Discussion

Conceptual frameworks for identification and treatment of women with perinatal psychiatric disorders are evolving. Screening may focus on depression or other disorders or alternatively on the identification of women at high psychosocial risk for mental illness and adverse maternal and infant outcomes. The latter is a concept that parallels research in schizophrenia that mental illnesses have identifiable prodromal characteristics which provide opportunities for prevention or early intervention (Addington et al., 2012).

Studies that document that such interventions may be cost-effective are emerging. Differences in approaches to perinatal mental health care appear to be driven by societal investment in the transition to parenthood and parallel resource allocation (Oates et al., 2004). Differing views of the importance of childbearing, infant attachment, and early child development are reflected in services. Examples are perinatal specialists and joint admission mother–baby units in the United Kingdom, France, and Australia, which are rare experiments in the United States and Canada (Glangeaud-Freudenthal et al., 2013). Such differences are also reflected in the law, such as a maximum charge of manslaughter with a 1-year maximum sentence for a woman in the United Kingdom who kills her child if the killing is within one year after birth. Reviews of the causes of maternal death in the United Kingdom and Australia (Kildea, Sullivan, & King, 2006) and multidisciplinary regional case reviews in France are powerful tools to bring attention to the personal and societal costs of perinatal mental illness.

Most studies in perinatal mental health are focused on depression, the most common primary disorder. However, the risk for bipolar disorder was reported to be a striking 23 times greater in the initial 30 days post birth (Munk-Olsen, Laursen, Pedersen, Mors, & Mortensen, 2006). Anxiety disorders are prevalent in childbearing-aged women and are predictors of postpartum depression (Bowen, Bowen, Maslany, & Muhajarine, 2008; Sutter-Dallay, Giaccone-Marcesche, Glatigny-Dallay, & Verdoux, 2004). Women with any serious mental illness and/or active substance use are appropriate for identification and treatment. Whether screening should be universal or targeted to women identified as having risk factors continues to be debated. Psychosocial screening may be more acceptable and inclusive, but broader psychosocial problems are difficult to remedy (poverty, community, and interpersonal violence). Screening for diagnoses is also challenging. Although recurrent major depression with comorbid anxiety disorder is the most common diagnosis in screen-positive postpartum women, multiple other diagnoses and comorbidities co-occur (Milgrom, Ericksen, Negri, & Gemmill, 2005; Wisner et al., 2013). A conundrum is the differentiation of unipolar from bipolar disorder *at the screening level* rather than through psychiatric diagnostic interviewing, which requires substantial expertise (Sharma & Xie, 2011).

Recommendations from most countries suggest screening both during pregnancy (to identify chronic and pregnancy-onset conditions) and postpartum. Instruments developed specifically for the perinatal period initially were intended to screen for depression, such as the EPDS (Cox et al., 1987). A two-question depression screen has also been advocated for use in the perinatal setting (National Institute for Clinical Excellence, 2007; Whooley et al., 1997). Screening for depression serves the goal of identifying women who urgently need treatment. An approach from a different theoretical framework is to screen for maternal psychosocial risk with a measure such as the Antenatal Risk Questionnaire (Austin, Colton, Priest, Reilly, & Hadzi-Pavlovic, 2013; Johnson et al., 2012), which targets women who are at high risk for preventive interventions. A relatively neglected option is to screen for positive maternal attributes, such as utilizing measures that tap adaptive function, exemplified by the Inventory of Functional Status after Childbirth (Fawcett, Tulman, & Myers, 1988) or the Barkin Index of Maternal Functioning (Barkin et al., 2010). Evaluation of adaptive function after birth may be less stigmatizing to childbearing women and families and suggests "skill building" rather than "treatment."

What is the "screening unit?" Support is often provided to not only the woman but also her infant and family. Other potential targets include the quality of mother–infant interaction, the woman's partner, and other children and family members who are part of her support system. The inclusion of the father is in the recommendations for interviews in France and if the mother has a positive screen in Saskatchewan (Canada).

Potential venues for screening and treatment are obstetrical, maternity, family practice and pediatric clinics, as well as insurers' care management programs. Just as lack of communication across systems is a barrier to optimal care, information sharing and consultation is a powerful mechanism among agencies that collaborate to improve maternal mental health and achieve functional recovery goals.

The International Marcé Society for Perinatal Mental Health strongly advocates for universal psychosocial evaluation of perinatal women in its position statement, Psychosocial Assessment and Depression Screening in Perinatal Women (2013). The society recognizes that universal screening is controversial. The need for data to support that the benefits of perinatal screening (whether broad or narrow) convincingly outweigh the cost is also recognized. Both the short- and long-term benefits of the screening process are considerations, since maternal mental illness during childbearing has impacts into adolescence (Halligan, Herbert, Goodyer, & Murray, 2004; Talge, Neal, & Glover, 2007). The conceptual underpinning of the Marcé Society position statement is the centrality of childbearing as a major adult developmental event with unparalleled potential for interventions to improve short- and long-term maternal, infant, and family health. The society also acknowledges that the enactment of screening procedures, although based upon a shared conceptual framework, depends upon local resources and preferred models of care, which shape the screening paradigm that is acceptable and feasible. Independent of diagnosis, women often request community-based, nonmedical interventions, social support, and self-help resources (Dennis & Hodnett, 2007; Dennis et al., 2009). The challenge is to screen broadly, which will yield a large group of screen-positive women, but to provide customized treatments relevant to the family being served.

Acknowledgment

The authors thank Ms. Emily Pinheiro for arranging the references.

References

Addington, J., Cadenhead, K. S., Cornblatt, B. A., Mathalon, D. H., McGlashan, T. H., Perkins, D. O., … Woods, S. W. (2012). North American prodrome longitudinal study (NAPLS 2): Overview and recruitment. *Schizophrenia Research, 142*(1–3), 77–82. doi:10.1016/j.schres.2012.09.012.

Agency for Healthcare Research and Quality. (2005). Perinatal depression: Prevalence, screening accuracy, and screening outcomes summary. Rockville, MD: Author. Retrieved form http://archive. ahrq.gov/downloads/pub/evidence/pdf/peridepr/peridep.pdf. Accessed December 10, 2014.

Agency for Healthcare Research and Quality. (2013). *Comparative Effectiveness Review Number 106: Efficacy and Safety of Screening for Postpartum Depression.* Rockville, MD: Author.

Alder, E. M., Reid, M., Sharp, L. J., Cantwell, R., Robertson, K., & Kearney, E. (2008). Policy and practice in the management of postnatal depression in Scotland. *Archives of Women's Mental Health, 11*(3), 213–219. doi:10.1007/s00737-008-0015-8.

American Academy of Pediatrics, and American College of Obstetricians and Gynecologists. (2007). *Guidelines for Perinatal Care.* Washington, DC: Author.

American College of Obstetricians, and Gynecologists Committee on Obstetric Practice. (2010). Committee opinion no. 453: Screening for depression during and after pregnancy. *Obstetrics and Gynecology, 115,* 394–395. doi:10.1097/AOG.0b013e3181d035aa.

Ammerman, R. T., Putnam, F. W., Altaye, M., Teeters, A. R., Stevens, J., & Van Ginkel, J. B. (2013). Treatment of depressed mothers in home visiting: Impact on psychological distress and social functioning. *Child Abuse and Neglect, 37*(8), 544–554. doi:10.1016/j.chiabu.2013.03.003.

Austin, M.-P., Colton, J., Priest, S., Reilly, N., & Hadzi-Pavlovic, D. (2013). The antenatal risk questionnaire (ANRQ): Acceptability and use for psychosocial risk assessment in the maternity setting. *Women and Birth, 26*(1), 17–25. doi:10.1016/j.wombi.2011.06.002.

Bales, M., Pambrun, E., Melchior, M., Glangeaud-Freudenthal, N. M.-C., Charles, M.-A., Verdoux, H., & Sutter-Dallay, A.-L. (2014). Prenatal psychological distress and access to mental health care in the ELFE cohort. *European Psychiatry,* in press.

Barkin, J. L., Wisner, K. L., Bromberger, J. T., Beach, S. R., Terry, M. A., & Wisniewski, S. R. (2010). Development of the barkin index of maternal functioning. *Journal of Women's Health (2002), 19*(12), 2239–2246. doi:10.1089/jwh.2009.1893.

Barnett, B., Glossop, P., Matthey, S., & Stewart, H. (2005). Screening in the context of integrated perinatal care. In C. Henshaw & S. Elliott (Ed.), *Screening for Perinatal Depression* (pp 68–82). London, UK: Jessica Kingsley Publishers.

Battle, C. L., & Howard, M. M. (2014). A mother–baby psychiatric day hospital: History, rationale, and why perinatal mental health is important for obstetric medicine. *Obstetric Medicine: The Medicine of Pregnancy, 7*(2), 66–70.

Bergink, V., Bouvy, P. F., Vervoort, J. S. P., Koorengevel, K. M., Steegers, E. A. P., & Kushner, S. A. (2012). Prevention of postpartum psychosis and mania in women at high risk. *American Journal of Psychiatry, 169*(6), 609–615. doi:10.1176/appi.ajp.2012.11071047.

Best Start. (2013). Resources. Retrieved form http://beststart.org/resources/ppmd. Accessed December 17, 2014.

Best Start and Ontario Prevention Clearinghouse. (2007). Postpartum mood disorders real. Retrieved from http://www.lifewithnewbaby.ca/resources/ppmd_bro_mood.pdf. Accessed January 7, 2015.

Beyondblue. (2008). *Perinatal Mental Health National Action Plan.* Hawthorn West, Australia: Author.

Beyondblue. (2011a). Beyond baby blues: Detecting and managing perinatal mental health disorders in primary care. Retrieved from http://thinkgp.com.au/beyondblue. Accessed December 17, 2014.

Beyondblue. (2011b). Clinical practice guidelines for depression and related disorders—Anxiety, bipolar disorder, and puerperal psychosis—In the perinatal period. A guideline for primary care health professionals. The National Depression Initiative. Retrieved form http://www.beyondblue.org.au/resources/health-professionals/clinical-practice-guidelines/perinatal-clinical-practice-guidelines. Accessed December 10, 2014.

Blondel, B., & Kermarrec, M. (2011). Les naissances en 2010 et leur évolution depuis 2003. In Inserm (Ed.), *Enquête Nationale Périnatale 2010.* Paris, France: DGS (Direction Générale de la Santé).

Bowen, A., Baetz, M., McKee, N., & Klebaum, N. (2008a). Optimizing maternal mental health within a primary health care centre: A model program. *Canadian Journal of Community Mental Health, 27*(2), 105–116.

Bowen, A., Bowen, R., Maslany, G., & Muhajarine, N. (2008b). Anxiety in a socially high-risk sample of pregnant women in Canada. *Canadian Journal of Psychiatry, 53*(7), 435–440.

Bowen, A., Duncan, V., Peacock, S., Bowen, R., Schwartz, L., Campbell, D., & Muhajarine, N. (2013). Mood and anxiety problems in perinatal Indigenous women in Australia, New Zealand, Canada, and the United States: A critical review of the literature. *Transcultural Psychiatry, 51*(1), 93–111.

British Colombia Perinatal Health Program. (2013). Celebrating the circle of life: Coming back to balance and harmony. An Aboriginal guide to emotional health in pregnancy and early motherhood: For women and their families, edited by Government of British Colombia. Victoria, BC: Author.

British Columbia Reproductive Mental Health Program. (2006). *Addressing Perinatal Depression: A framework for BC's Health Authorities.* Vancouver, BC: Author. Retrieved form http://www.health.gov.bc.ca/library/publications/year/2006/MHA_PerinatalDepression.pdf. Accessed December 10, 2014.

Bruce, L., Béland, D., & Bowen, A. (2012). MotherFirst: Developing a maternal mental health strategy in Saskatchewan. *Healthcare Policy (Politiques de sante), 8*(2), 46.

Cantwell, R., Clutton-Brock, T., Cooper, G., Dawson, A., Drife, J., Garrod, D., … Springett, A. (2011). Saving mothers' lives: Reviewing maternal deaths to make motherhood safer: 2006–2008. The Eighth Report of the Confidential Enquiries into Maternal Deaths in the United Kingdom. *BJOG: An International Journal of Obstetrics and Gynaecology, 118,* 1. doi:10.1111/j.1471-0528.2010.02847.x.

Chisholm, D., Conroy, S., Glangeaud-Freudenthal, N., Oates, M. R., Asten, P., Barry, S., … TCS-PND Group. (2004). Health services research into postnatal depression: Results from a preliminary cross-cultural study. *The British Journal of Psychiatry, 184*(46), s45–s52.

Clarke, P. J. (2008). Validation of two postpartum depression screening scales with a sample of First Nations and Metis women. *CJNR (Canadian Journal of Nursing Research), 40*(1), 112–125.

Cox, J. L., Holden, J. M., & Sagovsky, R. (1987). Detection of postnatal depression. Development of the 10-item Edinburgh Postnatal Depression Scale. *The British Journal of Psychiatry, 150*(6), 782–786.

Dennis, C.-L. (2010). Postpartum depression peer support: Maternal perceptions from a randomized controlled trial. *International Journal of Nursing Studies, 47*(5), 560–568. doi:10.1016/j.ijnurstu.2009.10.015.

Dennis, C.-L., Hodnett, E., Kenton, L., Weston, J., Zupancic, J., Stewart, D. E., & Kiss, A. (2009). Effect of peer support on prevention of postnatal depression among high risk women: Multisite randomised controlled trial. *BMJ: British Medical Journal, 338,* a3064. doi:10.1136/bmj.a3064.

Dennis, C.-L., & Hodnett, E. (2007). Psychosocial and psychological interventions for treating postpartum depression. *Cochrane Database of Systematic Reviews, 4,* CD006116.

Every Child Succeeds. (2013) Moving beyond depression. Retrieved from http://www.movingbeyond depression.org/. Accessed December 17, 2014.

Fawcett, J., Tulman, L., & Myers, S. T. (1988). Development of the inventory of functional status after childbirth. *Journal of Nurse-Midwifery*, *33*(6), 252–260.

Fung, K., & Dennis, C.-L. (2010). Postpartum depression among immigrant women. *Current Opinion in Psychiatry*, *23*(4), 342–348. doi:10.1097/YCO.0b013e32833ad721.

Glangeaud-Freudenthal, N., Howard, L., & Sutter-Dallay, A.-L. (2013). Mother-infant inpatient units. In M. W. O'Hara, K. L. Wisner, & J. Joseph (Eds.), *Best practice & research clinical obstetrics & gynaecology, perinatal mental illness: Guidance for the obstetrician-gynecologist*. Amsterdam, the Netherlands: Elsevier.

Glangeaud-Freudenthal, N. M.-C., Sutter, A.-L., Thieulin, A.-C., Dagens-Lafont, V., Zimmermann, M.-A., Debourg, A., … Khoshnood, B. (2011). Inpatient mother-and-child postpartum psychiatric care: Factors associated with improvement in maternal mental health. *European Psychiatry*, *26*(4), 215–223. doi:10.1016/j.eurpsy.2010.03.006.

Gluckman, P. D., Hanson, M. A., Cooper, C., & Thornburg, K. L. (2008). Effect of in utero and early-life conditions on adult health and disease. *New England Journal of Medicine*, *359*(1), 61–73. doi:10.1056/NEJMra0708473.

Halligan, S. L., Herbert, J., Goodyer, I. M., & Murray, L. (2004). Exposure to postnatal depression predicts elevated cortisol in adolescent offspring. *Biological Psychiatry*, *55*(4), 376–381.

Healthcare Improvement Scotland. (2011). Scottish woman held maternity record. Retrieved from http://www.healthcareimprovementscotland.org/our_work/reproductive,_maternal__child/woman_held_maternity_record/swhmr_maternity_record.aspx. Accessed December 17, 2014.

Hewitt, C. E., Gilbody, S. M., Brealey, S. D., Paulden, M., Palmer, S., Mann, R., … Richards, D. (2009). Methods to identify postnatal depression in primary care: An integrated evidence synthesis and value of information analysis. *Health Technology Assessment Reports*, *13*(36), 1–145. doi:10.3310/hta13360.

Hildebrandt, A. (2013). Winnipeg tragedy: Mothers lament postpartum depression stigma. *CBC News Canada*. Retrieved from http://www.cbc.ca/news/canada/winnipeg-tragedy-mothers-lament-postpartum-depression-stigma-1.1382546. Accessed December 17, 2014.

Isserlis, C., Sutter-Dallay, A.-L., Dugnat, M., & Glangeaud-Freudenthal, N. M.-C. (2008). Guide pour la pratique de l'entretien prénatal précoce et l'accompagnement psychique des femmes devenant mères. In Erès (Ed.), *Collection Petite enfance et parentalité*. Toulouse, France: Erès.

Joffres, M., Jaramillo, A., Dickinson, J., Lewin, G., Pottie, K., Shaw, E., … Tonelli, M. (2013). Recommendations on screening for depression in adults. *Canadian Medical Association Journal*, *185*(9), 775–782. doi:10.1503/cmaj.130403.

Johnson, M., Schmeid, V., Lupton, S. J., Austin, M.-P., Matthey, S. M., Kemp, L., … Yeo, A. E. (2012). Measuring perinatal mental health risk. *Archives of Women's Mental Health*, *15*(5), 375–386. doi:10.1007/s00737-012-0297-8.

Kaplan, L. A., Evans, L., & Monk, C. (2008). Effects of mothers' prenatal psychiatric status and postnatal caregiving on infant biobehavioral regulation: Can prenatal programming be modified? *Early Human Development*, *84*(4), 249–256.

Kildea, S., Sullivan, E. A., & King, J. F. (2006). Maternal deaths in Australia 2000–02. In *National Perinatal Statistics Unit (Maternal Deaths Series #2)*. Sydney, Australia: Australian Institute for Health and Welfare (AIWH).

Kroenke, K., Spitzer, R. L., & Williams, J. B. W. (2001). The PHQ-9: Validity of a brief depression severity measure. *Journal of General Internal Medicine*, *16*(9), 606–613.

La Société Marcé Francophone. (2011). Les adresses des unités mère-enfant. Retrieved from http://www.marce-francophone.fr/adresses-ume.html. Accessed December 17, 2014.

Milgrom, J., Ericksen, J., Negri, L., & Gemmill, A. W. (2005). Screening for postnatal depression in routine primary care: Properties of the Edinburgh Postnatal Depression Scale in an Australian sample. *Australian and New Zealand Journal of Psychiatry*, *39*, 833–839.

Miller, L., Shade, M., & Vasireddy, V. (2009). Beyond screening: Assessment of perinatal depression in a perinatal care setting. *Archives of Women's Mental Health, 12*(5), 329–334. doi:10.1007/s00737-009-0082-5.

Ministry of the Attorney General. (1985). Canada Health Act. In R.S.C., 1985, c. C-6. Ottawa, Canada: Government of Canada.

Misra, D. P., Guyer, B., & Allston, A. (2003). Integrated perinatal health framework. A multiple determinants model with a life span approach. *American Journal of Preventive Medicine, 25*(1), 65–75.

Morrell, C. J., Slade, P., Warner, R., Paley, G., Dixon, S., Walters, S. J., … Nicholl, J. (2009). Clinical effectiveness of health visitor training in psychologically informed approaches for depression in postnatal women: Pragmatic cluster randomised trial in primary care. *BMJ: British Medical Journal, 338*, a3045. doi:10.1136/bmj.a3045.

MotherFirst. (2010). *Maternal Mental Health Strategy: Building Capacity in Saskatchewan.* MotherFirst: Saskatchewan, Canada.

Munk-Olsen, T., Laursen, T. M., Pedersen, C. B., Mors, O., & Mortensen, P. B. (2006). New parents and mental disorders: A population-based register study. *JAMA: The Journal of the American Medical Association, 296*(21), 2582–2589. doi:296/21/2582 [pii] 10.1001/jama.296.21.2582.

Murray, L., & Cooper, P. J. (1997). Effects of postnatal depression on infant development. *Archives of Disease in Childhood, 77*(2), 99–101.

National Institute for Clinical Excellence. (2007). Antenatal and postnatal mental health (CG45). Retrieved from http://www.nice.org.uk/guidance/CG45. Accessed December 17, 2014.

National Institute for Health Care Management. (2010). Identifying and treating maternal depression: Strategies & considerations for health plans. Retrieved from http://www.nihcm.org/pdf/FINAL_MaternalDepression6-7.pdf. Accessed December 17, 2014.

Oates, M. R, Cox, J. L., Neema, S., Asten, P., Glangeaud-Freudenthal, N., Figueiredo, B., … Kammerer, M. H. (2004). Postnatal depression across countries and cultures: A qualitative study. *The British Journal of Psychiatry, 184*(46), s10–s16.

Pugh, N. (2012). Maternal depression online. Retrieved from https://www.onlinetherapyuser.ca/intro/mdo/. Accessed December 17, 2014.

Ross, L. E., Villegas, L., Dennis, C.-L., Bourgeault, I. L., Cairney, J., Grigoriadis, S., … Yudin, M. H. (2011). Rural residence and risk for perinatal depression: A Canadian pilot study. *Archives of Women's Mental Health, 14*(3), 175–185. doi:10.1007/s00737-011-0208-4.

Royal College of Obstetricians and Gynaecologists. (2011). Management of women with mental health issues during pregnancy in the postnatal period (Good Practice No 14). London, UK: RCOG.

Scottish Intercollegiate Guidelines Network (SIGN). (2002). *Postnatal depression and puerperal psychosis.* Edinburgh, Scotland: Author.

Scottish Intercollegiate Guidelines Network (SIGN). (2012). Management of perinatal mood disorders. Edinburgh, Scotland: Author. Retrieved from http://www.sign.ac.uk/pdf/sign127.pdf. Accessed December 17, 2014.

Sharma, V., & Xie, B. (2011). Screening for postpartum bipolar disorder: Validation of the Mood Disorder Questionnaire. *Journal of Affective Disorders, 131*(1–3), 408–411. doi:10.1016/j.jad.2010.11.026.

Stewart, D. E., Klompenhouwer, J.-L., Kendell, R. E., & Van Hulst, A. M. (1991). Prophylactic lithium in puerperal psychosis. The experience of three centres. *The British Journal of Psychiatry, 158*(3), 393–397.

Sutter-Dallay, A.-L., Giaccone-Marcesche, V., Glatigny-Dallay, E., & Verdoux, H. (2004). Women with anxiety disorders during pregnancy are at increased risk of intense postnatal depressive symptoms: A prospective survey of the MATQUID cohort. *European Psychiatry, 19*(8), 459–463.

Talge, N. M., Neal, C., & Glover, V. (2007). Antenatal maternal stress and long-term effects on child neurodevelopment: How and why? *Journal of Child Psychology and Psychiatry, 48*(3–4), 245–261.

U.S. Preventative Services Task Force. (2009). Screening for depression in adults. Retrieved from http://www.uspreventiveservicestaskforce.org/uspstf/uspsaddepr.htm. Accessed December 17, 2014.

University Health Network. (2013). Women's mental health program. Retrieved from http://www.uhn.ca/MCC/PatientsFamilies/Clinics_Tests/Women_Mental_Health. Accessed December 17, 2014.

University of North Carolina. (2014). North Carolina Center for women's mood disorders, perinatal psychiatry inpatient program—Program description. Retrieved from http://www.med.unc.edu/psych/wmd/patient_care/Program%20Description%208-5-11.pdf. Accessed December 17, 2014.

Whooley, M. A., Avins, A. L., & Browner, W. S. (1997). Case-finding instruments for depression. *Journal of General Internal Medicine, 12*(7), 439–445.

Wisner, K. L., Scholle, S., & Stein, B. D. (2008). Perinatal disorders. *The Journal of Clinical Psychiatry, 69*(10), 1602–1605.

Wisner, K. L., Sit, D. K. Y., McShea, M. C., Rizzo, D. M., Zoretich, R. A., Hughes, C. L., … Hanusa, B. H. (2013). Onset timing, thoughts of self-harm, and diagnoses in postpartum women with screen-positive depression findings. *JAMA Psychiatry, 70*(5), 490–498. doi:10.1001/jamapsychiatry.2013.87.

Wisner, K. L., Sit, D. K. Y., Reynolds, S. K., Altemus, M., Bogen, D. L., Sunder, K. R., … Perel, J. M. (2007). Psychiatric disorders. In S. G. Gabbe, J. R. Neibyl, & J. L. Simpson (Eds.), *Obstetrics: Normal & Problem Pregnancies*. Philadelphia, PA: Churchill Livingstone/Elsevier.

Yawn, B. P., Dietrich, A. J., Wollan, P., Bertram, S., Graham, D., Huff, J., … Pace, W. D. (2012). TRIPPD: A practice-based network effectiveness study of postpartum depression screening and management. *The Annals of Family Medicine, 10*(4), 320–329. doi:10.1370/afm.1418.

13

Training Health-Care Professionals for the Assessment and Management of Perinatal Depression and Anxiety

C. Jane Morrell, Jan Cubison, Tom Ricketts,
Anne Sved Williams, and Pauline Hall

Introduction

A diverse range of health-care professionals may be involved in the identification and management of perinatal depression and anxiety, such as midwives, health visitors (HVs), child and family health nurses, clinical psychologists, community mental health nurses, mental health social workers, counselors, general practitioners (GPs), and nurse practitioners. Any of these health-care professionals could benefit from relevant training.

While health-care professionals provide individual health care for pregnant and postnatal women, they also have a wider public health role in identifying health-care issues and referring on appropriately for management. A woman may have prepregnancy health problems or those arising from her pregnancy, labor, or delivery which may be simple, complex, minor or life threatening, physical, or emotional. Frontline health-care professionals need to have the skills and knowledge to identify relevant health issues, including perinatal depression and anxiety often while working under considerable time pressures. Any training program to implement a successful screening policy needs to be deliverable within this context, clear to understand, quick and easy to administer, and able to provide awareness of appropriate pathways for onward referral.

Two contrasting approaches to the training of health-care professionals are described in this chapter. The POstNatal Depression Economic evaluation and Randomised (PoNDER) trial training provided HVs with assessment skills and the skills to deliver psychologically informed approaches within a large randomized controlled trial (RCT) (Morrell et al., 2009a). In contrast, the training within the Australian National Perinatal Depression Initiative (NPDI) focused on the screening and referral skills of midwives (antenatally) and child and family health nurses (postnatally). Practice-based evidence for this approach is provided. The appropriate approach for any particular jurisdiction will be determined by factors such as the organization of health-care systems and the ease of access to different professional groups, particularly specialist mental health workers.

Identifying Perinatal Depression and Anxiety: Evidence-Based Practice in Screening, Psychosocial Assessment, and Management, First Edition. Edited by Jeannette Milgrom and Alan W. Gemmill.
© 2015 John Wiley & Sons, Ltd. Published 2015 by John Wiley & Sons, Ltd.

Strategies for Effective Training of Health-Care Professionals

Health-care professionals have expressed a need for more information to improve their confidence in identifying mental health problems (Jomeen, Glover, & Davies, 2009) because of the complexities they face in assessing psychological health (Jomeen, Glover, Jones, Garg, & Marshall, 2013). They have suggested that performance could be improved by continuing medical education, professional development, and learning with colleagues (Grol, 2002).

A number of issues make it difficult to examine the effectiveness of educational interventions, such as problems in standardizing the intervention, contamination of the control study arm within RCTs, and inadequately validated outcome assessment measures (Coomarasamy & Khan, 2004).

While it is widely accepted that teaching improves health-care professionals' knowledge (Gilbody, Whitty, Grimshaw, & Thomas, 2003), educational interventions do not necessarily result in the necessary changes to attitudes, skills, and behavior needed to improve care, which are more likely to occur when teaching is integrated into clinical practice (Coomarasamy & Khan, 2004).

A meta-analysis of teaching strategies to manage depression in primary care found that training worked best when it was part of an organizational intervention using a range of strategies, including collaborative care, particularly when offered in conjunction with the trainers (Gilbody et al., 2003).

Altering the professional practice of experienced health professionals generally requires multifaceted approaches that engage the practitioner in viewing the potential change as important and appropriate to their patients. The process of implementation of evidence-based practice is often termed "knowledge translation," and there are numerous theoretical frameworks available to support this endeavor (Rycroft-Malone & Bucknall, 2010). One common form of knowledge translation is through educational meetings. In a Cochrane review of continuing education meetings and workshops, Forsetlund et al. (2009) identified 81 studies addressing the relative effect of different combinations of educational interventions on professional practice and patient outcomes. They found that educational meetings and workshops could improve both professional behavior and patient outcomes but that effects were generally small. Mixed interactive and didactic approaches were more effective than either didactic meetings or interactive meetings alone.

Educational studies addressing depression recognition and management have tended to have rather weak effects. The Hampshire Depression Project (Thompson et al., 2000) evaluated the effectiveness of an educational program to aid the implementation of a depression clinical practice guideline within general practices across an English health district. While positive feedback was received regarding the training, there was no improvement in the recognition of, or recovery from, depression (defined by the Hospital Anxiety and Depression Scale) among a sample of 21,409 patients.

Similar negative findings were identified by King et al. (2002) in a study of the effects of training GPs in brief psychological management of depression. In contrast, a pilot RCT evaluating training and supervision of GPs regarding the recognition and psychological management of panic disorder indicated both a change in skills and practice (Heatley, Ricketts, & Forrest, 2005). It was hypothesized that the inclusion of a practice-focused supervisory component may have enhanced the impact of the brief educational intervention.

Trainers

Training programs appear to be more successful when they have charismatic leaders and active education strategies such as interactive workshops, and teaching combined with practical implementation and outreach visits. All are likely to be more effective than passive strategies such as didactic teaching and printed educational material (Epstein, 2008; Weeks, Robinson, Brooks, & Batalden, 2000). It is helpful for trainers to make statements about what participants will be able to do by the end of course (i.e., set learning objectives), ensure relevancy, explain how evidence relates to participants' work environment, and then ask participants how they would apply the evidence to their own work setting.

The quality of the training will depend in part upon the qualifications, skills, and experience of the trainers. Trainers require a formal professional or clinical qualification and preferably will also have a teaching qualification in order to employ a variety of teaching techniques. Trainers who are clinicians with years of experience in working with women with perinatal mental health problems will bring clinical case examples which, typically, are easily remembered by trainees. Most important is an enthusiastic delivery to motivate the trainees to listen and to implement their learning.

The Context of Training

UK context

In the United Kingdom, midwives care for women from pregnancy through to delivery and for up to 4 weeks postnatally. HVs see each woman for a mental health assessment, usually once in pregnancy for a first baby, twice postnatally for standard care, or more frequently if there are complex or maternal–infant issues. In England and Wales, the National Institute for Health and Care Excellence (NICE) guidelines for antenatal and postnatal mental health (NICE, 2007) recommend the use of the Whooley questions (Whooley, Avins, Miranda, & Browner, 1997). These were controversial because of their lack of validation in a perinatal context (Hewitt et al., 2009). However, they are simple and quick to administer and have been used widely in practice (The Patient's Association, 2011), particularly by midwives. The Whooley questions are recommended in the widely used *Perinatal Institute's National Standardised Pregnancy and Postnatal Notes*, with local variations in the handheld maternity records which accompany women throughout their pregnancy (The Maternity Notes, 2013). The key recommended times to screen are at a woman's first contact with primary care, at her booking visit, and postnatally, usually at 4–6 weeks and 3–4 months (NICE, 2007).

The Edinburgh Postnatal Depression Scale (EPDS) (Cox, Holden, & Sagovsky, 1987) was widely used by many HVs throughout the United Kingdom in local protocols and care pathways until the National Screening Committee (NSC) report of 2000 questioned its use as a screening tool (Shakespeare, 2001). The report did not entirely oppose the use of the EPDS, but recommended that it should only be used following training, used as a checklist as part of a mood assessment for postnatal mothers, used alongside professional judgment, and used as a clinical interview and not used as a pass/fail screening tool.

In Scotland, the Scottish Intercollegiate Guidelines Network (2012) states in its advice that "there is insufficient evidence to recommend the use of the EPDS or the Whooley Questions" for screening women but that "their use is likely to have benefit in facilitating discussion of emotional issues and aiding ongoing clinical monitoring."

It was in this context that the EPDS was used within the PoNDER trial (Morrell et al., 2009a).

More recently, in the United Kingdom, the maternal mental health pathway aims to support the delivery of the Healthy Child Program (Shribman, 2009) which recommends the use of the Whooley questions. Its resource for e-Learning for Healthcare (e-LfH) module "Mental Health Promotion in the Perinatal Period" (Adams, 2011) has the following four learning objectives:

1   Explain the significance of early screening and intervention for mental ill health during pregnancy and the first postnatal year.
2   Recognize the signs of common and more complex perinatal mental health disorders and describe the effect of anxiety and depression on the developing fetus, the mother, and the rest of the family.
3   Identify emotional distress by using a range of techniques including clinical judgment and evidence-based screening tools.
4   Distinguish sound judgments regarding appropriate health promotion actions that aim to enhance mental health.

Australian context

The Australian context for screening is quite different. Factors such as the Australian Government's NPDI, the differences in the organization of health systems (e.g., child and maternal health workers in Australia rather than HVs), and the distribution of the population over a vast geographical area combine to necessitate that modes and contents of training differ between Australia and the United Kingdom.

Face-to-face training days, which are held in some well-resourced capital cities, allow ample time for discussion and reflection and are popular and well attended. Furthermore, excellent free e-learning packages have simplified the provision of basic information about screening for many practitioners, both metropolitan and rural. Video-conferencing has also become increasingly popular as this enables remote practitioners to partake in two-way discussions with city-based presenters. Offering varied approaches, where possible, provides different benefits to different populations. For example, midwives working in many small rural communities have wider roles than their metropolitan counterparts and face issues of holding personal and professional relationships with women. This can cause difficulties when asking about sensitive issues such as thoughts of harm or domestic violence and therefore needs to be addressed within the content of face-to-face or video-conference training. e-learning, on the other hand, has enormous advantages in terms of cost, ease of dissemination geographically, and reduction of burden for trainers.

Under the NPDI framework, *beyondblue* in collaboration with the National Health and Medical Research Council (NHMRC) released clinical guidelines in 2011 (*beyondblue*, 2011c). *beyondblue* is a "not-for-profit" organization which aims to increase awareness and improve the treatment of depression, bipolar disorder, anxiety disorders, and related mental disorders, with a particular focus on perinatal health disorders and puerperal psychosis.

National perinatal mental health guidelines make recommendations based on best quality evidence including recommendation of routine, universal screening for depression (both in the antenatal and postnatal period) using the EPDS (Cox et al., 1987). This extensive review then provides information about the management of depression and related disorders in the perinatal period (see Chapter 12). A full copy or the executive summary can be ordered free of charge or downloaded (*beyondblue*, 2011c).

Training Aims

Training relevant health-care practitioners to assess women and to identify common mental health problems aims to ensure that women appropriately receive the best available support at the earliest possible time during their pregnancy or after their baby is born.

The training of health-care practitioners to undertake their role in perinatal mental health has four main purposes:

- To help practitioners acquire the skills in assessment of perinatal women and their mental health
- To improve practitioners' knowledge about common mental health conditions and increase their competence and confidence in discussing these issues with women
- To develop practitioners' interpersonal skills so that they can undertake sensitive assessments
- To provide practitioners with knowledge of available local mental health providers and services and to facilitate the practitioners' collaboration in care networks with mental health specialists

Training promotes consistency in adherence to assessment procedures and the use of evidence-based practice, resulting in greater equity in access to mental health services for perinatal women. Training also has the potential to develop skills which enhance the relationship between women and their practitioners, so women feel more able to trust their practitioner. When interviewed, women in the PoNDER trial, who had a 6-week EPDS score of 12 or more, indicated that the relationship with the HV was key to whether they would accept the offer of support from the HV (Slade et al., 2010). The HV–client relationship is considered especially important in enabling uptake by families who sometimes find services hard to access (Cowley et al., 2013).

Training to Develop Perinatal Screening Skills

Effective assessment requires training that provides skills including:

- Promoting a suitable screening environment
- Introducing a standardized, universal screening questionnaire
- Asking for consent for screening
- Delivering routine procedures and respecting individual responses and nuances
- Assessing risk
- Reassuring women to promote trust and honesty
- Minimizing stigma
- Interpreting and acting on true or false positives or true or false negatives
- Communicating the results to women
- Sensitively discussing management options with the woman and partner if appropriate

Accessing options for pathways to care, according to locally developed and available guidelines and policies, depends on multiple factors including the availability of appropriately trained (perinatal) mental health professionals, the severity and urgency of any problems identified, the expertise and confidence of staff, and the woman's wishes for further input.

Assessing Risk

Detail on assessing risk is provided in Chapters 2 and 4 of this book. As well as training to focus on depression or anxiety symptoms, training stresses the importance of exploring responses to the EPDS' question 10 on suicidal thinking and risk of harm. Staff are trained to understand that a positive response to this question necessitates further probing and discussion with the woman. Example probing questions include:

- Can you tell me a bit more about your thoughts? (Frequency, persistence)
- Have you thought about whether you would act on your thoughts? (Plans)
- What do you have available to you that you would need to do this? (Means)
- What is stopping you? (Protective factors)
- Have you ever harmed yourself before? What happened? How do feel about this now? (Risk factors)
- What are you looking forward to in the future? (Protective factors)
- What people are there who can support and help you? (Protective factors)

Training HVs in the PoNDER Trial

The following description details the training preparation for HVs who took part in the intervention arm of a prospective pragmatic cluster RCT and economic evaluation of training for HVs—the PoNDER trial. This was the largest conducted trial both of a HV training intervention and of PND. The training manuals developed for the HVs and their trainers are available via the University of Nottingham electronic links (Ricketts & Curran, 2009; Tudor, 2010).

The PoNDER trial summary

The experimental HV training examined in the PoNDER trial built upon promising work on the potential for a psychological intervention as an alternative to pharmaceutical management. HVs in 101 GP practices (clusters) in England and 4084 women consented to take part in the trial. HVs in the usual care (control) clusters did not receive training, while HVs in the training (intervention) clusters received group training for six full days plus four half days. The trial aim was to identify any differences in outcomes for postnatal women, child, or family, attributed to training HVs in systematically identifying depressive symptoms and delivering psychologically informed sessions (up to eight sessions of 1 h/week), based on either cognitive behavioral principles (CBA) or on person-centered principles (PCA) in primary care for women at greater risk of postnatal depression (PND).

Clinical outcomes

The published trial outcomes indicated the pragmatic effectiveness of the package of training for HVs to assess all women on their caseload, identify depressive symptoms, and provide a psychologically informed intervention (Morrell et al., 2009a) where indicated. There were no differences between the outcomes for women in the CBA training group and the PCA training group (Figure 13.1).

The training was associated with a reduction in depressive symptoms at 6 months post-natally among all intervention group women and some evidence of benefit for the intervention group for some of the secondary outcomes at 12 and 18 months follow-up. Hence, the trial generated evidence of the pragmatic cost-effectiveness of a package of training for HVs to 12 months postnatally (Morrell et al., 2009b). Further analysis of the PoNDER trial follow-up data reinforced the finding of a preventive effect of the HV training (Brugha, Morrell, Slade, & Walters, 2011).

Introductory training day in the PoNDER trial

HVs were trained to develop skills to undertake a clinical assessment and to appropriately administer the EPDS. This included training in how to assess a mother's mood, how to assess depressive symptoms and suicidal thoughts, and how to explore feelings about their baby.

The full-day introductory training covered:

1   A summary of the evidence for the causes, consequences, and treatment of PND
2   The skills of identification of symptoms and the use of the EPDS
3   Clinical interviewing and risk management

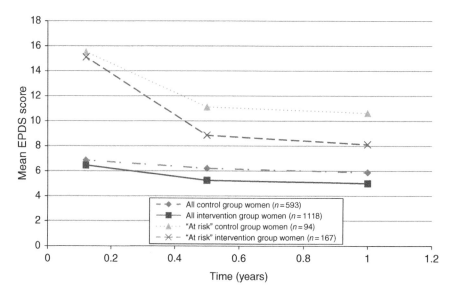

Figure 13.1   Mean EPDS scores for "at-risk" women (with a 6-week EPDS score $\geq$ 12) and for "all" women in the PoNDER trial from 6 weeks to 12 months postnatally.

The morning session included a PowerPoint presentation of research evidence to date, followed by in-depth discussion of each EPDS question. Although the rudiments of the use and misuse of the EPDS can be delivered quickly, a challenging aspect of screening procedures as part of policy is the prevention of "routine" outcomes, that is, the danger of implementing the procedure correctly but missing the subtleties involved in an effective clinical assessment (Gilbody, House, & Sheldon, 2001).

Next, there was an explanation of the EPDS and the rationale and protocol for its use, followed by small group discussions working through case examples. Three cases were used:

Case one, where the score was high
Case two, where the score was zero
Case three, where there was a positive response to question 10

The case studies were designed so that emerging issues would include risks to self, risk to baby and others, denial of mood, and thresholds for referring on. These issues were discussed in small groups initially, then in the larger group.

The afternoon covered clinical perspectives, the core features of depression, and assessing risk plus training in conducting a clinical interview.

The HVs were all asked to play three roles: that of a mother, an HV, and then an observer. This was to gain experience in the practical use of the EPDS and then report back their experience, both practically and emotionally.

The key features of the training were:

- Use of the evidence base and real-life case examples, some from the UK Confidential Enquiries into maternal deaths (Cantwell et al., 2011)
- Understanding the context of screening for depression, the rationale for HVs identifying symptoms of depression
- Knowledge of UK guidelines on the use of screening tools and local protocols, including details of the EPDS administration
- Small and large group discussions about screening issues
- Information about depression and clinical interview practice
- Knowledge of risk and understanding when and how to refer
- Varied teaching techniques including learning through experience
- Takeaway postcard-sized prompt cards to assist in the EPDS questions, clinical interview, and assessment of suicide risk (Appendix 13.A)

Training for psychologically informed sessions

The five-day HV training in psychological approaches conformed to the requirements of appropriate methods for comparative psychotherapy research (Hill & Lambert, 2004; Kendall & Holmbeck, 2004). A Training Reference Group (TRG) was established comprising experienced psychotherapy and counseling trainers representing CBA and PCA approaches to make sure that the training was rigorous, effective, and comparable for both approaches in order to minimize any potential bias in the head-to-head comparison of the training for the two approaches. The TRG also aimed to minimize the potential impact of the trainers' therapy allegiance (Luborsky et al., 1999) by inviting contributions from CBA and PCA experts to the training design.

Up to that point, previous trials had examined the effectiveness of "a brief training in the principles of person-centred counselling" for HVs in Edinburgh (Holden, Sagovsky, & Cox, 1989) and tested cognitive behavioral counseling against fluoxetine in Manchester (Appleby, Warner, Whitton, & Faragher, 1997). In the PoNDER trial, rather than training HVs to deliver psychotherapy or become mental health workers, therapists, or counselors (which would have taken much longer than 5 days), the brief training was to prepare HVs to deliver the critical elements derived from one of the two approaches (CBA and PCA). The training was designed to engage and enthuse the HVs through overt linkage to their existing skills. The aims were to develop their theoretical knowledge, skills, and confidence so they could support women with psychological difficulties. It was intended that the training would be accessible and easily distinguished, theoretically congruent, and reproducible with key skills. The terms "PCA" and "CBA" were used to avoid the use of the terms therapy and counseling. The trainers avoided using unfamiliar language and jargon, such as "negative automatic thoughts." The content of the training was adapted to the needs of postnatal women with little time or energy to do too much "homework" between visits.

The common aim for both the CBA and the PCA to psychotherapeutic training was to enable HVs to acquire further generic skills in developing warm, therapeutic, helpful relationships, such as unconditional positive regard and empathy. In addition, the respective trainings developed the HVs' skills in delivering either a CBA or a PCA for eligible women. The details of the training have been published (Morrell et al., 2011).

Training manuals in the PoNDER trial

The two main trainers were specialist practitioners, trainers and supervisors. They prepared a manual for each HV to refer to throughout the trial and a separate trainer's manual to promote consistency and reproducibility. To make sure the training could be replicated, the manuals covered the theoretical basis for the approach and the training plan. Although the ethos and style of the two approaches were different, the TRG verified that the training manuals were comparable. The training was planned to be similar and balanced, as far as possible. No more than 12 HVs were included in each training cohort so that four small groups of three HVs could work together. The training rooms were safe and not interrupted and consistent with what could be delivered in the UK National Health Service.

Five-day training evaluation

When each training cohort was finished, the HVs were asked to complete a questionnaire to provide feedback on the training delivery. The replies of these indicated a high level of satisfaction with the content and methods of the training (Morrell et al., 2009a).

Clinical supervision, reflective practice, and availability of follow-up support

Clinical supervision is a practice-focused professional relationship involving a clinician reflecting on practice, guided by a skilled supervisor. It can be distinguished from managerial supervision in that the primary purpose is to develop rather than evaluate competence. Clinical supervision and support pathways for practitioners implementing screening and intervention programs are core components of training. Practitioners learning a new skill benefit from employing that new skill and also from accessing trainers or relevant clinicians who can reinforce good practice and provide advice and support when questions arise in practice.

In the PoNDER trial, the HVs received clinical supervision and support through reflective practice groups at regular intervals after the training. These sessions used case material brought by participants in small groups of five to seven HVs. Skills were developed through the use of discussion, reflection on learning, and the rehearsal of skills in a safe, supportive setting. These sessions included training in peer supervisory methods, and HVs also attended locally organized peer supervisory sessions. In order to facilitate HVs being involved in their own development and to aid reflection on practice, each course participant was asked to complete a "record of learning experiences" for the duration of the course, including the reflective practice sessions.

The Australian NPDI

In Australia, training has been incorporated as part of a wider program run under the auspices of a Commonwealth and State funded NPDI (2008/9 to 2014/15). The general aim of the NPDI is *To improve the prevention and early detection of antenatal and postnatal depression; and to provide better care, support and treatment for expectant and new mothers experiencing perinatal depression* (Department of Health and Ageing, 2009).

The key objectives of the NPDI are:

- Routine and universal screening throughout Australia for antenatal and PND and psychosocial risk
- Workforce training and development for health professionals
- Clear and agreed pathways of care and follow-up support for women at risk of or experiencing perinatal depression
- Research and data collection
- National guidelines for screening for perinatal depression
- Increased community awareness regarding perinatal mood disorders

NPDI training programs in Australia

Federal and state governments in Australia have invested in the NPDI by providing funding to achieve key objectives including implementation of training programs for routine and universal perinatal screening for depression and psychosocial risk and to help ensure the development of pathways to care. This screening is predominantly conducted by midwives (antenatally) and maternal–child and family health nurses (postnatally). GPs are commonly involved in pathways to care in the first instance.

An expert committee working under the auspices of *beyondblue* established four levels of training appropriate for different health-care professionals and their role. The task of the Workforce Training and Development Committee was the development of a matrix which indicates the skills, knowledge, and expertise that practitioners who work with perinatal women and their families might expect to have acquired on completion of each level (*beyondblue*, 2011b). The four levels are:

1   "Basic knowledge": This may be obtained via an online training program covering how to assess perinatal women and information about common mental health conditions which can be identified by screening, how to screen, plus pathways to care. *beyondblue*, working with experts in the field, scoped the training needs of health professionals working in different levels of maternity care and then developed a free online training package entitled "Beyond babyblues: Detecting and managing perinatal mental health disorders in primary care." This includes a focus specifically on the use of the EPDS as a screening tool with perinatal populations (*beyondblue*, 2011c).
2   "Basic skills plus": Following completion of the "basic knowledge," practitioners require further training to develop their skills in the management of mild depression and anxiety. Training is provided either face-to-face, ideally in multiagency or multidisciplinary settings, or by accessing further online programs.
3   "Intermediate skills": For this level, clinicians require further training to enable them to carry out an assessment and complete a management plan and in some cases manage more complex perinatal mental health issues. Training is face-to-face with supervision during the course and beyond the training period. Such training programs have been developed in many states, for example, as certificate courses, and have depended on the knowledge, energy, and passion of local "champions."
4   "Advanced assessment and intervention": The highest level trainees are likely to be mental health professionals undertaking specialized training in the management of complex or severe perinatal mental health problems, providing care for a woman and her infant, within her whole family setting. This training involves in-depth study and supervised practice which may include mother–infant therapy.

The matrix was developed to assist with safe implementation of screening and facilitate adequate staff training for nonmental health professionals to undertake such screening. Each state employed staff centrally to coordinate training at the levels described, and in many jurisdictions, a large number of multidisciplinary clinicians have attended face-to-face training programs (e.g., SA Health, 2011).

Training at any level consisted of various modes of delivery including e-learning and other digital resources such as DVDs, face-to-face, or use of video-conferencing technology.

In the 2 years and 9 months following the launch of the free accredited online training program in April 2011, it has been accessed by over 5500 professionals. In South Australia with a population of 1,600,000 and approximately 20,000 live births annually, over 3,500 professionals have accessed face-to-face training in the first three and a half years of running the training sessions. This includes sessions at various levels and of varying duration to meet the needs of different staff. Training has ranged from a 1-h screening information session, targeted sessions on use of the screening tools delivered to teams in their own workplace, and an 8-h session covering other topics including attachment, effects of domestic violence on infants, psychotropic medication, case study discussion, and referral pathways. The e-learning program "Introduction to Perinatal Mental Health" has also been developed in South Australia, which is free to access by any professional in any country (SA Health, 2011).

Multidisciplinary Training: The Management of Training Programs

Systematic evaluations and meta-analyses of large-scale studies in primary care mental health screening have shown a clear benefit both of multiagency training (Gilbody, 2004) and of attempting to ensure collaborative care among agencies (Gilbody et al., 2003). In addition, in Australia, management support and intergovernmental agreements have aimed to develop a public health system-wide approach with successful implementation for a large proportion of perinatal women. Organizational support for training is essential at a basic level to allow staff the opportunity to be relived from usual duties to engage in the training and then importantly to help facilitate the transfer of knowledge gained into organizational and workplace practices.

Several principles for effective training include:

- Training those who wish to be trained (i.e., not to mandate)
- Training a whole agency/team
- Training across disciplines to facilitate shared knowledge and awareness of others' work places and practices
- Modes of setting up training programs to maximize their benefits
- Central management support for both screening and training

Summary

In this chapter, we have highlighted:

- The aims of training and recommended features of trainers
- A summary of the PoNDER trial
- The PoNDER trial introductory training day to develop assessment skills
- The value of training in the identification of symptoms of depression alongside the skills in providing a psychotherapeutic intervention for mild to moderate PND
- The availability of the PoNDER trial training manuals for training for psychologically informed sessions
- Clinical supervision and reflective practice
- The importance of organizational and senior management support for training
- The benefits of multidisciplinary/multiagency training
- The Australian NPDI
- Examples of training implemented under the NPDI
- *beyondblue* training skills matrix levels
- Free to access e-learning packages available

Conclusions

All health professionals who come into contact with pregnant and postnatal women need training in the identification and management of PND (Cox, Holden, & Henshaw, 2014, p. 67). This chapter describes a training model for HVs in the United Kingdom for which there is evidence of clinical effectiveness and cost-effectiveness. Prior to the trial, HVs in the United Kingdom had been using this approach as a viable alternative to pharmacological management of depression when they had been trained in the use of the EPDS and "listening visits." The PoNDER trial outcomes indicate that the training appears to have a preventive as well as treatment effect, which was an unexpected bonus. Therefore, investment in training for HVs for which there is evidence of clinical and cost-effectiveness could have long-term positive outcomes for women and potentially for their infants and families. In the United Kingdom, we await the recommendation from the ongoing revision of the NICE guidance for antenatal and postnatal mental health. The remaining challenge is to ensure that all HVs are appropriately trained.

In contrast, under the auspices of the NPDI in Australia, the provision of free access to training has enhanced screening, as well as improved knowledge of mood disorders and pathways to care among midwives and child and family health nurses throughout most of the country with potential benefit to the majority of Australian perinatal women and their families. Since the introduction of the NPDI in 2008/2009, thousands of relevant health professionals have received training in perinatal and infant mental health content, delivered via a range of modes including face-to-face sessions, video-conferencing technology, and e-learning programs (Highet & Purtell, 2012; SA Health, 2011). This training has facilitated and embedded safe implementation of routine antenatal and postnatal screening for depression and psychosocial risk which is now occurring in all states and territories across Australia. Pathways to care are better known, and many local networks of professionals have been facilitated by bringing together multidisciplinary staff from a variety of public and private agencies at training sessions. Screening is well embedded into routine practice and a substantial proportion of the workforce has access to training, particularly at the level of "basic knowledge." However, there are still areas where training has not been comprehensive, and there are remaining implementation challenges as the NPDI now moves into a maintenance phase.

Appendix 13.A

EPDS Questions and clinical assessment

1 I have been able to laugh and see the funny side of things
    Pervasive mood
2 I have looked forward with enjoyment to things
    Views of the future
    Reduced energy and activity
3 I have blamed myself unnecessarily when things went wrong
    Ideas of guilt and unworthiness
4 I have felt worried and anxious for no very good reason
    Depressive and anxiety cognitions
5 I have felt scared and panicky for no very good reason
    Feelings of loss of control and panic
6 Things have been getting on top of me
    Hopelessness and despair
7 I have been so unhappy that I have had difficulty sleeping
    Sleeping pattern
    Appetite disturbed?

8 I have felt sad or miserable
   Feelings? How long?
9 I have been so unhappy that I have been crying
   How much and how often?
   Thoughts? Sense of purpose
10 The thought of harming myself has occurred to me
   Nature & quality of suicidal thoughts—intent, plans
   What prevents you from acting on your thoughts?
   What level of support is available and will it be accepted?

EPDS Questionnaire: Cox et al. (1987). Clinical questions: Cubison J

Clinical Interview

Appearance

Manner of dress, level of hygiene, posture, usual gait, facial expression, eye contact—pupils dilation/constriction, general state of health and nutrition

Speech

Rate, volume, characteristics

Motor activity (physical movements)

Lethargic, tense, restless, agitated tics, grimaces, or tremors. Unusual mannerisms or gestures.

Mood

Does the person report feeling sad, fearful, hopeless, euphoric or anxious?
   Ask the her to rate mood on a scale of 1–10. Ask about thoughts of self-harm at this point, if the patient is thought to be suicidal. ***Suicidal thoughts must be addressed without delay.**

Affect

The person's statement of emotion and their appropriateness.
   Do the emotions shift rapidly from one to another? Is the emotion out of keeping with the speech content? Are the emotions flat?

Perceptions

Only seen in the most severe depressions.
   Two types of perceptual problems:

Hallucinations—false sensory impressions or experiences—may occur in any of the five major senses—sight, sound, touch, taste smell. In postnatal illness can be a "presence," "seeing someone."

Delusions—are false beliefs, are usually extremely rigid and without factual basis i.e. Belief that you have no stomach and consequent refusal to take food.

Thoughts

Recurrent and persistent, excessive worry. Worrying thoughts of death, their own or their baby's, are common.

Do things feel strange and unreal, singled out, watched, talked about by others, thoughts/actions are being controlled externally.

Memory

Anxiety and depression can impair immediate retention and recent memory.

Concentration

Ability to pay attention throughout the assessment interview, Subjective reporting i.e. Ability to read a newspaper or watch a favorite TV programme.

Insight

The person's understanding of the nature of the problems or the illness. Acceptance or denial of the presence of problems or illness.

Assessment of suicide risk *(Aide memoire, not to indicate severity of risk)*

Background Factors
- Family history of suicide
- Recent bereavement
- Past history of self-harm

Current Factors
- Intrusive thoughts
- Depressive/anxiety cognitions
- Suicidal intent/plans

Any person with active plans for suicide requires urgent referral and action

Assessing risk to others, infants and children
- Psychosis—always a serious risk
- Psychiatric disturbance with high emotional or social stressors
- Intrusive thoughts leading to attachment difficulties

Additional Stressors
- Co-morbid drug and alcohol use
- History of violence
- Severe mental illness

Protectors
- Compliance with treatment/care plans
- Acceptance of emotional and social support

References

Adams, H. (2011). *Mental health promotion in the perinatal period: Module HCP-10-04. The Healthy Child Program e-Learning Curriculum*. London, UK: Royal College of Paediatrics and Child Health.

Appleby, L., Warner, R., Whitton, A., & Faragher, B. (1997). A controlled study of fluoxetine and cognitive-behavioural counselling in the treatment of postnatal depression. *British Medical Journal, 314*, 932–936.

beyondblue. (2011a). Beyond baby blues: Detecting and managing perinatal mental health disorders in primary care. Retrieved from http://thinkgp.com.au/beyondblue. Accessed December 17, 2014.

beyondblue. (2011b). *Matrix framework of perinatal depression and related disorders*. Melbourne, Australia: Author. Retrieved from http://www.beyondblue.org.au/docs/default-source/8.-perinatal-documents/bw0118-training-matrix-for-perinatal-mental-health-skills-and-knowledge.pdf. Accessed December 17, 2014.

beyondblue. (2011c). Clinical practice guidelines for depression and related disorders—Anxiety, bipolar disorder and puerperal psychosis—In the perinatal period. Retrieved from http://www.beyondblue.org.au/resources/health-professionals/clinical-practice-guidelines/perinatal-clinical-practice-guidelines. Accessed December 17, 2014.

Brugha, T. S., Morrell, C. J., Slade, P., & Walters, S. J. (2011). Universal prevention of depression in women postnatally: Cluster randomized trial evidence in primary care. *Psychological Medicine, 41*(4), 739–748. doi:10.1017/S0033291710001467.

Cantwell, R., Clutton-Brock, T., Cooper, G., Dawson, A., Drife, J., Garrod, D., … Springett, A. (2011). Saving mothers' lives: Reviewing maternal deaths to make motherhood safer: 2006–2008. The Eighth Report of the Confidential Enquiries into Maternal Deaths in the United Kingdom. *BJOG: An International British Journal of Obstetrics and Gynaecology, 118*, 1–203.

Coomarasamy, A., & Khan, K. S. (2004). What is the evidence that postgraduate teaching in evidence based medicine changes anything? A systematic review. *British Medical Journal, 329*, 1017.

Cowley, S., Whittaker, K., Grigulis, A., Malone, M., Donetto, S., Wood, H., … Maben, J. (2013). *Why health visiting? A review of the literature about key health visitor interventions, processes and outcomes for children and families*. London, UK: National Nursing Research Unit, King's College London.

Cox, J., Holden, J., & Henshaw, C. (2014). *Perinatal Mental Health. The Edinburgh Postnatal Depression Scale (EPDS) Manual* (2nd ed.). London, UK: RCPsych Publications.

Cox, J. L., Holden, J. M., & Sagovsky, R. (1987). Detection of postnatal depression: Development of the 10-item Edinburgh Postnatal Depression Scale. *British Journal of Psychiatry, 150*, 782–786.

Department of Health and Ageing. (2009). National perinatal depression framework. Retrieved from http://www.commcarelink.health.gov.au/internet/publications/publishing.nsf/Content/mental-pubs-f-perinat-toc.

Epstein, A. M. (2008). *Performance measurement and professional improvement: Approaches, opportunities and challenges. Health systems, health and wealth.* Copenhagen, Denmark: WHO Ministerial Conference on Health Systems.

Forsetlund, L., Bjørndal, A., Rashidian, A., Jamtvedt, G., O'Brien, M. A., Wolf, F.M., ... Oxman, A. D. (2009). Continuing education meetings and workshops: Effects on professional practice and health care outcomes. *Cochrane Database of Systematic Reviews, 2*: CD003030. doi:10.1002/1465 1858.CD003030.pub2.

Gilbody, S. (2004). *What is the evidence on effectiveness of capacity building of primary health care professionals in the detection, management and outcome of depression?* Copenhagen, Denmark: WHO Regional Office for Europe's Health Evidence Network.

Gilbody, S. M., House, A. O., & Sheldon, A. (2001). Routinely administered questionnaires for depression and anxiety: Systematic review. *British Medical Journal, 322*, 406–409.

Gilbody, S., Whitty, P., Grimshaw, J., & Thomas, R. (2003). Educational and organisational interventions to improve the management of depression in primary care: A systematic review. *Journal of the American Medical Association, 289*, 3145–3152.

Grol, R. (2002). Changing physicians' competence and performance: Finding the balance between the individual and the organisation. *The Journal of Continuing Education in the Health Profession, 22*, 244–251.

Heatley, C., Ricketts, T., & Forrest, J. (2005). Training general practitioners in cognitive behavioural therapy for panic disorder: Randomized-controlled trial. *Journal of Mental Health, 14*(1), 73–82.

Hewitt, C. E., Gilbody, S. M., Brealey, S., Paulden, M., Palmer, S., Mann, R., ... Richards, D., (2009). Methods to identify postnatal depression in primary care: An integrated evidence synthesis and value of information analysis. *Health Technology Assessment, 13*, 1–230.

Highet, N. J., & Purtell C. A. (2012) *The National Perinatal Depression Initiative: A synopsis of progress to date and recommendations for beyond 2013.* Melbourne, Australia: beyondblue, The National Depression and Anxiety Initiative.

Hill, C. E., & Lambert, M. J. (2004). Methodological issues in studying psychotherapy process and outcomes. In M. J. Lambert (Ed.), *Bergin and Garfield's handbook of psychotherapy and behavior change* (5th ed., pp. 84–135). New York, NY: John Wiley & Sons, Inc.

Holden, J. M., Sagovsky, R., & Cox, J. L. (1989). Counselling in a general practice setting: Controlled study of HV intervention in treatment of postnatal depression. *British Medical Journal, 298*, 223–226.

Jomeen, J., Glover, L. F., & Davies, S.-A. (2009). Midwives' illness perceptions of antenatal depression. *British Journal of Midwifery, 17*, 296–303.

Jomeen, J., Glover, L. F., Jones, C., Garg, D., & Marshall, C. (2013). Assessing women's perinatal psychological health: Exploring the experiences of health visitors. *Journal of Reproductive and Infant Psychology, 31*, 479–489.

Kendall, P. C., & Holmbeck, G. V. T. (2004). Methodology, design and evaluation in psychotherapy research. In M. J. Lambert (Ed.), *Bergin and Garfield's handbook of psychotherapy and behavior change* (5th ed., pp 16–43). New York, NY: John Wiley & Sons, Inc.

King, M., Davidson, O., Taylor, F., Haines, A., Sharp, D., & Turner, R. (2002). Effectiveness of teaching general practitioners skills in brief cognitive behaviour therapy to treat patients with depression: Randomised controlled trial. *British Medical Journal, 231*, 1–6.

Luborsky, L., Diguer, L., Seligman, D. A., Rosenthal, R., Krause, E. D., & Johnson, S. (1999). The researcher's own therapy allegiances: A 'wild card' in comparisons of treatment efficacy. *Clinical Psychology, 6*, 95–106.

Morrell, C. J., Ricketts, T., Tudor, K., Williams, C., Curran, J., & Barkham, M. (2011). Training HVs in cognitive behavioural and person-centred approaches for depression in postnatal women as part of a cluster randomised trial and economic evaluation in primary care: The PoNDER trial. *Primary Health Care Research and Development, 12*, 11–20. ISSN 1463-4236.

Morrell, C. J., Slade, P., Warner, R., Paley, G., Dixon, S., Walters, S. J., ... Nicholl, J. (2009a). Clinical effectiveness of HV training in psychologically informed approaches for depression in postnatal women—Pragmatic cluster randomised trial in primary care. *British Medical Journal, 338*, a3045. doi:10.1136/bmj.a3045.

Morrell, C. J., Warner, R., Slade, P., Dixon, S., Walters, S., Paley, G., & Brugha T. (2009b). Psychological interventions for postnatal depression: Cluster randomised trial and economic evaluation. The PoNDER trial. *Health Technology Assessment, 13*(30), iii–iv, xi–xiii, 1–iii–iv, xi–xiii, 153.

National Institute for Health and Care Excellence (NICE). (2007). Antenatal and postnatal mental health: Clinical management and service guidance (NICE Clinical Guideline 45). London, UK: National Institute for Health and Clinical Excellence.

Ricketts, T., & Curran, J. (2009). Training manuals for the PoNDER trial. Retrieved from http://www.nottingham.ac.uk/research/groups/mcph/documents/ponder-trial-health-visitors-training-manual-cba-2009.pdf; http://www.nottingham.ac.uk/research/groups/mcph/documents/ponder-trial-trainers-training-manual-cba-2009.pdf. Accessed December 17, 2014.

Rycroft-Malone, J., & Bucknall, T. (2010). Using theory and frameworks to facilitate the implementation of evidence into practice. *Worldviews on Evidence-Based Nursing, 7*(2), 57–58.

SA Health. (2011). "Introduction to Perinatal Mental Health" National Perinatal Depression Initiative. Retrieved from http://www.sahealth.sa.gov.au/wps/wcm/connect/Public+Content/SA+Health+Internet/Clinical+resources/Professional+development/Mental+health+training/SA+Mental+Health+Training+Centre+eLearning.

Scottish Intercollegiate Guidelines Network (SIGN). (2012). Management of perinatal mood disorders, A National Clinical Guideline (SIGN Publication no. 127). Edinburgh, Scotland: Author.

Shakespeare, J. (2001). *Evaluation of screening for postnatal depression against NSC handbook criteria.* London, UK: National Screening Committee.

Shribman, S. (2009). *Healthy child programme: Pregnancy and the first five years of life.* London, UK: Department of Health.

Slade, P., Morrell, C. J., Rigby, A., Ricci, A., Spittlehouse, J., & Brugha, T. S. (2010). Postnatal women's experiences of management of depressive symptoms: A qualitative study. *British Journal of General Practice, 60*(580), e440–e448. doi:10.3399/bjgp10X532611.

The Maternity Notes. (2013). The perinatal institute for maternal and child health. Retrieved from http://www.perinatal.org.uk/. Accessed December 18, 2013.

The Patient's Association. (2011). Postnatal depression services: An investigation into NHS service provision March 2011. London, UK: UNICEF.

Thompson, C., Kinmonth, A. L., Stevens, L., Pevele, R. C., Stevens, A., Ostler, K. J., … Campbell, M. J. (2000). Effects of a clinical-practice guideline and practice-based education on detection and outcome of depression in primary care: Hampshire Depression Project randomised controlled trial. *The Lancet, 355*(9199), 185–191.

Tudor, K. (2010). Training manuals for the PoNDER trial. Retrieved from http://www.nottingham.ac.uk/research/groups/mcph/documents/ponder-trial-health-visitors-training-handbook-pca-2010.pdf; http://www.nottingham.ac.uk/research/groups/mcph/documents/ponder-trial-trainers-training-handbook-pca-2010.pdf. Accessed December 17, 2014.

Weeks, W., Robinson, J., Brooks, W., & Batalden, P. (2000). Using early clinical experiences to integrate quality-improvement learning into medical education. *Academic Medicine, 75,* 81–84.

Whooley, M. A., Avins, A. L., Miranda, J., & Browner, W. S. (1997). Case-finding instruments for depression. Two questions are as good as many. *Journal of General Internal Medicine, 12,* 439–445.

14

An Overview of Health Economic Aspects of Perinatal Depression

Stavros Petrou, C. Jane Morrell, and Martin Knapp

Introduction

Perinatal depression can be defined as depression during pregnancy, around the period of childbirth or during the first 12 months postpartum (Milgrom & Gemmill, 2013). Epidemiological evidence suggests that at least 12% of women face the crippling effects of major depressive disorder during pregnancy (O'Hara & Wisner, 2013), while a recent systematic review suggests that ~14% (95% CI: 11 and 19%) experience more broadly defined depression during the first three months postpartum (Gavin et al., 2005). Risk factors constellating around history of psychiatric illness, life stress, and poor social relationships have been identified as highly predictive of perinatal depression (O'Hara & McCabe, 2013). The attendant problems and long-term consequences of perinatal depression are important not only for the mother but also for the father, child, and broader family. Depression during pregnancy is associated with an increased risk of poor maternal self-care, inadequate nutrition, preterm labor, and adverse obstetric outcomes (Milgrom & Gemmill, 2013), while depression during the postnatal period is associated with an increased risk of early termination of breastfeeding, poor nutrition and weight gain, substance misuse, relationship difficulties, and impaired interaction with the infant (Muzik & Borovska, 2010). Mother–infant relationship difficulties within this context can lead to suboptimal cognitive, social, and emotional development of the child, manifested as insecure attachment to the mother (Murray, 1992) and long-term impaired socioemotional functioning (Stein et al., 1991), cognitive deficit (Cogill, Caplan, Alexandra, Robson, & Kumar, 1986), and behavioral disturbance at home (Murray, 1992) and in school (Sinclair & Murray, 1998) and extending into adolescence (Hay, Pawlby, Waters, Perra, & Sharp, 2010). Although the cognitive, emotional, and behavioral consequences of perinatal depression are likely to affect several areas of the economy, little is known about the economic consequences of the condition or the cost-effectiveness (CE) of interventions aimed at prevention or alleviation of effects. This chapter examines health economic aspects of perinatal depression, beginning with an overview of methods, and moving on to discussion of key evidence.

Identifying Perinatal Depression and Anxiety: Evidence-Based Practice in Screening, Psychosocial Assessment, and Management, First Edition. Edited by Jeannette Milgrom and Alan W. Gemmill.

An Overview of Health Economic Methods

Cost-of-illness studies estimate the economic costs of a particular disease or condition (Byford, Torgerson, & Raftery, 2000) but tell us little about prioritizing finite resources, as they do not look at interventions to address health or related needs or well-being associated with the disease or condition. In contrast, health economic evaluation compares alternative interventions or programs in terms of their costs and consequences.

Economic evaluations of interventions for perinatal depression can be conducted using observational evidence, but prospective economic evaluations conducted within randomized controlled trials (RCTs) possess highest internal validity (Ramsey et al., 2005). Trial-based economic evaluations of interventions targeting the prevention or treatment of perinatal depression have been conducted (Morrell, Spiby, Stewart, Walters, & Morgan, 2000; Morrell et al., 2009; Petrou, Cooper, Murray, & Davidson, 2006). The RCT is considered to act as the primary vehicle for collecting unbiased information on both the costs and consequences of the interventions being evaluated. However, a single RCT may be an inadequate and partial basis for decision-making for several reasons. For example, the sample may be too small for true between-group differences in outcomes to be recognized or too small for subgroup analyses; follow-up periods may be too short to capture all relevant differences in economic outcomes because of ethical or practical considerations; not all relevant intervention options may be compared; or the findings might not be generalizable outside the particular setting of the trial or the particular group of women. An alternative (or supplementary) basis for economic evaluation is provided by decision-analytic modeling, which involves application of mathematical techniques that synthesize data from multiple sources, including RCTs, or studies with other designs.

Four broad approaches can be delineated for health economic evaluations: cost-minimization analysis (CMA), CE analysis (CEA), cost–utility analysis (CUA), and cost–benefit analysis (CBA). Each approach characterizes the inputs or costs associated with an intervention in monetary units, where the costs can be estimated from alternative perspectives, such as the health-care system (including direct medical costs incurred directly by the health ministry or health insurance provider, sometimes referred to as the "payer" perspective), or the government (including all relevant public expenditure), or the whole society (broader in scope and including all direct and indirect costs associated with an intervention, irrespective of whether borne by the health-care system or by other parties, such as families or unpaid carers).

The alternative forms of economic evaluation differ in how consequences are measured and valued. A CMA assumes that the perinatal strategies under consideration are equal with respect to outcome and that the study design allows the equivalence of outcomes to be tested (Briggs & O'Brien, 2001). By implication, only costs are important in CMA and the least costly strategy is preferred. A CEA measures the consequences of competing interventions in natural units. A CEA generates an incremental cost-effectiveness ratio (ICER): the difference in costs between two interventions divided by the difference in effects. A CEA can only be used to compare interventions that produce the same kinds of consequences. It cannot be used to compare interventions whose primary outcomes are different; for example, it cannot compare prevention of postnatal depression with clinically defined consequences of schizophrenia treatment or cancer treatment. To make these broader comparisons, a common "currency" for measuring consequences is needed. This can be achieved in two different ways, one leading to CUA and the other to CBA. In both cases, by placing a value on the consequences of interventions, either through preference weighting (CUA) or monetary value weighting (CBA), the methods can address broader questions of the efficient allocation of scarce resources across different areas of health care.

In CUA, the consequences of health interventions are measured in terms of preference-based measures of health, such as quality-adjusted life years (QALYs), which attempt to capture health gains in a single metric combining life years gained and health-related life quality enhanced (Torrance & Feeny, 1989). The advantage of the QALY metric is that it allows interventions with diverse consequences to be compared, although not without methodological challenges (Petrou, 2003). As with CEA, a CUA can generate an ICER, but now, the denominator is the difference in QALYs between the two interventions.

In CBA, the consequences of health interventions are measured in monetary units. This can be achieved directly by using methods that ask individuals how much they are willing to pay for a health gain; this approach is called contingent valuation. The value of an effectiveness gain can also be monetized by eliciting individuals' preferences for alternative courses of action using a discrete choice experiment; willingness to pay for different interventions can then be quantified by deriving values of monetary equivalence. Contingent valuation and discrete choice methods have been applied to a number of perinatal issues and applications concerning children, but have not to our knowledge been applied in the context of perinatal depression. A CBA produces a summary measure of incremental cost (relative to the comparator) subtracted from incremental benefit. The reach of CBA in terms of informing resource allocation is the broadest of the evaluative approaches because it can inform decisions not only between health-care interventions but also between strategies that impact different sectors of the economy.

Regardless of the approach to economic evaluation used or the perspective adopted, costs and consequences should be discounted, and uncertainty surrounding the findings should be adequately reported (Drummond, O'Brien, Stoddart, & Torrance, 2005; Gold, Siefel, Russel, & Weinstein, 1996). Applying a discount rate to cost and consequences reflects the notion of time preference: it is generally better to receive health benefits from interventions earlier and to incur costs later (Drummond et al., 2005; Gold et al., 1996).

A number of different types of uncertainty can arise in economic evaluations. In trial-based economic evaluations, sampling (or stochastic) uncertainty is most commonly reported as a confidence interval, depending on variation in both the numerator and the denominator of the ICER. A common method for estimating confidence intervals for the ICER is the nonparametric bootstrap, which resamples with replacement cost–effect pairs from the trial data under the assumption that the trial population is a valid representation of the underlying population of interest (Briggs, Wonderling, & Mooney, 1997). In modeling-based economic evaluations, parameter uncertainty deals with the statistical precision of model variables (e.g., the probability of an event or the mean cost associated with a health state) (Briggs, Claxton, & Schulpher, 2006). Parameter uncertainty can be incorporated into the decision model by assigning each variable an empirical distribution; Monte Carlo simulation techniques can then be used to propagate parameter uncertainty throughout the model (Briggs et al., 2006).

The results of economic evaluations are often presented on the CE plane (Black, 1990). In Figure 14.1, incremental effectiveness (relative to the comparator) is shown on the horizontal axis, while the vertical axis shows the incremental cost, and the origin of the graph (C) represents the point of comparison or control. It is common for the ICER to fall in the northeast (NE) quadrant of the CE plane, where the new intervention is more effective but more costly, or the southwest quadrant (SW) where the intervention is less effective but less costly. In these circumstances, there is a trade-off between effect and cost: additional health benefit can be obtained but at higher cost (NE) or savings can be made but only by surrendering some health benefit (SW). To assess whether these trade-offs are acceptable,

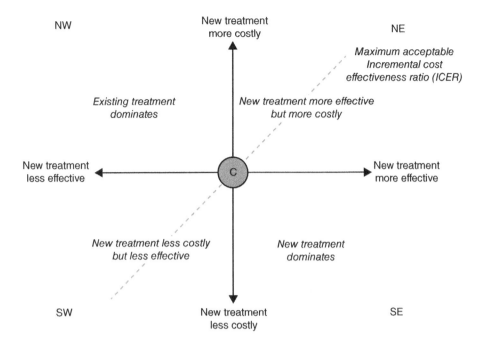

Figure 14.1 The cost-effectiveness plane. NW, denotes northwest; NE, denotes northeast; SW, denotes southwest; SE, denotes southeast.
Source: Gray, Clarke, Wolstenholme, and Wordsworth (2010). Reproduced with permission from Oxford University Press.

a maximum acceptable ICER (CE threshold), in effect a maximum willingness to pay for a unit of effect (λ or *lambda*), is required. The dashed diagonal line running through Figure 14.1 depicts one possible maximum willingness to pay for a unit of effect (or λ). ICERs falling to the right of this line would be considered cost-effective, while ICERs falling to the left would not. Decision rules surrounding the value of λ are available in many jurisdictions, although they have tended to evolve historically and with little scientific basis (Devlin & Parkin, 2004; Grosse, 2008). In England and Wales, for example, a maximum acceptable ICER of £20,000 to £30,000 per QALY gained is recommended for regulatory and reimbursement decisions (NICE, 2013). Decision uncertainty (uncertainty surrounding the value of λ) is commonly represented using the CE acceptability curve (CEAC) (Fenwick, O'Brien, & Briggs, 2004). The CEAC (van Hout, Al, Gordon, & Rutten, 1994) uses the bootstrapped or Monte Carlo replications to predict the percentage of ICER draws that are cost-effective at a given willingness to pay for a unit of effectiveness or QALY gain. Finally, standards of good reporting practice are available for health economic evaluations (Husereau et al., 2013).

We now turn to the health economic evidence surrounding perinatal depression.

Economic Costs Associated with Perinatal Depression

Studies of the economic costs of perinatal depression have focused on the postnatal period. Petrou and colleagues estimated the economic costs of postnatal depression in a geographically defined cohort of 206 women identified as at high risk of developing the condition and in their children (Petrou, Cooper, Murray, & Davidson, 2002). The women were recruited from antenatal clinics in the town of Reading in 1997–1999: 70 (34%) were subsequently diagnosed with postnatal depression, using the Structured Clinical Interview for DSM diagnoses (SCID) (Spitzer, Williams, Gibbon, & First, 1992) during the study period, and 136 (66%) were not diagnosed with postnatal depression. Information on health and social care resources received by these women and their infants was obtained during face-to-face interviews with the women at 18 weeks, 12 months, and 18 months postpartum and subsequently valued using unit costs estimated from primary and secondary sources. Mean mother–infant dyad costs over the first 18 months postpartum were £2419 for women with postnatal depression and £2027 for women without postnatal depression (UK £ sterling, 2000 prices), generating a mean cost difference of £392 ($P = 0.17$). The difference in mean cost between women with and without postnatal depression reached statistical significance for community care services ($P = 0.01$), but not for other categories of services. The study excluded direct nonmedical costs (e.g., travel and child care costs) and indirect costs (e.g., lost productivity), and the study's time horizon was limited to the first 18 months postpartum, and the authors suggested that a broader study perspective and longer time horizon would have widened the cost differences between the comparison groups.

A more recent economic study from the United States investigated the association between postnatal depression and health service expenditures (Dagher, McGovern, Dowd, & Gjerdingen, 2012). A total of 817 employed women, aged at least 18 years, were recruited from three Minnesota hospitals in 2001 and followed up to 11 weeks postpartum. Approximately 5% of the sample was identified as postnatally depressed using a threshold score of 12.5 on the Edinburgh Postnatal Depression Scale (EPDS) (Cox, Holden, & Sagovsky, 1987). The authors did not clarify whether the health service expenditures included in their analyses reflected costs or provider charges; the latter have been shown to include elements arising from corporate financial decisions (Finkler, 1982). Nevertheless, they reported that depressed women incurred 87% more health service expenditures than nondepressed women.

Depressive symptoms experienced by fathers following birth the of a child may also have economic consequences. Edoka and colleagues estimated health-care costs of paternal depression in the postnatal period for a sample of 192 fathers recruited when their partner was on one of two postnatal hospital wards in southern England (Edoka, Petrou, & Ramchandani, 2011). Mean father–infant dyad costs over the first 12 months postpartum were £1104 (£ sterling, 2008 prices) for fathers with depression (diagnosed using SCID) ($n = 31$), £1075 for fathers at high risk of developing depression (previous history of depression or scored highly (≥ 10) on the EPDS) ($n = 67$), and £945 for fathers without depression ($n = 94$). Of particular note, however, was the difference in cost between the comparator groups in particular areas of service provision. As with the study of maternal postnatal depression by Petrou and colleagues (2002), paternal depression was associated with significantly increased community care costs even after controlling for potentially confounding factors, highlighting the importance of primary care services in the management of the condition.

A recent study reported by Bauer and colleagues looked at the effects of perinatal depression on child development outcomes of children at 11 and 16 years of age, using data from the South London Child Development Study, and the associated costs (Bauer, Plant, King, Pariante, & Knapp, in press). Simple decision modeling, building on previous studies of epidemiology, health-related quality of life, public sector costs, and employment, suggested that the additional risks that children exposed to perinatal depression develop emotional, behavioral, or cognitive problems ranged from 5 to 21%. Tracing through the knock-on implications, the public sector costs for each child exposed to perinatal depression exceeded £3,030 (£ sterling, 2010–2011 prices), costs due to reduced earnings were £1,400, and health-related quality of life loss was valued at £3,760, emphasizing the wide-ranging and enduring consequences of postnatal depression for women, their families, and society.

CE of Prevention Strategies

The attendant problems and adverse personal, family, and economic sequelae of perinatal depression have heightened interest in prevention strategies and their CE (Ogrodniczuk & Piper, 2003). Strategies that involve identifying women during the antenatal period at high risk of developing postnatal depression are constrained by low positive predictive values of existing antenatal screening tools (Lumley & Austin, 2001). Petrou and colleagues (2006) estimated the CE of a health visitor preventive intervention (counseling and specific support for the mother–infant relationship) targeted at women at high risk of developing postnatal depression (score of ≥24 on the Cooper antenatal predictive index (Cooper, Murray, Hooper, & West, 1996)) in the context of a RCT in Reading, England. Mean health and social care costs during the first 18 months postpartum were £2397 per mother–infant dyad in the preventive intervention group compared to £2278 per dyad in a comparison routine primary care group (UK £ sterling, 2000 prices). Mean duration of depression was 2.21 months during the study period for women in the preventive intervention group and 2.70 months for women in the comparison group. At a CE threshold of £1000 per month of postnatal depression avoided, the probability that the preventive intervention was cost-effective was 0.71. However, these (Petrou et al., 2006) and other investigators (Dukhovny et al., 2013) have noted that the economic value placed on the benefits of prevention, expressed in terms of morbidity such as reduction in severity or duration of postnatal depression, remains to be elucidated through stated-preference studies.

Other analysts have examined CE of prevention strategies targeted at the *postnatal* period. Morrell and colleagues estimated the CE of community postnatal support in the form of up to 10 home visits (of up to 3 hours duration) during the first month postpartum, among 623 women aged 17 years or over in a RCT in Sheffield, England. At 6 weeks postpartum, mean total costs to the National Health Service were £635 (£ sterling, 1996 prices) for the intervention group compared to £456 for a control group receiving standard postnatal care ($P = 0.001$), while there was some evidence of a difference in mean EPDS scores in favor of the control group ($P = 0.05$) (Morrell et al., 2000). In contrast, MacArthur and colleagues found that a redesigned program of individualized, community-based postnatal care delivered in the former West Midlands Health Region in England, which extended postnatal care from the usual 10–14 days to 28 days and which was provided by a midwife, led to a significant reduction in EPDS scores at 4 and 12 months postpartum in an unselected population with no concomitant effect on health-care costs compared with a usual care control (MacArthur et al., 2003). Dukhovny and colleagues estimated the CE of a telephone-based peer support program targeted at high-risk women (EPDS score >9) participating in a RCT in Ontario, Canada (Dukhovny et al., 2013). Mean societal cost between randomization (which occurred at 2 weeks postpartum or less) and 12 weeks postpartum was estimated at $4,497 (Can$, 2011 prices) in the peer support group, compared to $3,380 in the usual care comparison group (mean difference of $1,117, $P<0.0001$). The peer support program had a 95% probability of CE if Canadian decision-makers are willing to pay approximately $20,000 to avert a case of postnatal depression. Finally, an economic evaluation conducted on the basis of the PoNDER trial in the Trent area of England, which evaluated a health visitor training intervention for identifying depressive symptoms and providing psychological intervention methods, indicated that for the cohort of *all* women included in the study, for whom there was a preventive effect, the intervention was cost-effective at CE thresholds used by the National Institute for Health and Care Excellence (NICE) in England and Wales (Morrell et al., 2009). Further analysis of the PoNDER trial data indicated that the CE for the women scoring <12 on the EPDS at 6 weeks postpartum reached 99% at CE thresholds of between £20,000 and £30,000 per QALY gained, reinforcing the CE of the preventive effect of the health visitor training (Brugha, Morrell, Slade, & Walters, 2011).

More generally, recent systematic reviews have identified a number of psychosocial and psychological interventions that may be effective in the prevention of postnatal depression (Dennis & Dowswell, 2013b; Ogrodniczuk & Piper, 2003; Sockol, Epperson, & Barber, 2013). Estimates of the CE of these interventions are clearly needed to inform regulatory and reimbursement decisions.

CE of Identification Strategies

A recent health technology assessment (Hewitt et al., 2009) delineated approaches aimed at improving identification of postnatal depression into five broad categories: (i) postnatal screening using a specialized depression screening questionnaire, for example, the EPDS (Cox et al., 1987); (ii) postnatal screening using a generic depression instrument, for example, the Beck Depression Inventory (BDI) (Beck, Ward, Mendelson, Mock, & Erbaugh, 1961); (iii) antenatal screening using a standardized depression questionnaire to identify preexisting depression or risk of developing significant depression in the postnatal period; (iv) antenatal screening based on known risk factors to identify those women likely to subsequently develop depression; and (v) targeted training of health-care professionals to enhance symptom recognition and ensure thorough psychosocial assessment. The authors found no published economic evaluations of these alternative identification approaches (Hewitt & Gilbody, 2009). Although some economic evaluations have encompassed a screening component, the strategies evaluated were accompanied by additional enhancements to health care, and consequently, it was not possible to estimate the CE of the screening component per se (Morrell et al., 2009; Petrou et al., 2006). The authors therefore developed a decision-analytic model (Hewitt et al., 2009; Paulden, Palmer, Hewitt, & Gilbody, 2009). The main strategies considered involved single screening with the EPDS (cut points 7–16) or BDI (cut point 10) at 6 weeks postpartum compared with case identification without the formal use of a diagnostic instrument. The results suggested that the use of formal identification strategies did not represent value for money based on CE thresholds of £20,000 to £40,000 per QALY gained. However, the results were primarily driven by the costs of false positives assumed in the model. Alternative assumptions employed in sensitivity analyses suggested that the use of the EPDS as a strategy for identifying women with postnatal depression may be cost-effective under some circumstances. For example, when the cost of a false-positive diagnosis was restricted to that associated with a single GP attendance, use of the EPDS at a cut point of 10 emerged as the optimal strategy in terms of CE.

Definitive evidence on the CE of formal identification strategies is dependent upon more robust data on the costs of managing false positives, for example, through the inclusion of a second administration of the EPDS. Moreover, there may be considerable value associated with obtaining more reliable data from a range of alternative symptom identification approaches or diagnostic approaches not considered as part of this decision modeling work and in extending the existing model to encompass effects on the infant and other family members.

CE of Treatment Strategies

A number of pharmacological, psychosocial, psychological, and other interventions have been developed for the management of depression during pregnancy, although recent RCTs have been too small and based on nongeneralizable samples to offer recommendations in their favor (Dennis & Dowswell, 2013a; Dennis, Ross, & Grigoriadis, 2007). Moreover, no economic evaluations of these interventions have, to our knowledge, been conducted, either through trials or decision-analytic models. In contrast, evidence from RCTs suggesting that psychosocial and psychological interventions may be effective treatment options for mothers with postnatal depression has accumulated in recent years (Dennis & Hodnett, 2007). This accumulation of evidence on clinical effectiveness has been accompanied by a limited number of economic evaluations of these treatment options. Boath and colleagues extracted evidence from a prospective cohort study in Staffordshire, England, with the aim of estimating the CE of treating postnatal depression in a psychiatric day hospital compared with routine primary care (Boath, Major, & Cox, 2003). Although prone to selection biases inherent to observational studies, the study showed that routine primary care is associated with lower overall health-care costs, but worse outcomes, compared to psychiatric day hospital care. Morrell and colleagues conducted a prospective economic evaluation using an RCT design with 18-month follow-up (PoNDER) in 101 GP practices in Trent, England. They evaluated training health visitors to assess women and deliver two psychologically informed interventions based on cognitive behavioral and person-centered principles (Morrell et al., 2009). Training led to significant reductions in EPDS score at 6 and 12 months postpartum among women with 6-week postpartum EPDS scores ≥ 12 (who were the focus of the trial). Notably, training was also associated with lower mean health and social care costs and higher mean QALYs, although neither difference was statistically significant. The probability that training was cost-effective was estimated at 0.79 at a CE threshold of £20,000 per QALY gained. It should be noted, however, that although the economic evaluation was subject to a large amount of missing data with data available for the primary analysis at 6 months postpartum in only 47% of women, the baseline EPDS scores were no different in the women without missing data and those in the overall at risk group of women.

More recently, Stevenson and colleagues conducted a systematic review and economic evaluation of group cognitive behavioral therapy (CBT) compared with routine primary care for women with postnatal depression (Stevenson, Scope, & Sutcliffe, 2010). The evaluation was based on a mathematical model and reliant on data from secondary sources, including the PoNDER trial. The study generated an ICER associated with group CBT of £46,462 per QALY gained, relatively high compared with recommended thresholds (NICE, 2013). Moreover, the investigators did not compare group CBT with individual CBT, which could be considered a more appropriate comparator.

Future Research Directions

Perinatal depression is a common problem which affects women all over the world, with potentially enormous consequences for the mother, father, infant, and other family members. Studies of the economic costs associated with perinatal depression have focused on the postnatal period, with no published studies on the economic consequences of depression during pregnancy and the intrapartum period. Moreover, studies of depression during the postnatal period have been limited in perspective and in time horizon. Ideally, economic costs associated with perinatal depression would be estimated from a broad, societal perspective, allowing estimation of direct nonmedical costs (e.g., travel and child care costs) and indirect costs (e.g., lost productivity) associated with the condition, including those experienced by fathers and other family members. Incorporating economic measures into longitudinal studies with extended periods of follow-up time would also allow valuation of the sequelae into midchildhood and beyond.

Turning to economic evaluation, there are several aspects of the management of perinatal depression for which CE evidence is lacking, for example, enhanced peer support or partner support, home visits by mental health nurses, or collaborative models of care. Future RCTs of intervention strategies should ideally incorporate prospective economic evaluations, and measure and value both costs and health consequences over long periods. Such evidence is required to inform the efficient allocation of scarce resources. However, there will clearly be circumstances where RCTs will not be feasible and assessments of CE will have to be based on evidence from decision-analytic models.

The chapter highlights the paucity of evidence on the value that pregnant women and new mothers, fathers, health-care professionals, and other groups in society place on interventions aimed at prevention of perinatal depression or alleviation of its severity, duration, and effects. We are not aware of preference elicitation studies in this area: particular attention should be paid to ensuring the attributes valued in future such studies reflect women's views of relevant health and nonhealth outcomes and process attributes. Synthesizing these preferences within a broader economic evaluation framework will be a challenge, particularly if they reflect concerns around attributes generally overlooked by economic evaluations, such as perceptions of the quality of care provided.

Conclusions

Future research on the economic consequences of perinatal depression should focus on using data from large-scale longitudinal studies to estimate costs from a broad perspective and over long time horizons. Prospective economic evaluations of prevention, identification, or treatment of perinatal depression should *routinely* be included in future RCTs in this area and should measure and value long-term costs and health consequences. Finally, techniques such as contingent valuation or discrete choice experiments should play a role in future assessments of the value that pregnant women and new mothers, fathers, health-care professionals, and other stakeholders place on intervention strategies.

Acknowledgments

The authors would like to thank work colleagues in our respective departments and the book editors, Professor Jeannette Milgrom and Dr Alan Gemmill, for their helpful comments on earlier drafts of this chapter.

References

Bauer, A., Plant, D., King, D., Pariante, C., & Knapp, M. (in press). Perinatal depression and child development: Exploring the economic consequences from a South London cohort. *Psychological Medicine, 45*(1), 51–61.

Beck, A. T., Ward, C. H., Mendelson, M., Mock, J., & Erbaugh, J. (1961). An inventory for measuring depression. *Archives of General Psychiatry, 4*, 561–571.

Black, W. C. (1990). The CE plane: A graphic representation of cost-effectiveness. *Medical Decision Making, 10*, 212–214.

Boath, E., Major, K., & Cox, J. (2003). When the cradle falls II: The cost-effectiveness of treating postnatal depression in a psychiatric day hospital compared with routine primary care. *Journal of Affective Disorders, 74*, 159–166.

Briggs, A. H., Claxton, K., & Schulpher, M. (2006). *Decision modelling for health economic evaluation.* Oxford, UK: Oxford University Press.

Briggs, A. H., & O'Brien, B. J. (2001). The death of cost-minimization analysis? *Health Economics, 10*, 179–184.

Briggs, A. H., Wonderling, D. E., & Mooney, C. Z. (1997). Pulling cost-effectiveness analysis up by its bootstraps: A non-parametric approach to confidence interval estimation. *Health Economics, 6*, 327–340.

Brugha, T. S., Morrell, C. J., Slade, P., & Walters, S. J. (2011). Universal prevention of depression in women postnatally: Cluster randomized trial evidence in primary care. *Psychological Medicine, 41*, 739–748.

Byford, S., Torgerson, D. J., & Raftery, J. (2000). Economic note: Cost of illness studies. *BMJ, 320*, 1335.

Cogill, S. R., Caplan, H. L., Alexandra, H., Robson, K. M., & Kumar, R. (1986). Impact of maternal postnatal depression on cognitive development of young children. *British Medical Journal (Clinical Research Ed.), 292*, 1165–1167.

Cooper, P. J., Murray, L., Hooper, R., & West, A. (1996). The development and validation of a predictive index for postpartum depression. *Psychological Medicine, 26*, 627–634.

Cox, J. L., Holden, J. M., & Sagovsky, R. (1987). Detection of postnatal depression. Development of the 10-item Edinburgh Postnatal Depression Scale. *The British Journal of Psychiatry, 150*, 782–786.

Dagher, R. K., McGovern, P. M., Dowd, B. E., & Gjerdingen, D. K. (2012). Postpartum depression and health services expenditures among employed women. *Journal of Occupational and Environmental Medicine, 54*, 210–215.

Dennis, C. L., & Dowswell, T. (2013a). Interventions (other than pharmacological, psychosocial or psychological) for treating antenatal depression. *Cochrane Database of Systematic Reviews, 7*, CD006795.

Dennis, C. L., & Dowswell, T. (2013b). Psychosocial and psychological interventions for preventing postpartum depression. *Cochrane Database of Systematic Reviews, 2*, CD001134.

Dennis, C. L., & Hodnett, E. (2007). Psychosocial and psychological interventions for treating postpartum depression. *The Cochrane Database of Systematic Reviews, (4)*, CD006116.

Dennis, C. L., Ross, L. E., & Grigoriadis, S. (2007). Psychosocial and psychological interventions for treating antenatal depression. *The Cochrane Database of Systematic Reviews, (3)*, CD006309.

Devlin, N., & Parkin, D. (2004). Does NICE have a cost-effectiveness threshold and what other factors influence its decisions? A binary choice analysis. *Health Economics, 13*, 437–452.

Drummond, M. F., O'Brien, B. J., Stoddart, G. L., & Torrance, G. W. (2005). *Methods for the economic evaluation of health care programmes.* Oxford, UK: Oxford University Press.

Dukhovny, D., Dennis, C. L., Hodnett, E., Weston, J., Stewart, D. E., Mao, W., & Zupancic, J. A. (2013). Prospective economic evaluation of a peer support intervention for prevention of postpartum depression among high-risk women in Ontario, Canada. *American Journal of Perinatology, 30*, 631–642.

Edoka, I. P., Petrou, S., & Ramchandani, P. G. (2011). Healthcare costs of paternal depression in the postnatal period. *Journal of Affective Disorders, 133*, 356–360.

Fenwick, E., O'Brien, B. J., & Briggs, A. (2004). Cost-effectiveness acceptability curves—Facts, fallacies and frequently asked questions. *Health Economics, 13*, 405–415.

Finkler, S. A. (1982). The distinction between cost and charges. *Annals of Internal Medicine, 96*, 102–109.

Gavin, N. I., Gaynes, B. N., Lohr, K. N., Meltzer-Brody, S., Gartlehner, G., & Swinson, T. (2005). Perinatal depression: A systematic review of prevalence and incidence. *Obstetrics & Gynecology, 106*, 1071–1083.

Gold, M. R., Siefel, J. E., Russel, L. B., & Weinstein, M. C. (1996). *Cost-effectiveness in health and medicine*. New York, NY: Oxford University Press.

Gray, A., Clarke, P., Wolstenholme, J., & Wordsworth, S. (2010). *Applied methods of cost-effectiveness analysis in health care*. Oxford, UK: Oxford University Press.

Grosse, S. D. (2008). Assessing cost-effectiveness in healthcare: History of the $50,000 per QALY threshold. *Expert Review of Pharmacoeconomics & Outcomes Research, 8*, 165–178.

Hay, D. F., Pawlby, S., Waters, C. S., Perra, O., & Sharp, D. (2010). Mothers' antenatal depression and their children's antisocial outcomes. *Child Development, 81*, 149–165.

Hewitt, C. E., & Gilbody, S. M. (2009). Is it clinically and cost effective to screen for postnatal depression: A systematic review of controlled clinical trials and economic evidence. *BJOG, 116*, 1019–1027.

Hewitt, C., Gilbody, S., Brealey, S., Paulden, M., Palmer, S., Mann, R., … Richards, D. (2009). Methods to identify postnatal depression in primary care: An integrated evidence synthesis and value of information analysis. *Health Technology Assessment, 13*(1–145), 147–230.

Husereau, D., Drummond, M., Petrou, S., Carswell, C., Moher, D., Greenberg, D., … ISPOR Health Economic Evaluation Publication Guidelines-CHEERS Good Reporting Practices Task Force. (2013). Consolidated Health Economic Evaluation Reporting Standards (CHEERS)—Explanation and elaboration: A report of the ISPOR Health Economic Evaluation Publication Guidelines Good Reporting Practices Task Force. *Value in Health, 16*, 231–250.

Lumley, J., & Austin, M. P. (2001). What interventions may reduce postpartum depression. *Current Opinion in Obstetrics & Gynecology, 13*, 605–611.

Macarthur, C., Winter, H. R., Bick, D. E., Lilford, R. J., Lancashire, R. J., Knowles, H., … Gee, H. (2003). Redesigning postnatal care: A randomised controlled trial of protocol-based midwifery-led care focused on individual women's physical and psychological health needs. *Health Technology Assessment, 7*, 1–98.

Milgrom, J., & Gemmill, A. W. (2013). Screening for perinatal depression. *Best Practice & Research. Clinical Obstetrics & Gynaecology, 28*(1), 13–23.

Morrell, C. J., Spiby, H., Stewart, P., Walters, S., & Morgan, A. (2000). Costs and effectiveness of community postnatal support workers: Randomised controlled trial. *BMJ, 321*, 593–598.

Morrell, C. J., Warner, R., Slade, P., Dixon, S., Walters, S., Paley, G., & Brugha, T. (2009). Psychological interventions for postnatal depression: cluster randomised trial and economic evaluation. The PoNDER trial. *Health Technology Assessment, 13*, iii–iv, xi–xiii, 1–153.

Murray, L. (1992). The impact of postnatal depression on infant development. *Journal of Child Psychology & Psychiatry, 33*, 543–561.

Muzik, M., & Borovska, S. (2010). Perinatal depression: Implications for child mental health. *Mental Health in Family Medicine, 7*, 239–247.

National Institute for Health and Care Excellence (NICE). (2013). *Guide to the methods of technology appraisal 2013*. London, UK: Author.

O'Hara, M. W., & McCabe, J. E. (2013). Postpartum depression: Current status and future directions. *Annual Review of Clinical Psychology, 9*, 379–407.

O'Hara, M. W., & Wisner, K. L. (2013). Perinatal mental illness: Definition, description and aetiology. *Best Practice & Research. Clinical Obstetrics & Gynaecology, 28*(1), 3–12.

Ogrodniczuk, J. S., & Piper, W. E. (2003). Preventing postnatal depression: A review of research findings. *Harvard Review of Psychiatry, 11*, 291–307.

Paulden, M., Palmer, S., Hewitt, C., & Gilbody, S. (2009). Screening for postnatal depression in primary care: Cost effectiveness analysis. *BMJ, 339*, b5203.

Petrou, S. (2003). Methodological issues raised by preference-based approaches to measuring the health status of children. *Health Economics, 12*, 697–702.

Petrou, S., Cooper, P., Murray, L., & Davidson, L. L. (2002). Economic costs of post-natal depression in a high-risk British cohort. *The British Journal of Psychiatry, 181*, 505–512.

Petrou, S., Cooper, P., Murray, L., & Davidson, L. L. (2006). Cost-effectiveness of a preventive counseling and support package for postnatal depression. *International Journal of Technology Assessment in Health Care, 22*, 443–453.

Ramsey, S., Willke, R., Briggs, A., Brown, R., Buxton, M., Chawla, A., … Reed, S. (2005). Good research practices for cost-effectiveness analysis alongside clinical trials: The ISPOR RCT-CEA Task Force report. *Value in Health, 8*, 521–533.

Sinclair, D., & Murray, L. (1998). Effects of postnatal depression on children's adjustment to school. Teacher's reports. *The British Journal of Psychiatry, 172*, 58–63.

Sockol, L. E., Epperson, C. N., & Barber, J. P. (2013). Preventing postpartum depression: A meta-analytic review. *Clinical Psychology Review, 33*, 1205–1217.

Spitzer, R. L., Williams, J. B., Gibbon, M., & First, M. B. (1992). The structured clinical interview for DSM-III-R (SCID). I: History, rationale, and description. *Archives of General Psychiatry, 49*, 624–629.

Stein, A., Gath, D. H., Bucher, J., Bond, A., Day, A., & Cooper, P. J. (1991). The relationship between post-natal depression and mother-child interaction. *The British Journal of Psychiatry, 158*, 46–52.

Stevenson, M. D., Scope, A., & Sutcliffe, P. A. (2010). The cost-effectiveness of group cognitive behavioral therapy compared with routine primary care for women with postnatal depression in the UK. *Value in Health, 13*, 580–584.

Torrance, G. W., & Feeny, D. (1989). Utilities and quality-adjusted life years. *International Journal of Technology Assessment in Health Care, 5*, 559–575.

Van Hout, B. A., Al, M. J., Gordon, G. S., & Rutten, F. F. (1994). Costs, effects and C/E-ratios alongside a clinical trial. *Health Economics, 3*, 309–319.

15

The Future of Perinatal Depression Identification

Can Information and Communication Technology Optimize Effectiveness?

Tara Donker, Pim Cuijpers, David Stanley,
and Brian Danaher

Introduction

Background

Because of the adverse consequences of untreated perinatal depression on mother, fetus/
child, and family (e.g., poor birth outcomes, poor health behaviors, poor infant outcomes
etc), early detection and treatment of perinatal depression are important. Universal perinatal screening for depression has been implemented widely, although there is limited and
inconclusive evidence that this affects perinatal maternal morbidity (Byatt, Simas,
Lundquist, Johnson, & Ziedonis, 2012; Gilbody, Sheldon, & House, 2008; Laios, Rio, &
Judd, 2013; Yonkers et al., 2009). A recent review (Myers et al., 2013), however, indicated
low-to-moderate strength of evidence that well-conducted and well-resourced screening
programs resulted in decreased depressive symptoms and improved mental health in perinatal women. Innovative methods now available through information technology may have
the potential to further optimize effectiveness of both the identification and treatment of
perinatal depression. Online screening for depression can be reliable and valid (Buchanan,
2002) and is low in cost (Austin, Carlbring, Richards, & Andersson, 2006) and time efficient
(Buchanan, 2002). Online psychological interventions have demonstrated efficacy in
decreasing depressive symptoms (Andrews, Cuijpers, Craske, McEvoy, & Titov, 2010;
Andersson & Cuijpers, 2009) and can facilitate the dissemination of therapies among the
public, in a way that is convenient, private, and inexpensive. These programs offer a source
for population-based approaches to reducing depression in the community.

*Identifying Perinatal Depression and Anxiety: Evidence-Based Practice in Screening, Psychosocial
Assessment, and Management*, First Edition. Edited by Jeannette Milgrom and Alan W. Gemmill.
© 2015 John Wiley & Sons, Ltd. Published 2015 by John Wiley & Sons, Ltd.

Definition of online screening

Detailed descriptions of mental health screening and psychometric properties of screening questionnaires are described elsewhere (Chapters 2, 4, and 5). In short, mental health screening involves the use of reliable (the measure is internally consistent or gives consistent results over time) and validated (the measure actually measures what it claims to measure) questionnaires or instruments to identify symptoms or positive "cases" of a mental health disorder. It can be used to indicate the prevalence or the probability of a mental health disorder in a patient or evaluate symptom severity. Screening can be conducted via self-report as well as by ratings made by a health professional and can be delivered via paper–pencil, telephone, face-to-face, or online. Online self-report screening questionnaires can be delivered by the Internet via technological tools, such as desktop/laptop computers, cell phones (including smartphones), and tablets.

Areas of application

Several widely used standard paper–pencil self-administered depression screening questionnaires have been evaluated for online purposes and have been shown to be equally reliable and valid (e.g., Holländare, Andersson, & Engström, 2010). Screening serves a range of purposes. For example, people can use online questionnaires on mental health websites to quickly and easily check whether they have symptoms of a specific disorder. This may lead to earlier detection, increased awareness, and recognition of symptoms. Interpretation should be cautious, however, given the limitations of online screening without professional input. Furthermore, online screening may be used by health professionals as routine outcome monitoring prior, during, and after treatment. See Donker, van Straten, and Cuijpers (2010) for an overview.

Outline of the Chapter

In this chapter, we discuss the current availability, advantages, and challenges of online and other computerized screening questionnaires for perinatal depression. We also outline state-of-the-art examples of how information technology can assist in perinatal depression screening and treatment. We address innovative methods to improve mental health screening, and describe online interventions for perinatal depression. We conclude by recommendations for further research.

Online Screening for Perinatal Depression

In a recent exploratory study examining the feasibility of online recruitment in women with postpartum depression (PPD), Maloni, Przeworski, and Damato (2013) concluded that the Internet is a promising means to recruit a national sample of women with PPD symptoms with high-risk pregnancies. Despite these promising results, however, to the best of our knowledge, only the Edinburgh Postnatal Depression Scale (EPDS; Drake,

Howard, & Kinsey, 2013; Le, Perry, & Sheng, 2009) and the Postpartum Depression Screening Scale (PDSS; Le et al., 2009) have been validated for online perinatal depression screening.

Current availability of online perinatal depression screening instruments

The psychometric properties of the online version of the EPDS demonstrated good internal consistency ($\alpha = 0.81, 0.87$) (Drake et al., 2013; Le et al., 2009), which is congruent with reliability estimates from the paper–pencil version ($\alpha = 0.81$–0.88) (Dennis, 2004; Logsdon et al., 2013). The online version of the PDSS showed excellent internal consistency ($\alpha = 0.97$) and content validity ($r = 0.80$, $p < 0.01$ with the online EPDS; $r = 0.79$, $p < 0.01$ with the in-person PDSS) in a study by Le et al. (2009) among a convenience sample of 142 postpartum women. However, the Drake et al. (2013) study used a very small sample size ($N = 18$), and both studies used a convenience sample of healthy volunteers. Therefore, generalizability to depressed subjects is limited. Furthermore, no diagnostic interview as a "gold standard" was used to test predictive validity.

Further research is needed to examine the reliability and validity of the online EPDS and other perinatal-specific tools in perinatal and postpartum depressed women. Further examination into the development of an evidence base for generic depression tools used in perinatal depression is also required.

Lastly, the reliability and validity of the PHQ-9 for diagnosing depression in perinatal women is showing promising results (Flynn, Sexton, Ratliff, Porter, & Zivin, 2011; Yawn et al., 2009). The PHQ-9 has also been administered online (Titov et al., 2010) but the psychometric properties of the PHQ-9 when delivered online need to be further established before this instrument can be used online in perinatal populations.

Advantages

How could information technology optimize identification of perinatal depression? Potential benefits are:

Improved detection and increased awareness   Especially during the last trimester when pregnant women are occupied with birth preparations and during the first months after birth when they are busy with child care responsibilities and physical recovery, women may be less willing to be involved with traditional in-person screening, due to the time-consuming nature and organizational difficulties associated with it. Online screening questionnaires have the potential to overcome these barriers, since they are easily accessible. Perinatal women can rate their mood online from home or any other preferred location and in their own time since online questionnaires can be filled in 24/7. The easy accessibility of online screening instruments therefore has the potential to increase willingness of perinatal depressed women to rate their mood. Larger samples sizes from a population otherwise hard to reach may lead to improved detection of perinatal depression, which in turn may lead to increased awareness of the disease. Online screening could even be further enhanced through delivery on mobile devices, such as mobile phones and tablets, because of its flexible and mobile usage. Repeated measurement of mood on mobile phones or tablets may improve detection of perinatal depression, given the differing peaks in the onset of perinatal depression (Gaynes et al., 2005; Sheeder, Jeanelle, Kabir, & Stafford, 2009).

Improved reach to help underserved depressed individuals   Innovative information technology offers promise to extend the reach of mental health programs so that they can assist a greater breadth of depressed individuals. It can improve detection of perinatal depression and increase access to treatment by groups who have higher rates of mental health and related problems than other antenatal women, such as indigenous Australians (Chan, Scott, Nguyen, & Sage, 2009) and adolescent mothers (Laios et al., 2013; Quinlivan, Petersen, & Gurrin, 1999; Quinlivan, Tan, Steele, & Black, 2004). Other potential advantages include the ability to better connect with cultural and linguistically diverse communities by screening in all languages in a potentially cost-effective manner. This may facilitate the development of culturally appropriate engagement strategies for ethnic and indigenous populations for maternal perinatal mental health. However, changing language does not guarantee that the assessment will incorporate—and accurately reflect—underlying cultural differences (see also "challenges").

More sensitive screening   With traditional perinatal depression screening instruments in particular, sensitivity coefficients are low (ranging from 0.43 to 0.71) (Gaynes et al., 2005; Paulden, Palmer, Hewitt, & Gilbody, 2009). A screening instrument is sensitive when it is usually positive in the presence of a disease. In general, a highly sensitive test is desirable when the consequence of missing a disease would be a clearly bad outcome (Gaynes et al., 2005). People tend to disclose more personal information in online assessments compared to face-to-face interviews (Buchanan, 2002; Donker, van Straten, Marks, & Cuijpers, 2010), and this may lead to more sensitive screening (Carlbring, Westling, Ljungstrand, Ekselius, & Andersson, 2001). Findings from Donker, van Straten, Marks, et al. (2010) show that sensitivity is indeed higher for online assessments compared to paper–pencil administration.

Improved interpretation of test results   Because much research with postpartum depressed women is characterized by small numbers of participants (Gaynes et al., 2005), interpretation of results on psychometric properties of screening instruments is limited. However, because of easy access at low dissemination costs, online screening may be better able to obtain larger groups of participants, which will increase statistical precision and may thus improve the interpretation of test results and the ability to draw valid conclusions. Furthermore, it may potentially be cost-effective, but this needs to be investigated in further research.

Avoidance of stigma   The stigma associated with being labeled as having a mental health condition may lead some women to underreport any symptoms or risk factors (Maloni et al., 2013; Shakespeare, Blake, & Garcia, 2003). Online screening can have the advantage of avoidance of stigma when it is anonymous or in circumstances when confidentiality is protected.

No human calculation errors   Online screening technology may play an important role in overcoming other challenges associated with universal perinatal screening using paper-based data gathering and identification tools. For example, given the likelihood of human calculation errors (Matthey, Lee, Črnčec, & Trapolini, 2013), electronic calculations have the advantage of providing an accurate threshold score for management decisions and seamless integration into a treatment management system.

The benefits are yet to be fully understood and include the possible use of self-screening followed by further electronic testing for early diagnosis and immediate provision of education and information to those that screen negative but show risk factors.

Challenges

Similar to traditional screening, there are also challenges to using online screening for at-home or out of care setting:

Accuracy   The physical experiences of pregnancy, such as fatigue, sleep disruption, weight change, and concentration difficulties, can overlap with the symptoms of depression and thus confuse the diagnostic picture (Klein & Essex, 1994). Since there is no medical doctor or obstetric nurse to rate symptoms with their professional knowledge, online self-rated screening in particular needs to be able to distinguish between pregnancy-related symptoms and depression. Furthermore, online screening should not focus on perinatal depression only but also on other mental health-related symptoms, such as anxiety, which is often comorbid with depression. Several leading authors in the field have asserted a need to screen for broader psychosocial risk factors (e.g., Laios et al., 2013). A stepped-care approach including follow-up of positive assessment results with additional diagnostic screens by health professionals might be recommended. A foundation tenet of screening is to identify those that need further investigation.

Heterogeneity   Prevalence rates of depression tend to be higher in women of culturally and linguistically diverse backgrounds than found in other antenatal women (Barnett, Matthey, & Gyaneshwar, 1999). These women often experience and label symptoms of anxiety, depression, and other mental disorders as something other than mental illness (Buist et al., 2007). In general, recruitment through the Internet can result in a more heterogeneous sample than from other recruitment methods (Bhui & Bhugra, 2002). With increased access and the capacity to reach a broader group of people not otherwise reached, online screening instruments in particular need to be culturally sensitive.

Computerized screening has been used by Wilkinson, Howard, and Stanley (2013) in Australia to conduct free, voluntary, and confidential health screening (e.g., alcohol-related harm, tobacco-related harm, and psychological health) of Aboriginal and Torres Strait Islanders, an underemployed or unemployed group who find it hard to access health care for a variety of reasons, such as geographical remoteness as well as financial, language, and cultural barriers. Wilkinson et al. (2013) found that 28.4% of the completed screen cohort ($n = 509$) provided a valid phone number for contact regarding their health screen and their health-related issues and 16.3% ($n = 292$) provided a valid email address for contacting regarding their health screen and health-related issues. The results gave encouragement that computerized screening could be used to reach from diverse cultural backgrounds.

Considerations to be made after online screening   Screening instruments are designed to identify people at risk for a certain disorder. They can give an indication of a disorder, but they cannot give a diagnosis of a mental disorder. Therefore, screening is not a substitute for full diagnosis. Considerations have to be made after a perinatal woman is screened positive for depression. An appointment could be scheduled with a mental health professional to conduct a diagnostic interview to confirm/disconfirm the diagnosis of perinatal depression, to conduct additional (online) assessment and follow-up, and/or to recommend necessary (online) treatment. The considerations involved in the decision to follow online assessment with confirmatory diagnostic testing are similar to those encountered in traditional screening, but because of its anonymous nature, these issues are particularly relevant for online screening.

Potential psychological harm after feedback of screening results   Potential harms from "traditional" routine screening for depression include, among others, the treatment of depression in patients who are incorrectly identified as having the disorder when there is no policy of following all positive screens with a diagnostic stage and the diversion of scarce resources from other endeavors, such as ensuring better care for patients already identified as having depression (Thombs et al., 2012). A clear distinction between screening tools and diagnostic tools is needed. Screening tools give an *indication* of a mental disorder, whereas diagnostic tools can *confirm* a diagnosis of a mental disorder. Despite the need for online diagnostic tools, previous research (Carlbring et al., 2002) reported unsatisfactory psychometric properties for online diagnostic instruments.

The PHQ-9, however, may be a useful alternative tool and is being used in primary medical settings without follow-up confirmatory diagnostic testing, as there is a literature in which the PHQ-9 has been validated against diagnostic tools (Davis, Pearlstein, Stuart, O'Hara, & Zlotnick, 2013).

Potential psychological harm related to online perinatal screening is another important consideration. For example, one concern is that strategies for responding to women who indicate suicidal ideation may be lacking in the online context (see Chapters 2 and 4 for risk assessment best practice). Further, messages from nonverbal communication, email in particular, can be interpreted in many different ways. It is unknown whether people interpret the feedback they receive from their online assessment in ways that could result in distress. Feedback needs to be delivered in a meaningful, unambiguous and sensitive manner (Buchanan & Smith, 1999) with clear statements about the extent to which the feedback should be applied. For example, screening results should indicate that they are only relevant on "this occasion" and may be influenced by the way the test was completed (Donker, van Straten, & Cuijpers, 2010). This is particularly true when evidence of the online screening instrument's reliability and validity is lacking (Buchanan, 2002). Benefits in excess of potential harms from depression screening should be consistently shown in well-conducted, randomized, controlled trials with sufficiently long follow-up to see important patient-oriented outcomes (Thombs et al., 2012). The advantages and disadvantages have to be examined in depth, before any advice can be given on whether or not to use screening tools for perinatal depression. Often, evidence of benefits is lacking (Thombs et al., 2012). See Donker, van Straten, and Cuijpers (2010) for additional discussion of these issues.

Overcoming Poor Screening Practices through Technology-Based Decision Support Systems

The usefulness of computer-based depression screening may well be enhanced by combining computer-based screening with decision support systems. Primary care clinicians are expected to be familiar with multiple health and mental health conditions and best-practice management. Simple prompts linked to screening results can be a valuable aid in assisting professionals to quickly respond appropriately (e.g., suicidal ideation requires a rapid risk assessment even if minimally positive). Carter et al. (2012) have described use of the QUICATOUCH program that combined screening with decision support system that was linked to clinician reports and referrals. When QUICATOUCH was used with oncology outpatients (over 29 months, 1778 patients), it was associated with a 40% increase in new patients receiving psychological treatment and contributed to a reduction in pain and distress (Carter et al., 2012). Similarly, the MHADRO program (Boudreaux et al., 2011) has been used to provide computerized assessment of physical and psychological functioning in cancer patients. The program provides personalized reports for patients and the provider, and it makes a referral to mental health facilities. This system might be particularly suited for patients with perinatal depression to encourage communication between the various treating health professionals (e.g., obstetricians, midwives, or community nurses) and to facilitate appropriate onward referral.

Based on experience in developing one of the first computer-assisted EPDS screening tools to assist in management using PC Tablets in waiting rooms in New Jersey, United States (New Jersey Department Human Services, 2006; New Jersey Department of Health and Senior Services, 2007), Gemmill, Milgrom, Highet, and Stanley (2013) have developed a perinatal screening and decision support system currently being trialed in Australia (see Box 15.1). This has also drawn on the comprehensive screen more recently developed for symptoms of diabetes using iPad technology which found high usability in low SES groups (Wilkinson et al., 2013).

Finally, at the time of writing, a large randomized trial of the feasibility and clinical and cost-effectiveness of mental health e-screening for perinatal depression, anxiety, and psychosocial risk is under way in Canada (Kingston, Austin et al., 2014; Kingston, McDonald et al., 2014).

New Developments: Innovative Information Technologies

Innovative strategies are now being developed to further optimize depression screening and intervention (e.g., Goodyear-Smith, Warren, & Elley, 2013; Warmerdam et al., 2012). Below, we briefly discuss two types of innovative information technologies: ecological momentary assessment (EMA) and computerized adaptive testing (CAT).

EMA and mobile phone applications

EMA (Shiffman, Stone, & Hufford, 2008) is an emerging assessment method to obtain ecologically valid data about behavior, thoughts, and feelings longitudinally over time while avoiding the pitfalls of retrospective recall (Shiffman, 2009). EMA involves repeated administration of assessments, in real time (or close to it, hence *momentary*) and in respondents' natural environments (hence *ecological*) (Shiffman et al., 2008). Ebner-Priemer and Trull (2009) concluded in his review that (i) real-time assessments increase accuracy and minimize retrospective bias; (ii) repeated assessments can reveal dynamic processes; (iii) multimodal assessments can integrate psychological, physiological, and behavioral data; (iv) setting- or context-specific relationships of symptoms or behaviors can be identified; (v) interactive feedback can be provided in real time; and (vi) assessments in real-life situations enhance generalizability. The development of mobile devices, such as smartphones

Box 15.1   Australian Pilot Study Based on New Jersey Model
with the Addition of a Decision Support System

Using a digital platform facilitates additional investigation for consumers who answer in the affirmative to specific questions, using conditional branching or skip logic. This is enhanced by raising further investigation flags to treating professionals (anxiety, psychosocial questions, and suicidal ideation):

- EPDS results are generated immediately in the health professional's secure-login management guide, saving time and eliminating errors in scoring.
- Additional tools for assessment and prompt questions based on national guidelines for management.
- Electronically generated report supports materials for care plan.
- Electronically generated materials for consumers.

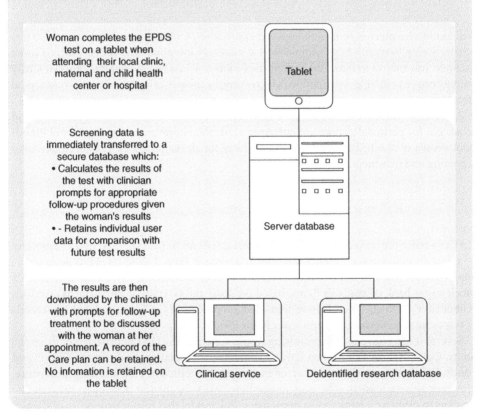

and tablets, has further facilitated the collection of EMA data. EMA questions can, for example, be delivered on a mobile device through short text message service (SMS) or a mobile application (app).

Large sample sizes are needed to answer important theoretical and clinical questions of which specific elements of a therapy are responsible for reducing symptoms of depression as

Box 15.2   Example: ICT4Depression

One innovative intervention using the Internet and mobile phones, the exploratory European FP7 project called "ICT4Depression" (Warmerdam et al., 2012), is currently being evaluated with depressed adults in primary care settings. The project aims to improve access to care as well as to enhance care delivery for depressed adults. Innovative technologies within the ICT4D system include (i) Internet and mobile phone self-help treatments for depression, (ii) Internet and mobile patient assessment, (iii) wearable biomedical sensor devices for monitoring activities and electrophysiological indicators, (iv) computational methods for determining the state of a patient and the risk of relapse (*reasoning engine*), and (v) a flexible system architecture for monitoring and supporting people using continuous observations and feedback via mobile phone and the web.

well as putative mechanisms of therapeutic approaches. Online interventions, in which it is relatively easy to recruit large sample sizes at relatively low costs, and EMA, which is more accurate, less subject to bias, and high in resolution so it can reveal dynamic processes, may therefore have a valuable contribution in increasing the theoretical knowledge of psychological treatments and enhance our ability to ameliorate depressive symptoms in patients (Box 15.2).

As far as we know, there are no such mobile interventions using EMA for screening and treatment for perinatal depression currently available. However, promising (unpublished) pilot results of the ICT4D project pave the way for development of improved perinatal screening and treatment methods.

CAT

CAT can tailor the online administration of test questions to the trait level of the responder by using an individual difference assessment approach (Segall, 2005). CAT is designed to adaptively present the respondent with a small set of assessment items excerpted from a much larger bank of available items, based on prior ability, trait, or impairment estimates (Gibbons et al., 2012). The adaptive item selection process of CAT can result in higher levels of test score precision while using fewer items (Segall, 2005).

Several studies have shown promising results for using the CAT approach. For example, Smits, Cuijpers, and Van Straten (2011) conducted a simulation study on the CES-D and concluded that it is a fruitful way of increasing the efficiency of a testing procedure. However, this increase in efficiency means more work for the test developer, since she/he first has to calibrate a bank of test items using IRT model that relates properties of the test items (e.g., their difficulty and discrimination) to the ability (or other trait) of the examinee. Gibbons et al. (2012) evaluated a Computerized Adaptive Test–Depression Inventory (CAT-DI) and resulted in increased precision of depression measurement yet required significant fewer assessment. CAT has the potential to decrease patient and clinician burden and increases measurement precision. Gibbons et al. (2012) also note that CAT has been less widely used in mental health measurement, because large item banks are generally unavailable for mental health constructs. Furthermore, mental health constructs (e.g., depression) are inherently multidimensional, and CAT has primarily been restricted to unidimensional constructs, such as mathematics achievement. Application of unidimensional models to multidimensional data can result in biased trait estimates (severity or impairment) and underestimates of uncertainty (Gibbons et al., 2012. Nevertheless, studies on CAT screening for depression show promising results and may eventually optimize screening in perinatal depression as well.

Internet-Based Interventions for Perinatal Depression

Background

An issue raised consistently across studies in perinatal or PPD is the gap between identification and treatment: specifically, the availability of adequate mental health services and successful linkage from health provider screening to these services (Byatt et al., 2012; Price, Corder-Mabe, & Austin, 2012). Besides limited resources of available treatments, especially for adolescents with PPD (Phipps, Raker, Ware, & Zlotnick, 2013), stigma, distance, and lack of maternal time due to child care responsibilities are reported barriers to care (Haga et al., 2012; Horowitz & Cousins, 2006; Maloni et al., 2013; Meyer et al., 2009). Online interventions, however, may be a promising means to overcome some of these barriers (Maloni et al., 2013). Internet interventions have (i) the potential to reach broad groups of people, independent of geographical distance; (ii) relatively low dissemination costs; (iii) potential for anonymity; (iv) 24/7 accessibility; (v) flexibility; and (vi) reduced likelihood of stigma.

Internet interventions have been shown to be effective for reducing depressive symptoms (e.g., Andrews et al., 2010; Spek et al., 2007; Warmerdam, van Straten, Twisk, Riper, & Cuijpers, 2008). Guided self-help interventions for depression have been shown to be as effective as face-to-face therapy (Cuijpers, Donker, van Straten, Li, & Andersson, 2010). Guided approaches may be more effective than unguided interventions (Spek et al., 2007), but these results are still inconclusive (Farrer, Christensen, Griffiths, & Mackinnon, 2011; Furmark et al., 2009). Maloni et al. (2013) showed in their exploratory study that half of their study sample of postpartum women with depressive symptoms had sought information about PPD in some manner and over 25% searched the Internet for information of PDD several times a week. Therefore, the Internet may be an ideal method to deliver convenient and flexible treatment for symptoms of PPD.

Current availability of online interventions for perinatal depression

As far as we know, web-based interventions for prevention or treatment of perinatal depression specifically are not yet widely available. However, recent research has focused on innovative web-based interventions for postnatal depression (Danaher et al., 2013a, 2013b; Logsdon et al., 2013; O'Mahen et al., 2013). O'Mahen et al. (2013) reported promising outcomes for postnatal depression in an online behavioral activation intervention (Netmums) with minimal support. Danaher et al. (2013a) developed the MumMoodBooster program, including innovative features supplementing 6 core CBT sessions, which include a partner's website, a library, and individual feedback by a personal coach. Details of the MumMoodBooster program are described in Box 15.3. A feasibility study (Danaher et al., 2013b) showed promising results and a pilot RCT has recently been completed.

Box 15.3   Example: MumMoodBooster

The web-based *MumMoodBooster* (MMB) program (Danaher et al., 2013a) is designed specifically to help women suffering with postpartum depression (PPD). Program content is based upon Milgrom's CBT program *Getting Ahead of Postnatal Depression* (Milgrom, Martin, & Negri, 1999; Milgrom, Negri, Gemmill, McNeil, & Martin, 2005), which draws upon Lewinsohn's *Coping with Depression* course (Cuijpers, Munoz, Clarke, & Lewinsohn, 2009; Lewinsohn, Antonuccio, Steinmetz, & Teri, 1984; Lewinsohn, Weinstein, & Shaw, 1969). In addition to the tailored, interactive 6-session MMB program, which includes videos and guidance by a personal coach through brief calls, the MMB program also includes a partner support website, a library of helpful articles, and an administrative website that offers a feature that enables personal coaches to review the progress each participant has made going through the program. A feasibility trial of MMB (Danaher et al., 2013b) showed that participants experienced significant improvement in their PHQ-9 scores from pretest to postest ($M = 12.6$ [SD $= 4.1$] vs. $M = 5.0$ [SD $= 4.4$]; $t = 8.66$, $p < 0.001$), an improvement that they maintained to the follow-up assessment ($M = 4.2$ [SD $= 3.9$]); pretest–follow-up ($t = 10.43$, $p < 0.001$). Analysis for minimal clinically important difference (MCID) defined as ≥ 5 point *decrease* in PHQ-9 scores (Lowe, Unutzer, Callahan, Perkins, & Kroenke, 2004) indicated that 77% of participants showed a MCID difference in their PHQ-9 scores from pretest to posttest. Participant engagement, ease of usability, and satisfaction were high (Danaher et al., 2013b). A pilot RCT testing the efficacy of the MMB treatment program for PPD depression has just been completed, and MMB is currently being evaluated against face-to-face CBT in a three-arm RCT in Australia funded by the NHMRC.

Another recent study investigated the feasibility and acceptability of a prototype web-based program targeting adolescent mothers with PPD (Logsdon et al., 2013). This program, aimed to persuade depressed adolescent mothers to seek and receive depression evaluation and treatment, was rated as easy to use, and users' attitudes related to depression and treatment improved. However, the impact of the website on subsequent depression treatment was not yet determined. Finally, MoodGYM, an online CBT program with known effectiveness in the wider community (Calear, Christensen, Mackinnon, Griffiths, & O'Kearney, 2009; Christensen, Griffiths, & Jorm, 2004), is currently being investigated for efficacy in the prevention of postnatal depression in at-risk women (Jones et al., 2013).

Final Remarks

E-mental health is a rapidly emerging and growing field. Emerging information and communication technology developments now make it possible to deliver online programs for screening and/or treatment. These programs are able to monitor emotions and arousal levels and to provide tailored support and recommendations. Online delivery of screening has the potential to increase detection and awareness of perinatal depression. Online perinatal depression treatment has the potential to decrease the barriers to treatment uptake, such as limited treatment availability, stigma, lack of child care, and the cost of treatment.

Applying Internet-based interventions for the prevention and treatment of perinatal depression may facilitate new ways in reaching out to people not yet reached. When online screening is followed by online treatment for perinatal depression, information technology can potentially have an enormous impact in reducing the prevalence of perinatal depression.

Future Directions

Future research is needed to examine psychometric properties of online perinatal depression screening questionnaires, the effectiveness and efficacy of online prevention interventions for perinatal depressed women, and whether guided Internet-delivered perinatal depression treatment is as effective as face-to-face perinatal depression treatment. It is important that future research investigates individual characteristics, such as sociodemographics that predict treatment response for online delivery of perinatal depression programs.

References

Andersson, G., & Cuijpers, P. (2009). Internet-based and other computerized psychological treatments for adult depression: A meta-analysis. *Cognitive Behaviour Therapy, 38,* 196–205. doi:10.1080/16506070903318960.

Andrews, G., Cuijpers, P., Craske, M. G., McEvoy, P., & Titov, N. (2010). Computer therapy for the anxiety and depressive disorders is effective, acceptable and practical health care: A meta-analysis and pilot implementation. *PLoS ONE, 5,* e13196. doi:10.1371/journal.pone.0013196.

Austin, D. W., Carlbring, P., Richards, J. C., & Andersson, G. (2006). Internet administration of three commonly used questionnaires in panic research: Equivalence to paper administration in Australian and Swedish samples of people with panic disorder. *International Journal of Testing, 6*(1), 25–39.

Barnett, B., Matthey, S., & Gyaneshwar, R. (1999). Screening for postnatal depression in women of non-English speaking background. *Archives of Women Mental Health, 2,* 67–74.

Bhui, K., & Bhugra, D. (2002). Explanatory models for mental distress: Implications for clinical practice and research. *British Journal of Psychiatry, 181,* 6–7. doi:10.1192/bjp.181.1.6.

Boudreaux, E. D., O'Hea, E. L., Grissom, G., Lord, S., Houseman, J., & Grana, G. (2011). Initial development of the Mental Health Assessment and Dynamic Referral for Oncology (MHADRO). *Journal of Psychosocial Oncology, 29*(1), 83–102.

Buchanan, T. (2002). Online assessment: Desirable or dangerous? *Professional Psychiatry, 33,* 148–154. doi:10.1037/0735-7028.33.2.148.

Buchanan, T., & Smith, J. L. (1999). Using the Internet for psychological research: Personality testing on the World-Wide Web. *British Journal of Psychology, 90,* 125–144. doi:10.1348/000712699161189.

Buist, A., Ellwood, D., Brooks, J., Milgrom, J., Hayes, B. A., Sved-Williams, A., … Bilszta, J. (2007). National program for depression associated with childbirth: The Australian experience. *Best Practice and Research Clinical Obstetrics and Gynaecology, 21,* 193–206. doi:10.1016/j.bpobgyn.2006.11.003.

Byatt, N., Simas, T. A. Lundquist, R. S., Johnson, J. V., & Ziedonis, D. M. (2012). Strategies for improving perinatal depression treatment in North American outpatient obstetric settings. *Journal of Psychosomatic Obstetrics and Gynecology, 33,* 143–161. doi:10.3109/0167482X.2012.728649.

Calear, A. L., Christensen, H., Mackinnon, A., Griffiths, K. M., & O'Kearney, R. (2009). The YouthMood Project: A cluster randomized controlled trial of an online cognitive behavioral program with adolescents. *Journal of Consulting and Clinical Psychology, 77,* 1021–1032. doi:10.1037/a0017391.

Carlbring, P., Forslin, P., Ljungstrand, P., Willebrand, M., Strandlund, C., Ekselius, L., & Andersson, G. (2002). Is the Internet-administered CIDI-SF equivalent to a clinician-administered SCID interview? *Cognitive Behaviour Therapy, 31,* 183–189. doi:10.1080/165060702321138573.

Carlbring, P., Westling, B. E., Ljungstrand, P., Ekselius, L., & Andersson, G. (2001). Treatment of panic disorder via the internet: A randomized trial of a self-help program. *Behaviour Therapy, 32,* 751–764. doi:10.1016/S0005-7894(01)80019-8.

Carter, G., Britton, B., Clover, K., Rogers, K., Adams, C., & McElduff, P.. (2012). Effectiveness of QUICATOUCH: A computerised touch screen evaluation for pain and distress in ambulatory oncology patients in Newcastle, Australia. *Psycho-Oncology, 21*(11), 1149–1157.

Chan, A., Scott, J., Nguyen, A.-M., & Sage, L. (2009). Pregnancy outcome in South Australia 2008. Adelaide, Australia: SA Health, Government of South Australia.

Christensen, H., Griffiths, K. M., & Jorm, A. F. (2004). Delivering interventions for depression by using the internet: Randomised controlled trial. *British Medical Journal, 328,* 265–267. doi:10.1136/bmj.37945.566632.

Cuijpers, P., Donker, T., van Straten, A., Li, J., & Andersson, G. (2010). Is guided self-help as effective as face-to-face psychotherapy for depression and anxiety disorders? A systematic review and meta-analysis of comparative outcome studies. *Psychological Medicine, 21,* 1–15. doi:10.1017/S0033291710000772.

Cuijpers, P., Muñoz, R. F., Clarke, G. N., & Lewinsohn, P. M. (2009). Psychoeducational treatment and prevention of depression: The "coping with depression" course thirty years later. *Clinical Psychology Review, 29,* 449–458. doi:10.1016/j.cpr.2009.04.005.

Danaher, B. G., Milgrom, J., Seeley, J. R., Stuart, S., Schembri, C., Tyler, M. S., … Lewinsohn, P. (2013a). Web-based intervention for postpartum depression: Formative research and design of the MomMoodBooster program. *Journal of Medical Internet Research Protocols, 2,* e18. doi:10.2196/resprot.2329.

Danaher, B. G., Milgrom, J., Seeley, J. R., Stuart, S., Schembri, C., Tyler, M. S., … Lewinsohn, P. (2013b). MomMoodBooster Web-based intervention for postpartum depression: Feasibility trial results. *Journal of Medical Internet Research, 15*(11), e242. doi:10.2196/jmir.2876.

Davis, K., Pearlstein, T., Stuart, S., O'Hara, M., & Zlotnick, C. (2013). Analysis of brief screening tools for the detection of postpartum depression: Comparisons of the PRAMS 6-item instrument, PHQ-9, and structured interviews. *Archives of Women's Mental Health, 16*(4), 271–277. doi:10.1007/s00737-013-0345-z.

Dennis, C.-L. (2004). Can we identify mothers at risk for postpartum depression in the immediate postpartum period using the Edinburgh Postnatal Depression Scale? *Journal of Affective Disorders, 78,* 163–169. doi:10.1016/S0165-0327(02)00299-9.

Donker, T., van Straten A., & Cuijpers, P. (2010a). Internet-based mental health screening and assessment. In J. Bennett-Levy, D. Richards, P. Farrand, H. Christensen, & K. Griffiths (Eds.), *Oxford guide to low CBT interventions* (pp. 241–245). New York, NY: Oxford University Press Inc.

Donker, T., van Straten, A., Marks, I. M., & Cuijpers, P. (2010b). Brief self-rated screening for depression on the Internet. *Journal of Affective Disorders, 122,* 253–259. doi:10.1016/j.jad.2009.07.013.

Drake, E., Howard, E., & Kinsey, E. (2013). Online screening and referral for postpartum depression: An exploratory study. *Community Mental Health Journal, 50*(3), 305–311. doi:10.1007/s10597-012-9573-3.

Ebner-Priemer, U. W., & Trull, T. J. (2009). Ecological momentary assessment of mood disorders and mood dysregulation. *Psychological Assessment, 21,* 463–475. doi:10.1037/a0017075.

Farrer, L., Christensen, H., Griffiths, K. M., & Mackinnon, A.. (2011). Internet-based CBT for depression with and without telephone tracking in a national helpline: Randomised controlled trial. *PLoS One, 6,* e28099. doi:10.1371/journal.pone.0028099.

Flynn, H. A., Sexton, M., Ratliff, S., Porter, K., & Zivin, K. (2011). Comparative performance of the Edinburgh Postnatal Depression Scale and the Patient Health Questionnaire-9 in pregnant and postpartum women seeking psychiatric services. *Psychiatry Research, 187,* 130–134. doi:10.1016/j.psychres.2010.10.022.

Furmark, T., Carlbring, P., Hedman, E., Sonnenstein, A., Clevberger, P., Bohman, B., ... Andersson, G.. (2009). Guided and unguided self-help for social anxiety disorder: Randomised controlled trial. *British Journal of Psychiatry, 195,* 440–447. doi:10.1192/bjp.bp.108.060996.

Gaynes, B. N., Gavin, N., Meltzer-Brody, S., Lohr, K. N., Swinson, T., Gartlehner, G., ... Miller, W. C.. (2005). Perinatal depression: Prevalence, screening accuracy, and screening outcomes. In *AHRQ evidence report summaries.* Rockville, MD: Agency for Healthcare Research and Quality. Retrieved from http://www.ncbi.nlm.nih.gov/books/NBK11854/. Accessed December 17, 2014.

Gemmill, A. W., Milgrom, J., Highet, N., & Stanley, D. (2013). Protocol for a feasibility and efficacy trial of a decision support and management system for electronic screening for perinatal depression (in preparation).

Gibbons, R. D., Weiss, D. J., Pilkonis, P. A., Frank, E., Moore, T., Kim, J. B., & Kupfer, D. J. (2012). Development of a computerized adaptive test for depression. *Archives of General Psychiatry, 69,* 1104–1112. doi:10.1001/archgenpsychiatry.2012.14.

Gilbody, S., Sheldon, T., & House, A. (2008). Screening and case-finding instruments for depression: A meta-analysis. *Canadian Medical Association Journal, 178,* 997–1003. doi:10.1503/cmaj.070281.

Goodyear-Smith, F., Warren, J., & Elley, C.R. (2013). The eCHAT program to facilitate healthy changes in New Zealand primary care. *Journal of American Board of Family Medicine, 26,* 177–182. doi:10.3122/jabfm.2013.02.120221.

Haga, S. M., Ulleberg, P., Slinning, K., Kraft, P., Steen, T. B., & Staff, A. (2012). A longitudinal study of postpartum depressive symptoms: Multilevel growth curve analyses of emotion regulation strategies, breastfeeding self-efficacy, and social support. *Archives of Women's Mental Health, 15,* 175–184. doi:10.1007/s00737-012-0274-2.

Holländare, F., Andersson, G., & Engström, I. (2010). A comparison of psychometric properties between internet and paper versions of two depression instruments (BDI-II and MADRS-S) administered to clinic patients. *Journal of Medical Internet Research, 12*(5), e49. doi:10.2196/jmir.1392.

Horowitz, J. A., & Cousins, A. (2006). Postpartum depression treatment rates for at-risk women. *Nursing Research, 55,* 23–27.

Jones, B., Griffiths, K. M., Christensen, H., Ellwood, D., Bennett, K., & Bennett, A. (2013). Online cognitive behaviour training for the prevention of postnatal depression in at-risk mothers: A randomised controlled trial protocol. *BMC Psychiatry, 13,* 265.

Kingston, D., Austin, M. P., Hegadoren, K., McDonald, S., Lasluk, G., McDonald, S., ... Biringer, A. (2014a). Study protocol for a randomized, controlled, superiority trial comparing the clinical and cost- effectiveness of integrated online mental health assessment-referral-care in pregnancy to usual prenatal care on prenatal and postnatal mental health and infant health and development: The Integrated Maternal Psychosocial Assessment to Care Trial (Impact). *Trials, 15,* 72.

Kingston, D., McDonald, S., Biringer, A., Austin, M. P., Hegadoren, K., Giallo, R., ... van Zanten, S. V. (2014b). Comparing the feasibility, acceptability, clinical-, and cost-effectiveness of mental health e-screening to paper-based screening on the detection of depression, anxiety, and psychosocial risk in pregnant women: A study protocol of a randomized, parallel-group, superiority trial. *Trials, 15,* 3.

Klein, M. H., & Essex, M. J. (1994). Pregnant or depressed? The effect of overlap between symptoms of depression and somatic complaints of pregnancy on rates of major depression in the second trimester. *Depression, 2,* 308–314. doi:10.1002/depr.3050020606.

Le, H.-N., Perry, D. F., & Sheng, X. (2009). Using the internet to screen for postpartum depression. *Maternal Child and Health Journal, 13,* 213–221. doi:10.1007/s10995-008-0322-8.

Lewinsohn, P. M., Antonuccio, D. O., Steinmetz, J.-L., & Teri, L. (1984). *The coping with depression course: A psycho-educational intervention for unipolar depression.* Eugene, OR: Castalia.

Lewinsohn, P. M., Weinstein, M. S., & Shaw, D. A. (1969). Depression: A clinical research approach. In R. D. Rubin & C. M. Franks (Eds.), *Advances in behavior therapy* (pp. 231–240). New York, NY: Academic Press.

Laios, L., Rio, I., & Judd, F. (2013). Improving maternal perinatal mental health: Integrated care for all women versus screening for depression. *Australasian Psychiatry, 21*, 171–175. doi:10.1177/1039856212466432.

Logsdon, C. M., Barone, M., Lynch, T., Robertson, A., Myers, J., Morrison, D., … Gregg, J. (2013). Testing of a prototype Web based intervention for adolescent mothers on postpartum depression. *Applied Nursing Research, 26*(3), 143–145. doi:10.1016/j.apnr.2013.01.005.

Lowe, B., Unutzer, J., Callahan, C. M., Perkins, A. J., & Kroenke, K. (2004). Monitoring depression treatment outcomes with the Patient Health Questionnaire-9. *Medical Care, 42*, 1194–1201.

Maloni, J. A., Przeworski, A., & Damato, E. G. (2013). Web recruitment and internet use and preferences reported by women with postpartum depression after pregnancy complications. *Archives of Psychiatric Nursing, 27*, 90–95. doi:10.1016/j.apnu.2012.12.001.

Matthey, S., Lee, C., Črnčec, R., & Trapolini, T. (2013). Errors in scoring the Edinburgh Postnatal Depression scale. *Archives of Women's Mental Health, 16*(2), 117–122.

Meyer, B., Berger, T., Caspar, F., Beevers, C. G., Andersson, G., & Weiss, M. (2009). Effectiveness of a novel integrative online treatment for depression (Deprexis): Randomized controlled trial. *Journal of Medical Internet Research, 11*, e15. doi:10.2196/jmir.1151.

Milgrom, J., Martin, P. R., & Negri, L. M. (1999). *Treating postnatal depression: A psychological approach for health care practitioners*. New York, NY: John Wiley & Sons, Inc.

Milgrom, J., Negri, L. M., Gemmill, A. W., McNeil, M., & Martin, P. R. (2005). A randomized controlled trial of psychological interventions for postnatal depression. *British Journal of Clinical Psychology, 44*, 529–542. doi:10.1348/014466505X34200.

Myers, E. R., Aubuchon-Endsley, N., Bastian, L. A., Gierisch, J. M., Kemper, A. R., Swamy, G. K., … Sanders, G. D. (2013). *Efficacy and safety of screening for postpartum depression*. Comparative Effectiveness Review, No. 106. Rockville, MD: Agency for Healthcare Research and Quality.

New Jersey Department Human Services, Division of Mental Health Services. (2006). Post Partum Mood Disorders (PPMD) service provision: Fiscal year 2006 (July 2005–June 2006) (Internal Report). Trenton, NJ: Author.

New Jersey Department of Health and Senior Services, Division of Family Health Services. (2007). Postpartum depression summary, state fiscal year 2007 (Internal Report). Trenton, NJ: Author.

O'Mahen, H. A., Woodford, J., McGinley, J., Warren, F. C., Richards, D. A., Lynch, T. R., & Taylor, R. S. (2013). Internet-based behavioral activation treatment for postnatal depression (Netmums): A randomized controlled trial. *Journal of Affective Disorders, 150*(3), 814–822. doi:10.1016/j.jad.2013.03.005.

Paulden, M., Palmer, S., Hewitt, C., & Gilbody, S. (2009). Screening for postnatal depression in primary care: Cost-effectiveness analysis. *British Medical Journal, 339*, b5203. doi:10.1136/bmj.b5203.

Phipps, M. G., Raker, C. A., Ware, C. F., & Zlotnick, C. (2013). Randomized controlled trial to prevent postpartum depression in adolescent mothers. *American Journal of Obstetrics Gynecology, 208*, 192.e1–192.e6. doi:10.1016/j.ajog.2012.12.036.

Price S. K., Corder-Mabe, J., & Austin, K. (2012). Perinatal depression screening and intervention: Enhancing health provider involvement. *Journal of Women's Health, 21*, 447–455. doi:10.1089/jwh.2011.3172.

Quinlivan, J. A., Petersen, R. W., & Gurrin, L. C. (1999). Adolescent pregnancy: Psychopathology missed. *Australian New Zealand Journal of Psychiatry, 33*, 864–868. doi:10.1046/j.1440-1614.1999.00592.x.

Quinlivan, J. A., Tan, L. H., Steele, A., & Black, K. (2004). Impact of demographic factors, early family relationships and depressive symptomatology in teenage pregnancy. *Australian New Zealand Journal of Psychiatry, 38*, 197–203.

Segall, D. O. (2005). Computerized adaptive testing. In K. Kempf-Leonard (Ed.), *Encyclopedia of social measurement* (Vol. 1, pp. 429–438). Oxford, UK: Elsevier.

Shakespeare, J., Blake, F., & Garcia, J. (2003). A qualitative study of the acceptability of routine screening of postnatal women using the Edinburgh Postnatal Depression Scale. *British Journal of General Practice, 53,* 614–619.

Sheeder, J., Kabir, K., & Stafford, B. (2009). Screening for postpartum depression at well-child visits: Is once enough during the first 6 months of life? *Pediatrics, 123,* 982–988. doi:10.1542/peds.2008-1160.

Shiffman, S. (2009). Ecological momentary assessment (EMA) in studies of substance use. *Psychol Assessment, 21,* 486–497. doi:10.1037/a0017074.

Shiffman, S., Stone, A. A., & Hufford, M. R. (2008). Ecological momentary assessment. *Annual Reviews of Clinical Psychology, 4,* 1–32. doi:10.1146/annurev.clinpsy.3.022806.091415.

Smits, N., Cuijpers, P., & van Straten, A. (2011). Applying computerized adaptive testing to the CES-D scale: A simulation study. *Psychiatry Research, 188,* 147–155. doi:10.1016/j.psychres.2010.12.001.

Spek, V., Cuijpers, P., Nyklícek, I., Riper, H., Keyzer, J., & Pop, V. (2007). Internet-based Cognitive Behaviour Therapy for mood and anxiety disorders: A meta-analysis. *Psychological Medicine, 37,* 319–328. doi:10.1017/S0033291706008944.

Thombs, B. D., Coyne, J. C., Cuijpers, P., de Jonge, P., Gilbody, S., Ioannidis, J. P. A., ... Ziegelstein, R. C.. (2012). Rethinking recommendations for screening for depression in primary care. *Canadian Medical Association, 184,* 413–418. doi:10.1503/cmaj.111035.

Titov, N., Andrews, G., Davies, M., McIntyre, K., Robinson, E., & Solley, K. (2010). Internet treatment for depression: A randomized controlled trial comparing clinician vs. technician assistance. *PLoS One, 5*(6), e10939.

Warmerdam, L., Riper, H., Klein, M., van den Ven, P., Rocha, A., Henriques, M. R., ... Cuijpers, P. (2012). Innovative ICT solutions to improve treatment outcomes for depression: The ICT4Depression project. *Studies in Health Technology and Informatics, 181,* 339–343. doi:10.3233/978-1-61499-121-2-339.

Warmerdam, L., van Straten, A., Twisk, J., Riper, H., & Cuijpers, P. (2008). Internet-based treatment for adults with depressive symptoms: Randomized controlled trial. *Journal of Medical Internet Research, 4,* e44. doi:10.2196/jmir.1094.

Wilkinson, V., Howard, M., & Stanley, D. (2013). Indigenous Community Health Screening Project. Project report: Gender and Reproductive Health Section, Population Health Division. Melbourne, Australia Prevention Xpress.

Yawn, B. P., Pace, W., Wollan, P. C., Bertram, S., Kurland, M., Graham, D., & Dietrich, A.. (2009). Concordance of Edinburgh Postnatal Depression Scale (Epds) and Patient Health Questionnaire (Phq-9) to assess increased risk of depression among postpartum women. *Journal of the American Board of Family Medicine: JABFM, 22,* 483–491.

Yonkers, K. A., Smith, M. V., Lin, H., Howell, H. B., Shao, L., & Rosenheck, R. A. (2009). Depression screening of perinatal women: An evaluation of the healthy start depression initiative. *Psychiatric Services, 60,* 322–328. doi:10.1176/appi.ps.60.3.322.

16

Conclusion

Perinatal Depression: Looking Back, Moving Forward

Alan W. Gemmill, Jeannette Milgrom, and Nicole Highet

In writing the conclusions to this book, we have aimed to select some of the questions that reflect current dilemmas and to share something of our own journey to this point. We finish with presenting some ways we think the field can move forward including key recommendations that emerge from the contributed chapters. Screening tests for perinatal depression have been available for some years now, their psychometric properties are well studied, and their accuracy is reasonable. Should we use such tests to "sieve" the wider perinatal population and identify individual women with a high likelihood of having a depressive disorder? In what circumstances would such an activity reduce the suffering caused by perinatal depression? Could other disorders be screened for and what other, broader assessments are needed in routine care? How can we resource universal or targeted screening programs (including putting in place the necessary pathways to care)?

Our Own Journey So Far

As editors, we co-opted the help of Dr Nicole Highett to reflect on the evolution of perinatal depression identification policy in Australia. Together, the three of us worked alongside many other co-researchers and leaders[1] involved in Australia's first *beyondblue* National Postnatal Depression Program (NPDP) between 2001 and 2005 (NPDP: *beyondblue*, 2005). We have now been focused on the ongoing questions surrounding perinatal depression screening for some 14 years. In Australia, the advent of *beyondblue*, an independent, not-for-profit national depression initiative funded by the Commonwealth and Victorian state governments, had much to do with kick-starting a reinvigorated public and scientific consciousness of maternal mental health and, ultimately, a broad governmental commitment to tackle perinatal depression as a public health priority in 2008 (see Figure 16.1).

In 2001, the NPDP was novel in bringing together key perinatal depression researchers from around the country, and 43 health services, to collaborate in a feasibility study

Identifying Perinatal Depression and Anxiety: Evidence-Based Practice in Screening, Psychosocial Assessment, and Management, First Edition. Edited by Jeannette Milgrom and Alan W. Gemmill.
© 2015 John Wiley & Sons, Ltd. Published 2015 by John Wiley & Sons, Ltd.

Australia's perinatal journey

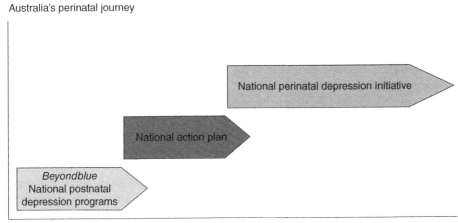

Figure 16.1 Timeline of the National Perinatal Depression Initiative (NPDI) in Australia. The Initiative involves psychosocial assessment, including depression screening, for every perinatal woman at least once in pregnancy and at least once in the first year postpartum.
Source: © Nicole Highet.

of antenatal and postnatal screening involving more than 40,000 women over 5 years (*beyondblue*, 2005). This culminated in a National Action Plan[2] focused on the detailed mapping of perinatal mental health needs in Australia at the time (led by the Perinatal Mental Health Consortium in 2008). Armed with the empirical results of the NPDP, the new plan recommended the resources and structures (both at policy and operational level) required to implement depression screening, psychosocial assessment, training, workforce development and to ensure effective pathways to care. A remarkably rapid translation of research to practice through lobbying by *beyondblue* and others resulted in an election promise of $85 million for a new national initiative. Since the initiation of the NPDP in Australia, over a decade of focused public health initiatives, research, strategic planning, advocacy, and government investment have ensued under the umbrella of what is now termed the National Perinatal Depression Initiative (NPDI:http://www.health.gov.au/internet/main/publishing.nsf/Content/mental-perinat).

Along the way, we encountered, in national microcosm, many of the global questions and issues addressed by the contributors to this international book: the prevalence of perinatal depression and anxiety symptoms was established based on large, prospective Australian cohorts; major risk factors specific to this population and the barriers to help and recovery were identified (Milgrom et al., 2008); research on screening was systematically reviewed and was found limited in various areas (*beyondblue*, 2011); a major problem with low help-seeking and treatment rates was identified which spurred national efforts to raise awareness and combat stigmatizing attitudes around depression and motherhood (Bilszta, Ericksen, Buist, & Milgrom, 2010; Highet, Gemmill, & Milgrom, 2011).

In developing best-practice national guidelines on identification and treatment (see also Chapter 12 of this book), important ideas such as psychosocial assessment were critically reviewed, recommendations for screening were formulated, and future research targets identified. Ultimately, agreement on a national recommendation for the implementation of routine perinatal depression screening emerged, with each element of its accompanying guidelines prudently qualified in terms of whether, when, how, by whom, and for what purpose a screening program should be conducted. Potential screening tests were considered—but only one had a sufficient history of validation and psychometric evaluation (the EPDS). With the "screening genie" out of the bottle, the issue of potentially screening for other disorders became unavoidable and the best-practice guidelines acknowledged both the limitations of screening and the need to balance limited evidence with expert clinical wisdom. Similarly, this ongoing process of public, scientific, and governmental engagement quickly shone a light on the lack of health economic data regarding the costs of both treated and untreated perinatal depression in Australia and provided the impetus for several important appraisals in this regard (PANDA, 2012; *beyondblue* and Price Waterhouse Cooper, 2012).

Whether a policy of universal perinatal depression screening and psychosocial assessment in Australia is justified and whether current universal screening activities satisfy criteria for a well-designed and resourced screening program are debatable. Australia has now embarked on this journey, and the effect on the mental health outcomes of Australian women remains to be measured. Nonetheless, the long process of questioning, research, debate, and advocacy has undoubtedly introduced a new awareness of perinatal mental health into routine healthcare practice, has been enthusiastically embraced by some State governments and clinicians, has sharpened the curiosity of researchers, won the sympathy of the public, and secured the commitment of government to acknowledge and tackle the problem at multiple levels on a national scale. Our own position as clinician-researchers and perinatal mental health advocates has been to focus on the controversy around screening tools themselves and how to improve their use. We established a research program (see http://www.piri.org.au) developing brief interventions for mothers, fathers, and babies in recognition that these need to be cost-effective, evidence based (through randomized controlled trials (RCTs)), and accessible (e.g., self-help and e-treatments). We, as well as others, continue to screen and offer management to hundreds of women each year. with building on evidence of acceptability (Gemmill, Leigh, Ericksen, & Milgrom, 2006), We remain invested in contributing to the outstanding questions through our research and collaborations. Both ourselves and the organizations in which we work remain committed to ongoing promotion of perinatal mental health, raising awareness and reducing stigma (http://www.cope.org.au).

Recurring themes

How is the experience in Australia mirrored in the current state of affairs around the globe?

Our curiosity on this question led us to propose the concept for this book to the publisher. Internationally, the state of the field reflected in this book suggests that we continue to lack reliable evidence to judge the effectiveness of perinatal depression screening programs one way or the other. On the other hand, the contributions to this book underline once again the great scope for harm through the continued nonidentification and nontreatment of the majority of cases of perinatal depression. This refocuses us on the continued importance of increasing identification rates. As eloquently outlined in Chapter 1, this is the one link in the care continuum where the single biggest difference can be made to ensure depressed women receive treatment. Finding ways to make an impact through some kind of screening or systematic early identification effort continues to present itself as a possible part of the solution. The contributions to the book show how some commonly cited potential harms connected with screening (misdiagnosis, labeling, stigma, etc.) can be deliberately and consciously minimized in practice by sensitive, appropriate use of tests and by an integrated health-care culture that never takes a clinical decision about initiating interventions for a mental disorder on the basis of a screening result alone. As all international guidelines emphasize, screening tests are not designed to diagnose, but assist in identifying a group of women who are likely to benefit from further psychosocial and clinical assessment. Effective training for health professionals in skillful, woman-centered psychosocial assessment are vital both to maximize the potential benefits to individual women and thereby impact on the alleviation of morbidity at a population level.

Which Way Forward?

Build the evidence base for effectiveness

In considering the utility of depression screening programs, professionals working in perinatal mental health need to make decisions about what to do in the here and now based on the best evidence available and on their clinical experience. To aid in this, more definitive and robust answers will only emerge through further RCTs capable of providing the relevant information on perinatal depression screening efficacy. Further, the design of such RCTs needs to take into account the necessary elements of a screening program beyond deployment of the screening test itself: if follow-up management and treatment resources in the program are superior to current "usual care," they would need to be matched in the control condition of an RCT (Gemmill, 2014; Thombs et al., 2014). Such design considerations must be addressed to reliably establish the efficacy of a screening program (so that we can be confident that any advantage detected is not due only to better management and treatment resources). The forthcoming US Preventive Services Task Force (USPSTF) Evidence Report on depression screening will soon provide a new update on the state of the evidence base by specifically reviewing perinatal screening in parallel with general adult screening (USPSTF, 2014).

Better health economic models

In the health economic sphere, future decision modeling efforts are likely to be important in providing guidance on issues where we lack evidence from empirical studies. In improving our estimates of cost-effectiveness ratios, it would be extremely valuable to be able to include both health utilities obtained directly from depressed perinatal women and a consideration of infant outcomes in such models. A recent analysis found that the costs of perinatal mental illness in the United Kingdom totaled more than £8 billion for every 1-year cohort of births (Bauer, Parsonage, Knapp, Iemmi, & Adelaja, 2014). Nearly three-quarters of these costs related to negative impacts on children rather than mothers.

Better clarity on the objectives of screening

Across those international jurisdictions where guidelines on the identification of perinatal mental health disorders have been developed, there is some lack of clarity about what, exactly, is the purpose of perinatal depression screening (this applies both to guidelines that recommend screening and those that do not). We take the view that if currently available screening tests are used, it should be with the limited purpose of increasing the rate of identification and treatment of a current depressive episode. The evidence for any other utility of screening tests for perinatal depression is currently limited, though this may change with new research.

Consideration of psychiatric illnesses other than depression in screening programs (bipolar and anxiety disorders) has also been proposed. In the case of low-prevalence disorders such as bipolar disorders, given the heightened risk of onset and recurrence in the perinatal period and the risks of both nondiagnosis and inappropriate treatment, it would be desirable to increase reliable identification as much as possible. However, it seems that an evidence base for using screening instruments to do this in low-prevalence disorders is lacking. For example, the Canadian Network for Mood and Anxiety Treatments, the International Society for Bipolar Disorders (Yatham et al., 2013), and the reviews by others (Kelly & Sharma, 2010) acknowledge that, based on critical review (Chessick & Dimidjian, 2010) of the properties of available instruments, a suitable test of known precision with an established cutoff has not been identified for bipolar disorders. The same is true for anxiety disorders although, like depression, anxiety disorders are highly prevalent in perinatal populations. The continued absence of a strong evidence base for the accuracy, acceptability, and clinical effectiveness of screening tests for perinatal anxiety makes firm recommendations difficult. Further, in practice, the more mental health screening instruments that are introduced, the greater the time burden on perinatal women and clinicians which may result in poorer compliance with screening.

In addition, most existing sources of guidance advocate that a positive depression screen should be followed by a full diagnostic interview based on gold standard criteria. This has been found to reveal relatively few psychiatric noncases among screen-positive women and a plurality of disorders other than unipolar depression, if properly conducted (Milgrom, Ericksen, Negri, & Gemmill, 2005; Wisner et al., 2013). For example, Wisner and colleagues (2013) report that in a cohort of 826 women with a positive depression screening result on the EPDS, while nearly 70% had a primary diagnosis of depression, a full 22% had a primary diagnosis of a bipolar disorder. Furthermore, in women with a primary diagnosis of unipolar depression, two-thirds had a comorbid anxiety disorder as a secondary diagnosis. Only 2% of women with positive screening results had no diagnosis of a mental disorder. Perinatal depression screening tools (in this case the EPDS) can clearly help capture a wider range of mental disorders than just depressive disorders, and with some success.

We take the view that, as currently recommended in some jurisdictions, all positive screens be followed by a diagnostic assessment (which would capture a range of other disorders) and, further, that screening be conducted in the context of a psychosocial assessment which includes personal and family history of all mental disorders as well as other concerning issues (e.g., domestic violence, eating disorders; see Chapter 8). Any vulnerability to bipolar or other low-prevalence disorders should trigger a further diagnostic assessment regardless of women's scores on depression screening tests (e.g., as recommended in Scotland; SIGN, 2012). Indeed, taking a full history is generally recognized as best practice in mental health assessment in order to set in place appropriate management plans for women with complex issues or significant but "subclinical" symptoms.

Finally, there is also space for ambiguity on who the "unit" of screening should be. As discussed elsewhere in this book, an important consideration is whether screening in perinatal populations should take a "universal" or a "targeted" approach. A potential area of future importance for improved performance of "targeted" screening lies in its connection with prevention programs. While treating existing depressive illness in pregnancy will impact on the prevalence of postnatal depression, there is now also evidence that interventions commenced in the postpartum period which are targeted to "high-risk" groups can have a measurable impact in prevention of new cases in the first year (Dennis & Dowswell, 2013). This raises the question of whether we might eventually devise improved methods of identifying perinatal "high-risk" populations to whom prevention programs could then be targeted with improved efficiency.

Improved screening performance

This book underlines the fact that many considerations around perinatal depression identification require further research. The optimal screening interval for perinatal depression is a subject that deserves much more sustained attention from researchers—currently, most recommendations seem to be based only on convenience of fit with other perinatal care considerations which (although important) surely cannot be the whole answer about how to optimize the timing of screening tests to maximize identification rates. Indeed, it is to be hoped that research continues into how to improve all aspects of the screening paradigm. Work should continue on the application and interpretation of optimal cutoff scores in varying contexts. Indeed, moving away from reliance on a single, optimal cutoff score may allow more clinically useful interpretation of an individual's results by establishing stratum-specific likelihood ratios, for example (Schmitz, Kruse, & Tress, 2000; Slade, Grove, & Burgess, 2011). New processes or new/adapted screening tests that improve predictive accuracy are always going to be welcome to the degree that they make a screening approach more viable. Apart from the EPDS, there is limited information on the utility of most other depression screening tests that could potentially be used in perinatal populations. Further work seems unavoidable, both in terms of producing improved individual tests and the possibilities of combining tests to improve accuracy. A better understanding of the performance of screening tests (including the EPDS) in pregnancy and better validation of ultrabrief screening tests both deserve attention.

Further assessment and diagnosis

Despite continuing questions over the adequacy of our formal classification systems (DSM and ICD) in terms of perinatal depression, arriving at a definitive diagnosis following a positive screening result remains paramount. Further work on making an accurate diagnosis of perinatal depression in the most reliable, rapid, and seamless manner would be of great value. This could potentially involve either clinician-administered or patient-completed structured assessments, such as was the intention behind the PRIME-MD (Spitzer, Kroenke, & Williams, 1999) which itself led to the development of briefer instruments such as the PHQ-9 (Kroenke & Spitzer, 2002).

In addition, some structured tools for conducting a broader psychosocial assessment have been developed, but their effectiveness remains largely unevaluated. Along with any expansion of the use of structured tools, care must be taken not to apply such psychosocial tools in a perfunctory "tick box" manner, which could result in merely assigning potentially stigmatizing "psychopathological labels to describe social suffering" (as the authors of Chapter 8 argue with considerable force).

Pathways to care

By necessity, a successful screening program requires available supports for women identified as depressed. Concerns have arisen in clinical practice regarding the ethics of screening without extensive professional treatment available. Given the growing evidence on the effectiveness of a broad range of interventions, there is an opportunity to further research types of support that extend beyond classical psychotherapy and pharmacotherapy. For instance, depressed women with different levels of symptom severity may benefit by being matched with more intensive or less intensive treatments or supports delivered by a range of professionals, semiprofessionals, or volunteers. In addition, self-help, e-treatments, complementary and alternative medicine, and social or family support may be enough to produce sufficient benefit for some women. An expansion of utilizing these kinds of supports could be coupled with further research on how to improve the poor treatment uptake and help-seeking seen in so many perinatal populations.

Screening in diverse communities

There are important questions around how to improve identification and how to translate that into better outcomes for women in resource-constrained settings, in ways that are culturally sensitive. Ongoing efforts should be aimed at cultural appropriateness of identification processes and at changing unhelpful or stigmatizing attitudes toward perinatal mental illness. Further, both patients' and providers' attitudes are significant in the success of screening and referral processes and engagement with treatment across all cultures.

Infants, fathers, and couples

It can be argued that a broad psychosocial assessment should include the family unit. Health professionals working with the mental health needs of new parents may benefit in being trained to systematically identify difficulties in parenting in the context of perinatal depression and anxiety. Where difficulties are identified, better interventions aimed at protecting and improving early mother–infant interactions are desirable given the limited evidence to date.

Better identification methods for paternal depression are also necessary in recognition of its potential impact on both men and their families. Different models of early identification will need to be developed, taking account of new research on male-specific expressions of depression (as discussed in Chapter 10). In addition, given the impact of either partner's mental health on the couple relationship, there may be a need to develop specific interventions in this area.

Final thoughts

Many of the prerequisites for perinatal depression screening to be worthwhile are already met (Chapters 1 and 2). Perinatal depression is prevalent and has serious consequences. At the same time, acceptable screening tools and effective treatments are both available. Albeit gradually, the evidence base needed for judging the effectiveness of screening continues to grow. The strength of the case both for and against its introduction is likely to vary across communities, regions, and countries depending in large measure on the availability and accessibility of resources for diagnosis, treatment, and alternative sources of support. If conducted, screening needs to be part of an integrated, sufficiently resourced screening program and rooted in a broader assessment of women's psychosocial contexts. New methods of achieving this integration will no doubt take advantage of e-technology and promise many new frontiers in screening, treatment, self-help, and peer support. We look forward to the next decade of research and to the implementation and evaluation of programs to increase identification of perinatal depression and anxiety and to improve the mental health care of all new families.

Editors' Acknowledgments

We would like to extend our deep and sincere thanks to all of the authors who contributed their valuable time and invaluable expertise to the production of this book. Our thanks also go to Dr Natalie Rose for offering to proofread and comment on a number of sections and to Barbara Frazer, Eliza Hartley and Vera Corbisieri for assistance in preparing parts of the manuscript.

Notes

1   The *beyondblue* CEOs Professor Ian Hickie and Ms Leonie Young; the *beyondblue* Board and its Chair, the Hon. Jeff Kennett; and the *beyondblue* staff led by Dr Nicole Highett. The project was made possible by 43 hospitals/area health services involved in the National Screening Program and by the involvement of many perinatal clinicians and researchers around Australia: **National Office**: A/Prof Anne Buist, National Coordinator (2001–2005); Dr Justin Bilszta, National Project Manager (2001–2005). **Victoria and Tasmania**: Prof Jeannette Milgrom, State Coordinator (2001–2005); Ms Jennie Ericksen, State Project Manager (2001–2005); Dr Alan Gemmill, Senior Research Officer (2001–2005); Ms Melina Ramp, Senior Research Assistant (Dec 2002–2005); Ms Kate Neilson, p/t Research Assistant (2001–2004); Mr Christopher Holt, p/t Research Assistant (2004–2005); Ms Bella Saunders, Clinical Psychologist (2001–2005); Ms Elizabeth Loughlin, Clinical Psychologist (2001–2005); Ms Yolanda Romeo, Clinical Psychologist (2001–2005); Ms Bronwyn Leigh, Health Psychologist (2001–2005); Ms Rachael McCarthy, Clinical Psychologist (2001–2005); *students* such as Bronwyn Leigh, Ying Zhi Gu, Melissa Tang, Eddie Tan, Jessica Rowe, Clare Heaney, Brooke Ellis, Michelle Puttick, Penny Koutsouridis, and Megan Andrews. **South Australia:** Prof John Condon, State Coordinator (2001–2005); Ms Ann Alder, State Project Manager (2001–2005); Ms Liz Gamble, Senior Research Midwife (2001–2005); Ms Carolyn Corkindale, Associate Researcher (2001–2005); Dr Anne Sved-Williams, Associate Researcher (2001–2005). **Western Australia:** Prof Sherryl Pope, State Coordinator (2001–Dec 2003); Dr Craig Speelman, State Coordinator (Jan 2004–2005); Ms Janette Brooks, State Project Manager (2002–2005); Ms Colleen Ball, Research Midwife (2001–Dec 2004); Ms Jocelyn Bristol, Research Midwife (2001–2005); Ms Sandy McClean, Research Midwife (2002–2005); Ms Monica Howard, Research Assistant (2003–2004); Ms Debbie Lien, Research Assistant (2003–2004); Mr James Humphreys, Data Management (2001–2005). **Queensland:** Prof Barbara Hayes, Queensland Director (2001–2005); Ms Beryl Buckby, Assistant Qld Project Manager (Nov 2003–Feb 2004) and Queensland Project Manager (Feb 2004–2005); Ms Renee McAllister, Queensland Project Manager (2002–Feb 2004); Ms Justine Doherty, Assistant Qld Project Manager (August–Dec 2003); Ms Janese McCulley, Assistant Qld Project Manager (April 2004–2005); Dr Alistair Campbell, IT Consultant (2003–2005); Ms Lynore Geia, Indigenous Consultant/Research Assistant (June 2002–Dec 2004); Ms Margaret Egan, Indigenous

Consultant/Research Assistant (Feb 2004–2005); Ms Annemarie Lawrence, Research Midwife (The Townsville Hospital) (Sept 2002–Dec 2004); Ms Jackie Bowen, Research Midwife (Cairns Base Hospital) (Nov 2002–June 2003); Ms Lesley Williams, Research Midwife (Cairns Base Hospital) (June 2003–Jan 2005); Ms Alison Thwaites, Research Midwife (Mackay Base Hospital) (Feb 2004–Sept 2004); Ms Justine Collins, Research Midwife (Mackay Base Hospital) (July 2004–Jan 2005); Ms Ruth McKitrick, Research Midwife (Ipswich Hospital) (April 2004–March 2005); Ms Cheryl Hewlett, Research Midwife (Logan Hospital) (June 2004–March 2005); Ms Lynda Steward, Research Assistant/Midwife (Townsville) (Sept 2004–2005); Ms Annette Kelly, Research and Admin Support (June 2003–Aug 2004); Ms Maryanne Martin, Research and Admin Support (Sept 2004–2005); Ms Tara MacDonald, Prof Hayes Admin Support (2003–2005); Ms Annette Riley, Research Assistant (Indigenous Initiative, Mt Isa) (April 2004–Dec 2004); Ms Claudinia Daley, Research Assistant (Indigenous Initiative, Townsville) (June 2003–March 2005); Ms Annie Eaton, Research Midwife, Birthcare-Mackay (Dec 2004–March 2005). **New South Wales:** Prof Bryanne Barnett, State Coordinator and Senior Investigator SWSHAS (2001–2005); Dr Stephen Matthey, Research Director (2001–2005); Ms Janan Karatas, Research and Liaison Officer (Sept 2003–2005); Ms Leanne Agius (August 2002–July 2003); Ms Robby Taouk, Project Officer Arabic Component (March 2002–Dec 2004); Ms Thu Tram Lee (March 2002–July 2003); Ms Hanh Tran (February 2004–Dec 2004); Ms Jane Phillips, Research Assistant IPC (2002–2003); A/Prof Marie-Paule Austin, Senior Investigator Royal Hospital for Women (2001–2005); Dr Susan Priest, Project Coordinator Royal Hospital for Women (2001–2005); Ms Sabine Merz, Research Assistant (2004–2005); Dr Nick Kowalenko, Senior Investigator Royal North Shore (2002–2005); Ms Yvonne McCann, Coinvestigator, Royal North Shore (2002–2005); Ms Karen Saint, Senior Research Assistant (2003–2005). **Australian Capital Territory:** Prof David Ellwood, State Coordinator (2003–2005); Ms Rebecca Reay, State Project Manager (2003–2005); Ms Maureen Scott, Research Officer (March 2004–2005).

2   The National Action Plan was developed by the *beyondblue* Perinatal Mental Health Consortium and its National Steering Committee, chaired by Prof Marie-Paule Austin and Barbara Wellesley, respectively, and managed by Carol Bennett (*beyondblue*). A large group of researchers and other key stakeholders were represented in the consortium and contributed their time and expertise.

References

Bauer, A., Parsonage, M., Knapp, M., Iemmi, V., & Adelaja, B. (2014). *The costs of perinatal mental health problems.* London, UK: London School of Economics and the Centre for Mental Health.

Bilszta, J., Ericksen, J., Buist, A., & Milgrom, J. (2010). Women's experiences of postnatal depression—Beliefs and attitudes as barriers to care. *Australian Journal of Advanced Nursing, 27*(3), 44–54.

beyondblue. (2005). Final report of the National Postnatal Depression Program, 2001–2005. Melbourne, Australia: Author.

beyondblue Perinatal Mental Health Consortium. (2008). Perinatal Mental Health National Action Plan, 2008–2010 (Full Report). Melbourne, Australia: Author.

beyondblue. (2011). Clinical practice guidelines for depression and related disorders—Anxiety, bipolar disorder and puerperal psychosis—In the perinatal period. A guideline for primary care health professionals. Melbourne, Australia: Author.

Chessick, C. A., & Dimidjian, S. (2010). Screening for bipolar disorder during pregnancy and the postpartum period. *Archives of Women's Mental Health, 13*(3), 233–248.

Dennis, C.-L., & Dowswell, T. (2013). Psychosocial and psychological interventions for preventing postpartum depression. *Cochrane Database of Systematic Reviews, 2013*(2), CD001134. doi:10.1002/14651858.CD001134.

Gemmill, A. W. (2014). The long gestation of screening programmes for perinatal depressive disorders. *Journal of Psychosomatic Research, 77,* 242–243.

Gemmill, A. W., Leigh, B., Ericksen, J., & Milgrom, J. (2006). A survey of the clinical acceptability of screening for postnatal depression in depressed and non-depressed women. *BMC Public Health, 6,* 211. doi:10.1186/1471-2458-6-211.

Highet, N. J., Gemmill, A. W., & Milgrom, J. (2011). Depression in the perinatal period: Awareness, attitudes and knowledge in the Australian population. *Australian & New Zealand Journal of Psychiatry, 45*, 223–231.

Kelly, E., & Sharma, V. (2010). Diagnosis and treatment of postpartum bipolar depression. *Expert Review of Neurotherapeutics, 10*(7), 1045–1051. doi:10.1586/ern.10.81.

Kroenke, K., & Spitzer R. L. (2002). The PHQ-9: A new depression diagnostic and severity measure. *Psychiatric Annals, 32*, 509–521.

Milgrom, J., Ericksen, J., Negri, L., & Gemmill, A. W. (2005). Screening for postnatal depression in routine primary care: Properties of the Edinburgh Postnatal Depression Scale in an Australian sample. *Australian and New Zealand Journal of Psychiatry, 39*, 833–839.

Milgrom, J., Gemmill, A. W., Bilszta, J. L., Hayes, B., Barnett, B., Brooks, J., … Buist, A. (2008). Antenatal risk factors for postnatal depression: A large prospective study. *Journal of Affective Disorders, 108*, 147–157.

Price Waterhouse Cooper. (2012). Valuing Perinatal Mental Health. The consequences of not treating perinatal depression and anxiety. Author. Retrieved from http://www.beyondblue.org.au/docs/default-source/8.-perinatal-documents/bw0079-report-valuing-perintal-health.pdf?sfvrsn=2. Accessed December 17, 2014.

Post and Antenatal Depression Association (PANDA) and Deloitte Economics. (2012). The cost of perinatal depression in Australia (Final Report). Melbourne, Australia: Post and Antenatal Depression Association (PANDA) and Deloitte.

Schmitz, N., Kruse, J., & Tress, W. (2000). Application of stratum-specific likelihood ratios in mental health screening. *Social Psychiatry and Psychiatric Epidemiology, 35*(8), 375–379.

Scottish Intercollegiate Guidelines Network (SIGN). (2012). Management of perinatal mood disorders 2012. Retrieved from http://www.sign.ac.uk/pdf/sign127.pdf. Accessed December 17, 2014.

Slade, T., Grove, R., & Burgess, P. (2011). Kessler psychological distress scale: Normative data from the 2007 Australian National Survey of Mental Health and Wellbeing. *Australian and New Zealand Journal of Psychiatry, 45*(4), 308–316. doi:10.3109/00048674.2010.543653.

Spitzer, R. L., Kroenke, K., Williams, J. B. W, & for the Patient Health Questionnaire Primary Care Study Group. (1999). Validation and utility of a self-report version of PRIME-MD: The PHQ Primary Care Study. *JAMA: The Journal of the American Medical Association, 282*, 1737–1744.

Thombs, B. D., Arthurs, E., Coronado-Montoya, S., Roseman, M., Delisle, V. C., & Leavens, A. (2014). Depression screening and patient outcomes in pregnancy or postpartum: A systematic review. *Journal of Psychosomatic Research, 76*, 433–446.

United States Preventive Services Task Force. (2014). Final research plan: Primary care screening for depression in adults. Retrieved from http://www.uspreventiveservicestaskforce.org/Page/Document/ResearchPlanFinal/depression-in-adults-screening1. Accessed December 17, 2014.

Wisner, K., Sit, D. Y., McShea, M. C., Rizzo, D. M., Zoretich, R. A., Hughes, C. L., … Hanusa, B. H. (2013). Onset timing, thoughts of self-harm, and diagnoses in postpartum women with screen-positive depression findings. *JAMA Psychiatry, 70*, 490–498. doi:10.1001/jamapsychiatry.2013.87.

Yatham, L. N., Kennedy, S. H., Parikh, S. V., Schaffer, A., Beaulieu, S., Alda, M., … Berk, M. (2013). Canadian Network for Mood and Anxiety Treatments (CANMAT) and International Society for Bipolar Disorders (ISBD) collaborative update of CANMAT guidelines for the management of patients with bipolar disorder: Update 2013. *Bipolar Disorders, 15*(1), 1–44.

Index

Note: Page numbers in *italics* refer to Figures; those in **bold** to Tables.

aggression
  children of postnatally depressed mothers,
    148
  fathers' perinatal mental health, 167
  independent assessments, 148
  and poor peer relationships, 148
Altman Mania Rating Scale (AMRS), 115
American College of Obstetricians and
    Gynecologists (ACOG), 48, 183
American Congress of Obstetricians and
    Gynecologists (ACOG), 202
AMRS *see* Altman Mania Rating Scale (AMRS)
ANRQ *see* Antenatal Risk Questionnaire
    (ANRQ)
antenatal acceptability, screening, 52
Antenatal Psychosocial Questionnaire, 125–6
Antenatal Risk Questionnaire (ANRQ),
    125–7
anxiety *see also* perinatal depression (PND)
  bipolar disorders, 114–15
  fathers'
    factor analysis, 168–9
    perinatal mental health, 168–9
    "postnatal distress", 168
  maternal, 83, 94
  perinatal *see* perinatal anxiety
  resource-constrained settings, 130
  transient *vs.* enduring, 96–7
attention regulation, 145

Australian National Perinatal Depression
    Initiative (NPDI)
  objectives, 219
  training programs, 219–20

barriers
  biological treatment, 57–8
  CAM therapy, 182
  culturally and linguistically diverse (CALD)
    families, 67
  depression, 55
  EPDS, as screening tool, 64
  father-inclusive model (FIM), 171–2
  mood symptoms, 55–7
  mother-infant difficulties, 57
  pregnancy, 181
  psychoeducational emotional health
    booklet, 55
  to screening and care, 199
BDI *see* Beck Depression Inventory (BDI)
Beck Depression Inventory (BDI), 78, 80–85,
    234
beyondblue, 53, 55, 65, 213, 219, 220, 256, 258
bipolar disorders
  and childbirth, 114–15
  low-prevalence disorders, 261
  mood and anxiety disorders, 114–15
  risk, perinatal mental health screening, 203
  screening, 261

*Identifying Perinatal Depression and Anxiety: Evidence-Based Practice in Screening, Psychosocial
Assessment, and Management*, First Edition. Edited by Jeannette Milgrom and Alan W. Gemmill.
© 2015 John Wiley & Sons, Ltd. Published 2015 by John Wiley & Sons, Ltd.

Bright light therapy, 18, 183
Bromley Postnatal Depression Scale (BPDS), 83

CAM *see* complementary and alternative
    medicine (CAM)
Canadian Network for Mood and Anxiety
    Treatments, 261
CE *see* cost effectiveness (CE)
childhood sexual abuse (CSA), 121, 123
CIDI *see* Composite International Diagnostic
    Interview (CIDI)
clinical interview, 21, 69, 94, 223–4
clinician-rated scales, 84
cognitive behavioral therapy (CBT), 235
collaborative care, 184–5
Community Practitioners' and Health Visitors'
    Association (CPHVA) stress, 69
complementary and alternative medicine
    (CAM)
  evidence-based treatments, 177
  exercise, 183
  massage, 184
  omega-3 fatty acid supplements, 183
  perinatal women, 183
  yoga intervention, pregnancy, 184
Composite International Diagnostic Interview
    (CIDI), 98–9, 117
Computerized Adaptive Test–Depression
    Inventory (CAT–DI), 248
computerized adaptive testing (CAT)
  adaptive item selection process, 248
  Computerized Adaptive Test–Depression
    Inventory (CAT–DI), 248
  restriction, 249
cost effectiveness (CE)
  identification strategies, 234–5
  prevention strategies, 233–4
  treatment strategies, 235
CSA *see* childhood sexual abuse (CSA)
culturally and linguistically diverse (CALD)
    groups, 55–6, 67, 68, 73

delusions, 224
depression *see also* generic self-report
    instruments
  antenatal, 178–9
  anxious women, 5
  barriers, 55
  characteristics, 14–15
  computer-based screening, 9
  maternal *see* maternal depression
  paternal *see* paternal depression

perinatal *see* perinatal depression (PND)
  postnatal, 178
  in pregnancy and postpartum, 110
  prevalence, 3
  screening
    computerized adaptive testing (CAT),
      248–9
    ecological momentary assessment (EMA),
      246–8
  in societies and cultures, 5
Diagnostic and Statistical Manual of Mental
    Disorders, Fifth Edition (DSM-5),
    108–111, **110**
  depressive episode, **110,** 110–111
  mood episodes, 109–110
  in pregnancy and postpartum depression, 110

ecological momentary assessment (EMA)
  description, 246
  "ICT4Depression", 248
  questions, 247
economic costs *see* health economic methods
Edinburgh Postnatal Depression Scale (EPDS),
    195, 232, 241, 242 *see also* screening
  administration, 64–5
  Clinical Practice Guidelines Good Practice
    Point 11, 65–6
  controversies, 3
  depression rate, 111
  EPDS-3A, 100–101
  false-negative result, 69
  father's depression and anxiety, 170
  and GMDS questionnaire items, **168**
  management plan development, 72
  motivational interviewing techniques, 73
  negative screening result, 70
  online screening, 65
  perinatal depression identification
    antenatal and postnatal populations, 77
    and anxiety, 17, 63–4, 70
    English language version, 77
    population mass screening program, 77
    in postnatal period, 76–7
    UK National Screening Committee, 77
  positive screening result, 70
  postnatal acceptability, 52
  primary care health professionals, 64
  questions and clinical assessment, 222–3
  responsible sites/resources, 65
  risk assessment, 70–72
  score and result interpretation, 68–9
  screening time, 65–6

Edinburgh Postnatal Depression Scale (EPDS)
  (*cont'd*)
  universal screening, 72
  woman-centered care, 66–7, 70
  women, diverse backgrounds, 67–8
emancipated decision-making (EDM), 58
e-mental health, 250
emotion dysregulation, 145
EPDS *see* Edinburgh Postnatal Depression Scale
  (EPDS)
evidence-based treatments
  CAM, 182–4
  collaborative care, 184–5
  home visiting and nontraditional providers
    high-income countries, 185–6
    low- and middle-income (LAMI) countries,
    186
  pharmacological treatment
    postpartum, 182
    pregnancy, 181–2
  postnatal depression prevention
    effective approaches, 180
    meta-analysis, 179
    moderator analyses, 180
    treatment, pregnancy, 180–181
  psychological interventions
    antenatal depression, 178–9
    perinatal anxiety, 179
    postnatal depression, 178

father-inclusive model (FIM), 171–2
fathers' perinatal mental health
  acceptability and engagement, 171
  anxiety, 168–9
  depression *see* paternal depression
  detection, 165
  father-inclusive model (FIM), 171–2
  maladaptive behaviors, 165
  maternal mental health disorders, 165–6
  with perinatal depression, 171–2
  recognition, 165
  sad dads, 169–70
  screening, 170, 172
"fetal programming", 193
FIM *see* father-inclusive model (FIM)

GAD *see* generalized anxiety disorder (GAD)
gender-sensitive screening, 167
General Health Questionnaire (GHQ), 78, 82
generalized anxiety disorder (GAD), 12–13, 17,
  94–5, 98, 99
generic self-report instruments

Beck Depression Inventory (BDI), 78, 80
Duke Anxiety-Depression Scale, 81
EPDS and, 80
examples, 78, **79**
General Health Questionnaire (GHQ), 78
Hospital Anxiety and Depression Scale
  (HADS), 81
Index of Depression, 81
Inventory of Depressive Symptomatology, 81
Patient Health Questionnaire (PHQ), 78, 80
in perinatal period, 78
perinatal-specific instruments, 82
Postpartum Depression Screening Scale
  (PDSS), 78, 80
Generalized Anxiety Disorder Scale-7 (GAD-7),
  17, 36
GHQ *see* General Health Questionnaire (GHQ)
Gotland Male Depression Scale (GMDS), 167–8,
  168

HADS *see* Hospital Anxiety and Depression
  Scale (HADS)
hallucinations, 224
The Hampshire Depression Project, 211
health-care provider attitudes, depression in
  perinatal period
  "champion" depression care processes, 59
  implementing reason, 54
  interpersonal style, 58
  in perinatal period, 54
  training programs, 54
  treatment engagement rates, 54–5
health-care settings
  in maternity, 127–8
  primary, 17, 20, 126–7, 184
  resource-constrained, 128–131
  women preferences, 58
health economic methods
  cost effectiveness (CE)
    identification strategies, 234–5
    prevention strategies, 233–4
    treatment strategies, 235
  decision uncertainty, 231
  Edinburgh Postnatal Depression Scale
    (EPDS), 232
  evaluation approaches, 229–30
  father's depressive symptoms, 232
  health economic models, 260
  health service expenditures and postnatal
    depression, 232
  incremental effectiveness and cost, 230, *231*
  modeling-based economic evaluations, 230

parameter uncertainty, 230
postnatal period, 231–2
randomized controlled trials (RCTs), 229
South London Child Development Study,
    232–3
trial based economic evaluations, 230
health visitors (HVs)
perinatal mental health screening, 197
training
    clinical outcomes, 216
    clinical supervision and support, 218–19
    five-day training evaluation, 218
    introductory training day, 216–17
    mean EPDS scores, "at-risk" women, 216,
    216
    psychological intervention, 215, 216
    psychologically informed sessions,
    217–18
Highs Scale, 115
Hopkins Symptom Check List 25-item version,
    111
Hospital Anxiety and Depression Scale (HADS),
    81, 82, 84, 100, 103
hypomania/mania, 115, 117

"ICT4Depression", 248
Immediate Action Protocol (IAP), 40, *41*
integrated care, 124
integrated perinatal care (IPC), **195**
International Classification of Diseases, Tenth
    Edition (ICD-10), 12, 81, 108, 109, 112,
    115
International Marce Society for Perinatal Mental
    Health, 204
International Society for Bipolar Disorders, 261
internet-based interventions, perinatal
    depression
adolescent mothers, PPD, 250
guided self-help interventions, 249
MumMoodBooster (MMB) program, 249,
    250
"Introduction to Perinatal Mental Health",
    e-learning program, 220

major depressive episode (MDE), 12, 13
maladaptive behaviors, 165
"male depressive syndrome", 167
maternal anxiety, 83, 94
maternal depression
and anxiety, 11, 16
attention regulation, 145
emotion regulation processes, 145

HPA axis functioning, 142
infants and toddlers born to, 16
mother–child *see* mother–child relationships
NICHD study, 145
parenting in, 142
and paternal mood symptoms, 17
and PND, 16
suicide, 16
maternal hostility and coercion, 150
maternal responsiveness, 141, 144, 145
Matthey Generic Mood Question (MGMQ),
    102, **103**
MDE *see* major depressive episode (MDE)
Mini-International Neuropsychiatric Interview
    (MINI), 98
minimal clinically important difference
    (MCID), 250
MMB program *see* MumMoodBooster (MMB)
    program
Mom's Opportunity To Access Help, Education,
    Research, and Support for Postpartum
    Depression Act (MOTHERS), 202
mood and anxiety disorders
bipolar disorder, 114–15
clinical evaluation, 116–17
Diagnostic and Statistical Manual of Mental
    Disorders, Fifth Edition (DSM-5),
    108–111, **110**
diagnostic tools, 116–17
International Classification of Diseases, Tenth
    Edition (ICD-10), 108, 109
perinatal symptoms unrelated to, 115
peripartum onset specifier, 112–14
physical disorders, 115
pregnancy and childbirth
    epidemiological studies, 111
    etiological studies, 112
    follow-up studies, 112
    obsessive–compulsive disorder, 114
    phenomenological studies, 111
Research Domain Criteria (RDoC) project,
    109
subthreshold symptoms, 115–16
mother–child relationships
difficulties, 57
perinatal mental health screening, 200
postnatal depression effect
    Campbell study, 141
    child responsiveness, 141
    depressed mothers, 140, 141
    early infancy, 140
    insecure infant attachment, 141

multidisciplinary training, health-care
    professionals, 221
MumMoodBooster (MMB) program, 249, 250

National Comorbidity Study, 167
National Health and Medical Research Council
    (NHMRC), 213, 250
National Institute for Health and Care
    Excellence (NICE), 11, 13, 21, 32, 122,
    185, 196, 212, 234
National Perinatal Depression Initiative (NPDI),
    256, *257*
National Postnatal Depression Program
    (NPDP), 256, 258
National Screening Committee (NSC), 2
NPDI training programs, Australia, 219–20

obsessive–compulsive disorder, 114, 115
online screening
    advantages
        detection and increased awareness, 242–3
        human calculation errors, 243–4
        sensitive screening, 243
        stigma avoidance, 243
        test results interpretation, 243
        underserved depressed individuals, 243
    challenges
        accuracy, 244
        considerations, after online screening,
            244–5
        heterogeneity, 244
        potential psychological harm, 245
    definition, 241
    Edinburgh Postnatal Depression Scale
        (EPDS), 65
    innovative information technologies
        CAT, 248–9
        ecological momentary assessment (EMA),
            246–8
    instruments, 242
    technology-based decision support systems
        MHADRO program, 246
        primary care clinicians, 245
        QUICATOUCH program, 246

PAS *see* Pregnancy Anxiety Scale (PAS)
paternal depression
    aggression, 167
    gender-sensitive screening, 167
    Gotland Male Depression Scale (GMDS),
        167–8, **168**
    indicators, 167–8

"male depressive syndrome", 167
    male-specific type, 167
    National Comorbidity Study, 167
    partners' scores, 166
    paternal, 166
    rate, 167
    Schedule for Affective Disorders and
        Schizophrenia (SADS), 166
Patient Health Questionnaire-9 (PHQ-9), 80
Patient Protection and Affordable Care Act, 202
PDS *see* Pitt Depression Scale (PDS)
PDSS *see* Postpartum Depression Screening
    Scale (PDSS)
perinatal anxiety
    child behavior problems, 94
    diagnostic interviews, assessment
        Composite International Diagnostic
            Interview (CIDI), 98–9
        Mini-International Neuropsychiatric
            Interview (MINI), 98
        Structured Clinical Interview for DSM-IV
            Axis I Disorders (SCID-I), 98
    generalized anxiety disorder (GAD), 94–5
    Matthey Generic Mood Question (MGMQ),
        102, **103**
    measurement
        purpose, 96
        screening timing, 97–8
        transient *vs.* enduring anxiety, 96–7
    perinatal women, standard diagnostic
        criteria, 95–6
    poor birth and infant outcomes, 94
    pregnancy-specific measures, 101–2
    in pregnant/postpartum women, 94
    questionnaire measures, 100–101
    symptoms, 94
perinatal depression (PND)
    adverse health effects, 15–17
    assessment and diagnosis, 262–3
    beyondblue, 256, 258
    care continuum, 13–14, *14*, 20, *21*
    clinical presentation, 12–13
    clinical recognition, 17–18
    combined identification and treatment, 4
    definition, 228
    Edinburgh Postnatal Depression Scale
        (EPDS), 63–4
    evidence base, effectiveness, 260
    health economic methods *see* health
        economic methods
    health economic models, 260
    infants, fathers, and couples, 263

information collection, 1
internet-based interventions, 249–50
National Perinatal Depression Initiative
    (NPDI), 256, *257*
National Postnatal Depression Program
    (NPDP), 256, 258
pathways, care, 263
perinatal psychiatry, 22
population-based screening, 20
pregnancy and postpartum period, 14–15
psychosocial assessment, 259
quality-adjusted life year (QALY), 21
recurring themes, 259–60
screening
    diverse communities, 263
    improved screening performance, 262
    internet-based interventions, 249–50
    objectives, 261–2
    online *see* online screening
    program, 2
    tests, 259
treatment
    availability and barriers, 19
    guidelines and practices, adherence,
      19–20
    hormonal therapy, 18
    pharmacotherapy, 18
Perinatal Mental Health National Action Plan,
    2009, 196
perinatal mental health screening
anxiety disorders, 203
Australia
    guidelines, 194, **195**
    The Medicare system, 196
    psychosocial assessment, 195, 196
    survey studies, 196
    training programs, 195
    words and phrasing, 194
bipolar disorder risk, 203
Canada, 199–200
"fetal programming", 193
France
    l'Enfance project, 201
    medical psychosocial interview, 201
    mother-baby units, mother-infant
      attachment, 201
    national insurance program, 200
    postpartum visits, 200, 201
screening, 203, 204
United Kingdom
    cost-benefit analyses, 199
    high risk, 198

interventions, 198
    NICE guideline, 196
    RCOG Good Practice Guideline, 197
    risk reduction and identification, 197
    SIGN guideline, 197
    Woman-Held Maternity Record, 197, **198**
United States
    home visiting programs, 203
    Melanie Blocker Stokes Act, 202
    postpartum suicide prevention, 202
    staff-assisted depression care supports, 202
    stepped-care depression management
      model, 202
perinatal mood screening policies
Australian Midwifery Association, 32
depression, 37
elevated screening scores, 38
evidence gaps, 40–44, **44**
health professionals, 34
partners in care, 39–40
patient engagement, 39
questions to answer before implementation,
    33
rescreening, AAP recommendation, 37–8
site for, 34–5
suicidal ideation, evaluation, 40, *41*
therapeutic approach selection, 39
tools
    characteristics, 35, **35**
    Edinburgh Postnatal Depression Scale
      (EPDS), 36
    Generalized Anxiety Disorder-7 (GAD-7),
      36
    maternal suicide and infanticide, 37
    PHQ-9, 36
    Pregnancy Report and Monitoring Survey
      (PRAMS), 36–7
universal *vs.* targeted, 34
US Women, Infant and Children (WIC)
    program, 34
perinatal-specific self-report instruments
Bromley Postnatal Depression Scale (BPDS),
    83
Pitt Depression Scale (PDS), 83
Postpartum Depression Screening Scale
    (PDSS), 83
Pregnancy Risk Assessment Monitoring
    System (PRAMS), 82
peripartum onset specifier, 112–14
physical disorders, mood and anxiety disorders,
    115
Pitt Depression Scale (PDS), 83–4

PND *see* perinatal depression (PND); postnatal depression (PND)
postnatal acceptability
  cultural groups, 53
  Edinburgh Postnatal Depression Scale (EPDS), 52–3
  health visitors, 53
  postnatal depression (PND), 52
  quantitative and qualitative studies, 53
postnatal depression (PND) *see also* perinatal mood screening policies
  behavioral problems
    independent assessments, 147–8
    maternal reports, 146–7
    psychiatric disturbance in adolescence, 148–9
  on biological outcomes
    HPA axis functioning, 142–3
    neural development, 141–2
  care continuum, *14*
  on cognitive development
    attention regulation, 145
    emotion dysregulation, 145
    maternal depression, 144
    outcome studies, 143–4
    poor mother–child interactions, 145
    responsiveness, 144–5
  maternal depression, 16
  maternal reports
    antenatal and postnatal depressive symptoms, 146
    Behavior Screening Questionnaire (BSQ), 146
    and child behavior disturbance, 146–7
    chronic depressive disorder, 147
    preschool-aged children, 146
    Rutter Scale, 147
  mother–child relationships, 140–141
  motherhood and, 56
  nondepressed populations, 138
  poor psychiatric outcomes, mediators, 150–151
  postnatal acceptability, 52
  during pregnancy, 12
  prevention
    effective approaches, 180
    meta-analysis, 179
    moderator analyses, 180
    treatment, pregnancy, 180–181
  screening, 32
  socioemotional outcomes
    contagion of distress, 149

    interactive repair failures, 149–50
    maternal hostility and coercion, 150
  treatment
    alternative care, 153
    intervention effects, 152–3
    screening, mother–infant interactions difficulties, 153–5
POstNatal Depression Economic evaluation and Randomised (PoNDER) trial *see* health visitors (HVs)
"postnatal mood disorder", 39, 64, 168
postpartum depression (PPD), 249, 250
Postpartum Depression Screening Scale (PDSS), 83, 242
postpartum obsessive–compulsive disorder (PP-OCD), 12–13, 15
postpartum/postnatal depression (PND) *see* postnatal depression (PND)
postpartum posttraumatic stress disorder (PP-PTSD), 13, 15
PRAMS *see* Pregnancy Risk Assessment Monitoring System(PRAMS)
PRAQ *see* Pregnancy-Related Anxiety Questionnaire (PRAQ)
Predictive Index of PND, 125–6
Pregnancy Anxiety Scale (PAS), 101–2
Pregnancy-Related Anxiety Questionnaire (PRAQ), 101
Pregnancy Risk Assessment Monitoring System(PRAMS), 82–3
Pregnancy-Specific Anxiety Scale (PSAS), 102
primary health-care setting, psychosocial assessment, 126–7
PSAS *see* Pregnancy-Specific Anxiety Scale (PSAS)
psychiatric disturbance in adolescence, 148–9
psychoeducational emotional health booklet, 55
psychological interventions
  antenatal depression, 178–9
  perinatal anxiety, 179
  postnatal depression, 178
psychosocial assessment
  anxiety and stress in pregnancy, 122–3
  e-screening, 132
  health education, 124
  integrated care, 124
  International Marcé Society Position Statement 2013, 122
  interpersonal violence (IPV), 123
  in maternity setting, 127–8
  mental illness, 122

morbidity, identification and management, 124

non-mental health-trained care providers, conversation with, 125

perinatal period, 121

postnatal depression, 122

practice summary, 127, **129**

pregnant women/mothers, awareness and education, 125

in primary health-care setting, 126–7

programs, 123–4, 132

psychiatric episodes, 121–2

Psychosocial Assessment and Depression Screening in Perinatal Women, 122

risk factors, 122, 123

routine assessment, 125

tools for clinicians, 125–6

woman's emotional state, 124–5

Psychosocial Assessment and Depression Screening in Perinatal Women, 122, 204

quality-adjusted life years (QALYs), 21, 230

randomized controlled trials (RCTs), 229

recurrent brief depressive disorder, 115–16

repetitive transcranial magnetic stimulation (rTMS), 18

Research Domain Criteria (RDoC) project, 109

resource-constrained settings

countries, 128

depression and anxiety, 130

health-care participation and infant health, associations, 130

indicators, 131

mental disorders

screening, 130–131

severe patterns and prevalence, 128–30

perinatal mental disorders, 128

pregnancy-related deaths, 128

questionnaires, 131

schizophrenia and, 128–9

suicide and suicidal behaviors, 130

Royal College of Obstetricians and Gynaecologists (RCOG), 196

sad dads, influence

on children, 169

on partners, 169–70

Schedule for Affective Disorders and Schizophrenia (SADS), 166

SCID-I *see* Structured Clinical Interview for DSM-IV Axis I Disorders (SCID-I)

Scottish Intercollegiate Guidelines Network (SIGN) Management of Perinatal Mood Disorders, 196

screening

benefits, 198

definition, 194

perinatal depression identification

clinician-rated scales, 84

Edinburgh Postnatal Depression Scale (EPDS), 76–7

generic self-report instruments, 78–82, **79**

self-report instruments, 82–3

program, 2–5

evidence-based recommendations, **44**

population-based, 11, 22

postnatal acceptability, 52

test

guidelines and training, 7–8

National Screening Committee (NSC) definition, 2

"selection into parenthood", 111

self-harm/suicidal ideation, 37, 70, 71

social interactions, failures, 149–50

South London Child Development Study, 232

State-Trait Anxiety Inventory (STAI), 17–18, 99–100

Structured Clinical Interview for DSM diagnoses (SCID), 232

Structured Clinical Interview for DSM-IV Axis I Disorders (SCID-I), 98, 117

subsyndromal GAD, 95

suicide

infanticide, 37

maternal, 16, 37, 116

postpartum prevention, 202

risk assessment, 224–5

and suicidal behaviors, 130

training, health-care professionals

aims, 214

Australian context, 213–14

Australian NPDI, 219–20

clinical interview, 223–4

educational meetings, 211

The Hampshire Depression Project, 211

health visitors (HVs), PoNDER trial *see* health visitors (HVs)

"knowledge translation", 211

mixed interactive and didactic approaches, 211

multidisciplinary training, 221

training, health-care professionals (*cont'd*)
  perinatal screening skills development, 214–15
  risk assessment, 215
  suicide risk assessment, 224–5
  trainers, 212
  UK context, 212–13
Training Reference Group (TRG), 217, 218
transient *vs.* enduring anxiety, 96–7

US Preventive Services Task Force (USPSTF), 32, 33, 36, 260

woman-centered care, 66–7
women
  anxious, 5
  complementary and alternative medicine (CAM), 183
  diverse backgrounds, 67–8
  health-care settings, preferences, 58
  health visitors (HVs), training, 216, *216*
  perinatal anxiety, 94, 95–6
  psychosocial assessment, 122
  in resource-constrained settings *see* resource-constrained settings

Printed and bound by CPI Group (UK) Ltd, Croydon, CR0 4YY

16/04/2025

14658460-0002

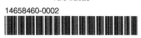